I dedicate this work to two people whose unwavering support allows me to discover and rediscover every day: Adelle, my wife, who makes the adage *Behind every good man there is a great woman* more true than ever, and my son, Elan, who will always be my ultimate teacher.

Equally I dedicate this book, and my practice each and every day, to my students around the globe, those whom I have met as well as those whom I will never meet—you all inspire me to be the best that I can be.

> We shall not cease from exploration, and the end of all our exploring will be to arrive where we started and know the place for the first time.
>
> —Little Gidding, T.S. Eliot, 1888-1965

Contents

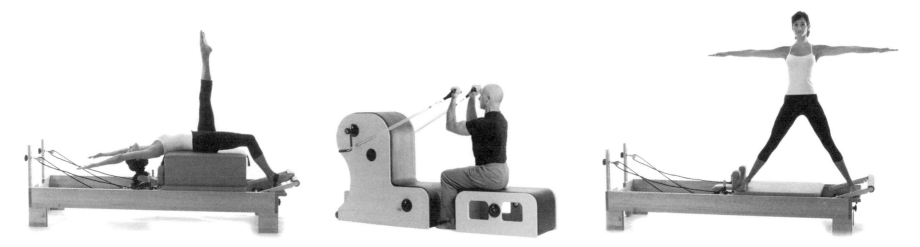

Pilates

SECOND EDITION

Rael Isacowitz

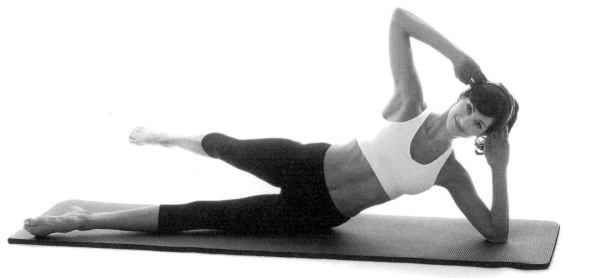

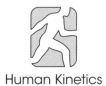

Human Kinetics

Library of Congress Cataloging-in-Publication Data

Isacowitz, Rael, 1955-.
 Pilates / Rael Isacowitz. -- Second edition.
    pages cm
 Includes bibliographical references and index.
  1. Pilates method. I. Title.
 RA781.4.I73 2014
 613.7'192--dc23

                                    2013019507

ISBN: 978-1-4504-3416-4 (print)

This publication is written and published to provide accurate and authoritative information relevant to the subject matter presented. It is published and sold with the understanding that the author and publisher are not engaged in rendering legal, medical, or other professional services by reason of their authorship or publication of this work. If medical or other expert assistance is required, the services of a competent professional person should be sought.

The web addresses cited in this text were current as of November 2013, unless otherwise noted.

Acquisitions Editor: Tom Heine; **Developmental Editor:** Carla Zych; **Assistant Editors:** Rachel Fowler and Elizabeth Evans; **Indexer:** Nan N. Badgett; **Permissions Manager:** Martha Gullo; **Graphic Designer:** Nancy Rasmus; **Graphic Artist:** Kim McFarland; **Cover Designer:** Keith Blomberg; **Photographer (cover and interior):** Kirk Fitzek; **Visual Production Assistant:** Joyce Brumfield; **Photo Production Manager:** Jason Allen; **Art Manager:** Kelly Hendren; **Associate Art Manager:** Alan L. Wilborn; **Illustrations:** © Human Kinetics; **Printer:** United Graphics

Human Kinetics books are available at special discounts for bulk purchase. Special editions or book excerpts can also be created to specification. For details, contact the Special Sales Manager at Human Kinetics.

Printed in the United States of America   10   9   8   7   6   5   4

The paper in this book is certified under a sustainable forestry program.

Human Kinetics
Web site: www.HumanKinetics.com

United States: Human Kinetics
P.O. Box 5076
Champaign, IL 61825-5076
800-747-4457
e-mail: info@hkusa.com

Canada: Human Kinetics
475 Devonshire Road Unit 100
Windsor, ON N8Y 2L5
800-465-7301 (in Canada only)
e-mail: info@hkcanada.com

Europe: Human Kinetics
107 Bradford Road
Stanningley
Leeds LS28 6AT, United Kingdom
+44 (0) 113 255 5665
e-mail: hk@hkeurope.com

Australia: Human Kinetics
57A Price Avenue
Lower Mitcham, South Australia 5062
08 8372 0999
e-mail: info@hkaustralia.com

New Zealand: Human Kinetics
P.O. Box 80
Mitcham Shopping Centre, South Australia 5062
0800 222 062
e-mail: info@hknewzealand.com

E5764

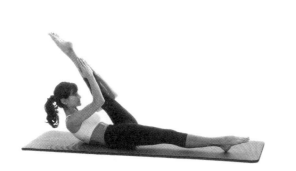

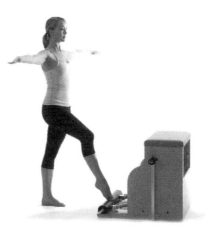

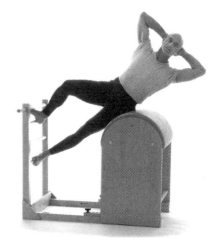

Foreword

Kathleen Stanford Grant (August 1, 1921–May 27, 2010) wrote the
following words for the first edition of this book. She will be desperately
missed by her family, her friends, and by the entire Pilates community.
She left an indelible mark on this industry.

When I first met Rael in Santa Fe, New Mexico, in 1991, the Pilates community was indeed very small. Upon the recommendation of John Claude West, who had studied with me and was running his own studio in New York, I was invited to teach a workshop on the Wunda Chair, a Pilates apparatus that I had worked on a lot with Joseph Pilates. Until then, I had not been consulted for professional advice by the Pilates community. The gathering in Santa Fe was a breakthrough; first and foremost, in recognizing the first generation of Pilates teachers and also in the sharing of information and drawing on our collective experience and expertise.

I was guided to Mr. Pilates by Pearl Lang, the renowned dancer and choreographer, after undergoing double knee surgery. He used the Wunda Chair extensively for my knee therapy, believing it to be most beneficial for that purpose. I learned a vast amount about the Wunda Chair during my rehabilitation and went on to develop my own repertoire. I continued to use the Wunda Chair in my teaching at Henri Bendel, from 1973 to 1988, and I still use it in my teaching today, including the Pilates program I run for the Tisch School of the Arts at NYU.

When I entered the studio in Santa Fe, I was immediately surrounded by a group of seasoned professionals who had come from far and wide, hungry for information and enthusiastic about spending time with me. I noticed a man in the group and when I asked for a volunteer to demonstrate some of the work, he eagerly jumped up. He got on the Wunda Chair and started demonstrating. I immediately recognized that he was an accomplished mover and that he knew Pilates well. As I started prodding and poking, making intricate adjustments to his alignment and movement, I could see a look of astonishment cross his face. The young male ego! This made me chuckle inside. He was clearly strong, but he relied too much on his strength and athletic ability rather than on his core.

We proceeded to work for several hours together as I taught, demonstrated, adjusted, and corrected. I respected his openness to learning and his humility in the presence of another teacher. That workshop was a pivotal point in the evolution of Pilates. From that point on the Wunda Chair, which had become all but obsolete, boomed in popularity.

Rael, for the young man was of course him, has often expressed to me that our meeting changed his career. It set him on a path of inner exploration and self-assessment. His work changed and his teaching changed; he discovered how to work from within. Rael and I went on to become, above all else, good friends. I am now regarded as one of the elders of the Pilates community, and Rael as a world-renowned teacher and a leader in his own right. He has developed a fine teacher training program, Body Arts and Science International (BASI Pilates), to which he invited me to serve as honorary advisor.

Back in 1991 Rael requested that I conduct a workshop at his center in Southern California. I made a promise to him that I would do it, but I could not say when. Thereafter, on every occasion we met, he would remind me of my promise. It took 14 years for me to fulfill it. In 2005 I came to Southern California from New York to give a workshop at On Center Conditioning. Although Rael also taught, the students got to witness their mentor being guided by his mentor. This in itself was a valuable lesson, possibly more valuable than the work itself.

Rael performs the work with unique mastery, and he certainly moves from within. At the same time he demonstrates an ever-present youthful desire to continue learning and growing. We need to keep the lineage of Pilates alive, preserving the past and respecting the future, upholding the values and principles of this system—and few have done as much toward that end as Rael. He is the male that Mr. Pilates wished for to continue his work.

Kathy Stanford Grant
First-generation Pilates teacher, Pilates Elder

When the first edition of this book was published, it was the culmination of 16 years of good intentions and 3 years of actual writing. I wanted to put my work as a teacher and student of Pilates into words, yet each time I attempted to do so the enormity of this system of physical and mental conditioning overwhelmed me. I knew that in order to offer something profound and valuable to Pilates enthusiasts, I needed more knowledge and experience. So back to the studio I went, to master the repertoire of movements, to explore the work further, and to teach another few thousand sessions. This process of ever-expanding education spanned five continents and more practice hours than I could ever recall.

Around 1990, when I first felt the urge to write a book, I had already been doing Pilates for more than 10 years. I had earned a bachelor's degree from the Wingate Institute of Physical Education in Israel, danced professionally, and completed my master's degree in dance studies in England. I had been an avid competitive athlete since my youth and had practiced yoga since my early teens. Yet, endeavoring to master Pilates felt like learning to crawl and walk again. This humbling experience, which taught me how to move with an ease and flow I had never before experienced, inspired me—and at times frustrated me. I had embarked on a lifelong journey of learning and practice that would deepen my understanding of movement and offer me a path to physical and mental well-being.

Now, with the publication of the second edition of *Pilates*, my initial agonizing over the writing of the book seems like time well spent. My own body of work, knowledge, and experience has continued to expand; the number of people who practice Pilates worldwide has continued to grow; and Pilates has further established itself in the mainstream of fitness, athletic training, and even therapy. As a result, the demand for well-trained teachers has also continued to increase, and teachers have become better educated and equipped to deal with the expanding scope of this method. The educational organization I founded in 1989, *Body Arts and Science International (BASI Pilates)*, now has a global reach of 30 countries and continues growing by the day.

Joseph Pilates dreamed of universal recognition and growth and believed it could happen; yet I doubt that even in his most ambitious dreams, he envisaged the popularity of the Pilates method that we are witnessing today. He wanted to see his method (which he called *Contrology*) taught in every school because he believed it could affect society as a whole in a positive way. He wanted the medical profession to embrace the method for the beneficial physical and mental effects it has on general wellbeing.

Today, Joseph Pilates' dreams are coming true. His method is indeed being used in schools, and it is increasingly found in clinics, hospitals, and research centers. Research is substantiating many of his principles and concepts and the medical profession is recognizing its value. I have long believed that if every person on earth did Pilates mat work every day, we would live in a far better world—it simply makes you feel so good!

Joseph Pilates died a disillusioned man, by many accounts. In his book *Your Health*, he expresses his disdain for the medical profession and people's closed-mindedness. Tragically, he and his wife Clara did not live to witness the development of their method into the phenomenon it has become. Yet the spirit of their teaching lives on, and I feel a deep, personal responsibility to uphold the integrity and high standard of their work. I hope this book makes a valuable contribution to keeping the flame burning strong.

Acknowledgments

This edition of *Pilates* is the culmination of a career that has spanned 35 years, and several pages of acknowledgments would not suffice to thank everyone who has helped me along the way. Many people have taught, inspired, and guided me: students, teachers, colleagues, peers, friends, and my dear family. All have influenced the outcome of this book and deserve my deepest gratitude.

A number of people made a huge contribution to the first edition: Martin Bernard, Julie Rhoda, Dr. Jason Cheng, Chris Murray, Carol Appel, and Karla Adams. Of course, my gratitude to them continues. They helped create the book that has touched so many lives—we share this ultimate reward.

Tom Heine of Human Kinetics honored me with a request to embark on writing a second edition. Tom has stood by me not only over the course of this second edition of *Pilates*, but also during the entire process of writing *Pilates Anatomy* together with my dear friend and colleague, Karen Clippinger. Tom managed to keep me on track and on schedule, which those who know me can attest is an incredible feat in itself.

I would like to thank Carla Zych, editor extraordinaire, for her genuine interest in the book and appreciation for the discipline. Her comments were always intelligent, thoughtful, and thought provoking. At times when I desperately wanted to simply be done, she guided me back to the drawing board and helped me to make what was good even better. Together with Tom, she held my feet to the fire and kept the project moving toward completion.

Kirk Fitzek, photographer, designer, and friend, again gave generously of his time, expertise, and enormous talent. He shot 1,000 photos for this second edition, in addition to the 2,500 pictures taken for the first edition. Kirk has a never-ending supply of patience and manages to be calming and encouraging, even when a shoot drags on longer than anticipated and energy resources are low. Kirk now understands as much about alignment and muscle recruitment as any excellent Pilates teacher.

It is with pride that I thank the talented models whose dedication and skill continue to inspire me: Lisa Hubbard, Leah Stewart, Kristi Cooper White, and Tracy Mallett. Each one of them has trained with me, is an accomplished teacher, and has developed a brand of her own. Each is an active member of Body Arts and Science International (BASI) and a devotee of the BASI system. Three of them modeled for the first edition, and all three look and perform better now than they did seven years ago—and they were spectacular then! (Leah has had 2 children in the interim, one only 6 weeks before the photo shoot.) Their accomplishments speak volumes for the system, and they represent the BASI family honorably. All are a testament to the power of Pilates.

The staff and faculty of BASI Pilates, the Pilates education organization that I founded in 1989 and continue to direct, and of BASI Academy and Studio, the beautiful Pilates center in Southern California that I established in 1991, are the backbone of everything I do. I am proud to work with you all. I can't possibly thank you enough, but for now—thank you!

I am honored to have traveled this path of exploration and practice and to have encountered so many soulful and generous people along the way. My hope is that in some small way, this book serves to thank you all.

This book is for people who are seeking a comprehensive understanding of the Pilates method—from the underlying philosophy and far-reaching benefits of the method to much of the vast Pilates repertoire. I have attempted to cover the widest possible ground, with the aim of providing a definitive textbook for those who teach and practice the method with commitment and dedication. At the same time, *Pilates* is not exclusively for the professional; my hope is that it will serve as an informative introduction for anyone interested in delving into the depths of this work.

In this second edition, I offer variations for many of the exercises, in order to make the material more widely accessible and usable to a broader audience, ranging from novices just starting their Pilates journey, to teachers using Pilates in a therapeutic environment, to veteran instructors working with athletes. Most of the variations make the exercises simpler to execute, while certain variations add challenge to the original exercise.

All references to Pilates and the Pilates method in this book refer to the system of physical and mental conditioning developed by Joseph Hubertus Pilates. Although some of the movements differ from the exact manner or sequence in which they were originally performed, the intent and text is inspired by, and closely aligned with, the original works of Mr. Pilates. The legacy of this man, whom the great choreographer George Balanchine called the "genius of the body" (according to first generation teacher Romana Kryzanowska), remains an invaluable resource for generations of teachers and enthusiasts.

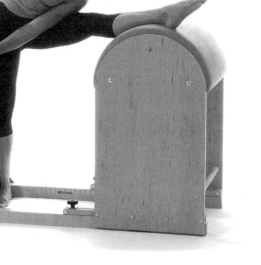

Joseph and his wife Clara set up the first Pilates studio in New York City soon after arriving from Germany in the mid-1920s. The rest is history—and an important and fundamental part of the method itself. Understanding the method's history allows us to understand the exercises and see them in the context of their time, taking into account the lifestyle and general activities of people in the 1920s. At that time, computers did not exist to encourage the development of round-shoulder syndrome, fast food was not available to hasten the advance of obesity, the relative scarcity of cars kept people more physically active, and lower back pain did not plague 80 percent of the population as it does today. It was a very different world!

Brief History of Pilates

Joseph Pilates was born near Düsseldorf, Germany, in 1880. He was a sickly child, plagued with rickets, asthma, and rheumatic fever. His drive to overcome these ailments led him to explore and practice body-building, gymnastics, diving, and other physical pursuits. He studied Eastern and Western philosophies and forms of exercise and was greatly influenced by ancient Greek and Roman regimens. This rich background provided him with the foundation to innovate a system that he developed throughout his life.

In 1912, Pilates traveled to England as a circus performer in a living Greek statue act. When World War I broke out, he was interned in a camp on the Isle of Man along with other German nationals. While there, he taught and practiced his physical fitness program and began devising apparatus to aid in the rehabilitation of the disabled and sick. A look at the apparatus of today reveals that certain pieces must have been fashioned around the frame of a hospital bed, most notably the Cadillac. Pilates is credited with assisting many victims of the influenza epidemic and helping others recover from wartime diseases.

After the war, Pilates returned to Germany and was invited by the German government to train the new army. Recognizing the implications of this, he decided to leave for America. (By certain accounts he was invited to the United States to help train world title holding boxer, Max Schmeling, from Germany.) The period before Pilates' immigration to the United States is not well documented, but he appears to have met some of the great European movement innovators of that time, such as Rudolf von Laban, Kurt Jooss, and Mary Wigman. Although Pilates was not a dancer, these early encounters may have set the stage for his profound involvement with the dance community later in his career.

On the way to the United States, Joseph met Clara, who soon became his wife and played an integral role in developing and teaching his method. She has been described as a compassionate, knowledgeable, and kind teacher, in some ways a superior teacher to Joseph Pilates himself. In 1926 they set up their first studio in New York City, which attracted a diverse population, including socialites, circus performers, gymnasts, and athletes.

But those who truly recognized the value of Pilates' system and his inherent, deep understanding of the workings of the human body were the members of the dance community, including luminaries such as Balanchine, Ted Shawn, Martha Graham, and Hanya Holm. They embraced the method, often integrating it into their dance technique and training, as they witnessed its positive effects on dancers' bodies in both rehabilitation and performance.

Pilates was a disciplined man, as his teaching and his physical condition and performance reveal. His work shows the influence of yoga, gymnastics, boxing, martial arts, and Eastern and Western philosophies. He taught and demonstrated his work in many environments, from the studio to his small New York apartment to the outdoors, where he seemed the most comfortable and inspired. He had the drive of a believer and the creativity of a genius. This was a man who believed deeply in his system as a way of life. He was convinced that it could affect every facet of one's being, and therefore society as a whole.

Pilates dreamed of seeing his work taught in every college and school. He believed that children should be given knowledge of the body, and that the information should be simple and accessible. He revered the simplicity of movement and the elegance of nature's design of the body, both human and animal. Many early articles on Pilates describe his passion for animals and animal-like movement, which is indicated by the names he gave to several of the exercises.

Over the course of his career Pilates developed more than 600 exercises for the various pieces of apparatus that he invented. His guiding philosophy was that achieving good health means that the whole being—body, mind, and spirit—must be addressed. Pilates equipment is designed to condition the entire body, using positions and movements that simulate functional activities and thereby correct body alignment and balance. An extensive repertoire of exercises, from fundamental to master level, can be done on each piece of apparatus. Using springs, pulleys, and gravity, the equipment challenges the musculature in diverse ways, with particular focus on the intrinsic muscles. These deep layers of muscle are encouraged to work to achieve optimum movement mechanics and maintain correct positioning and alignment.

Joseph Pilates was ahead of his time in his approach to well-being, in his creation of exercises, and in his invention of exercise equipment and its integration into everyday life. He created the wunda chair, which doubled as a piece of furniture and could arguably be considered the first home gym. The image of Joseph Pilates extolling the virtues of his equipment in his New York apartment, with Clara looking on, suggests that his presentations exceeded the bounds of mere demonstration. Rare footage corroborates this impression; Pilates produced a film that explains and promotes the many facets of his system, including personal health tips and even showering techniques. Something between an instructional guide and an infomercial, the film suggests that Pilates was forward thinking in his marketing methods as well as his approach to health, fitness, and well-being. Years after his death, his work spearheaded a revolution in the world of fitness and led to an evolution of the wellness industry.

The Pilates method offers a path to total health. It is not merely a physical fitness regimen of mindlessly repeated exercises. Pilates is a holistic approach to well-being and a lifelong process of refinement. In the opening paragraph of his book *Return to Life Through Contrology*, Pilates wrote, "Physical fitness is the first requisite to happiness. Our interpretation of physical fitness is the attainment and maintenance of a uniformly developed body with a sound mind fully capable of naturally, easily, and satisfactorily performing our many and varied daily tasks with spontaneous zest and pleasure."

Pilates covers the art and science of human movement as it relates to the Pilates method. I believe that every movement of this method can and should be substantiated both scientifically (through anatomy, physiology, biomechanics, and kinesiology), and artistically (through aesthetics, inner sensations, psychological components, and the flow of energy and life force). The significant overlap between the art and science of human movement has been recognized and explored through the ages. The mind and the body share a nourishing, symbiotic relationship that brings about profound and at times inexplicable results. This mind–body relationship lies at the heart of Pilates.

An in-depth exploration of each aspect of Pilates would far exceed the parameters of this book; for instance, it would take more than 100 pages to thoroughly cover breathing alone. Instead, I provide information about the Pilates method as a whole, emphasizing the repertoire and how to approach each exercise, via presentation, description, and analysis. Of course, a discussion of breathing is included, because it is one of the central principles of the method, and a breathing pattern is offered for each exercise. The subjects of anatomy, physiology, and biomechanics are not covered here in detail, though a working knowledge of these areas of study is important for Pilates professionals and serious enthusiasts, and therefore further study in these areas is highly recommended. See the selected resources list at the end of the book for suggestions.

Pilates takes you through a range of exercise levels, from fundamental through intermediate and finally touching on the advanced level. The book's 200-plus exercises are conveniently organized; each piece of apparatus is addressed in a separate chapter. The exercises in each chapter are grouped into blocks, based on regions of the body and the function of certain muscle groups. Within each block there are individual exercises and collections of exercises called series and groups. The description of each exercise includes its level of difficulty and a recommended resistance range. I also provide a muscle focus, objectives of the exercise, commentary, some ideas for imagery that may prove valuable in both executing and teaching the movements, and a checklist of points that help ensure a positive outcome. This book does not include the most advanced and master-level work, which warrant a separate book altogether.

Over the years, several approaches to the practice of the Pilates method have emerged. The classical approach advocates doing the work, manufacturing the apparatus, and sequencing the exercises exactly as Joseph Pilates did. Some other approaches deal primarily with rehabilitation; they have created protocols for specific treatments that use the Pilates apparatus but have changed the repertoire substantially. Often practitioners do not address the original repertoire or the holistic aspect of the work; and at times the relationship to the source is very loose indeed. Still other approaches deal with select populations, such as dancers or athletes, adapting the repertoire to their needs and, again, at times forgoing the original Pilates exercises and philosophy.

Throughout this book, and in my teaching and practice, I strive to remain true to the essence of Joseph Pilates' work while allowing an evolutionary process to take place. I call this approach *body arts and science*,

and it led to *Body Arts and Science International (BASI)*, an international organization that provides Pilates education. The approach incorporates the art and science of the Pilates method in a contemporary context, and the organization is a means of sharing this dynamic system with enthusiasts and professionals worldwide. Evolution is at times misconstrued as rejection of the classical work of Joseph Pilates. Nothing could be further from the truth. Evolution of Pilates, which I consider BASI to be, vindicates prior information and keeps the method as alive and relevant today as it was when Mr. Pilates was alive. Evolution is necessary, and as long as it is soundly grounded in the original works of Joseph Pilates and preserves his work and intent, it should be referred to as Pilates.

Joseph Pilates planted the seeds of a new approach to body conditioning, yet we can surmise that he did not define or even understand many of the concepts as we do today. Computers and sophisticated research methods enable us to scientifically substantiate notions that for Pilates and other innovators of that time were largely based on intuition. This modern substantiation of what was only intuited in the discipline's early days has given impetus to the adoption of Pilates in many arenas, such as therapeutic work, athletic training, pre- and postnatal exercising, and working with the elderly.

Therapists have long yearned for a system that could take patients from the early stages of rehabilitation to the long-term goal of a well-conditioned, efficiently functioning body. Athletes have searched for ways to gain an extra edge to peak their performance in competition. Dancers have looked for a system by which they could improve their strength, flexibility, and technique while maintaining the body type they are required to have. Actors, circus performers, musicians, singers— the list goes on— are constantly seeking to enhance their performance and extend their careers. Pilates is extremely well suited for all these groups.

Top performers in all disciplines are now keenly aware of the need to use the mind as well as the body.

Herein lies the essence of the Pilates method. Once an athlete has maximized physical capabilities such as speed, strength, and the skills required to perform the required actions, additional training and practice produce diminishing returns. It is tapping into the potential of the mind and its intricate connection to the body that will likely provide the elusive edge. Many have found the answer in Pilates; its credibility is now widely accepted.

Pilates not only offers a bridge between mind and body, between everyday life and optimal performance, between rehabilitation and healthy movement, it offers a system that, when used to its full potential, can enhance every aspect of life. It offers a solution to those with restricted mobility as well as to elite athletes. It is as beneficial for an 11-year-old as it is for an 80-year-old and as motivating for men as for women. It is adaptable and diverse, and that is its magic—not that it can transform the body in a few sessions or offer a perfect physique at the wave of a wand (which unfortunately is sometimes claimed).

Pilates is for the elderly who cannot find an environment, equipment, or system suited to their needs. It is for the young who want to look and feel better. It is for the fit and the nonfit who want to function at an optimal level, without pain. It is for people who seek balance in life, who want to change their lives for the better. Pilates, in other words, is for anyone (but not necessarily for everyone). As long as there is an ambition to be better, a world of discovery and untapped potential awaits.

Enhancing the Mind and Body

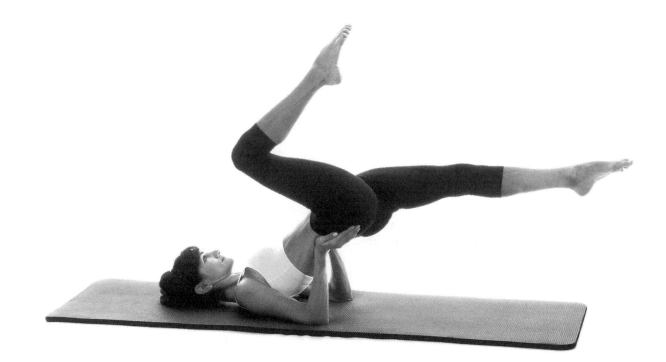

Is the exponential growth of Pilates—a method known by few people before the year 2000—merely hype? Why this sudden growth spurt, which would be characterized as nothing short of an epidemic by the author of the widely-read book *The Tipping Point*, Malcolm Gladwell? The reasons for the enormous popularity of Pilates lie in its far-reaching, diverse benefits, which include but are not limited to improved fitness and athletic performance, enhanced appearance, and a heightened sense of well-being.

The dance community has long benefited from Pilates, and for good reason. Dancers are supreme athletes, as measured by the feats they perform and the level of physical fitness they exhibit. Yet the demand on their bodies is enormous, and they suffer a very high incidence of injury—some studies suggest even higher than among football players. Dancers need an exceptional conditioning regimen that supplements their dance training and assists with injury prevention and rehabilitation. A dancer myself, I have often maintained that Joseph Pilates is the unsung hero of the dance world, given that many a dance career has been enhanced or saved by his method. Now everyone can benefit from the method that dancers have used as a form of cross-training for so many years, and enjoy many of the same results.

Athletes were the first to cross-train extensively and to recognize the far-reaching rewards of doing so. Now they are awakening to Pilates and embracing it as a legitimate form of cross-training to enhance performance and prevent injury. Many athletes have at their fingertips any form of conditioning they choose to improve their performance. The fact that so many elect to use Pilates is a testament to its value. It is good for the highest-ranked golfers and the best swimmers in the world; the most elite dancers, figure skaters and tennis players; the fastest, highest-jumping ball players; and a host of actors, singers, and musicians. At the same time, it is also the best possible choice for people who have never exercised before and is an excellent foray into the world of fitness.

In 2000 I gave a presentation on enhancing athletic performance using the Pilates method. In preparation I informally surveyed some Olympic-level swimmers, asking them what they looked for in a cross-training regimen and how they thought Pilates could help their performance. The answers varied, but most respondents identified two goals: to improve core strength and to explore the benefits of mind–body control and power. These two concepts encapsulate the essence of Pilates; very few, if any, training regimens are as effective as Pilates in achieving these goals.

Is Pilates for anyone? Yes. Will everyone select Pilates as their fitness regimen of choice? No. Not everyone will relate to the Pilates approach, and for certain training goals it may not be the most effective choice. For instance, bodybuilders interested in increasing muscle mass are better served by weight training. Sprinters who wish to gain speed and agility may prefer plyometrics or another form of resistance training. (Although, I believe that even bodybuilders and sprinters will benefit greatly from certain aspects of Pilates, such as the core strength it develops, the heightened awareness it provides, and the flexibility and control it offers.)

Still, the adaptability and wide appeal of Pilates is astounding. It can serve a broad spectrum of the population, because its benefits are not limited to the young or the super-fit or super-athletic. It has long been my view that the two populations that will ultimately benefit the most from Pilates are the youth and the elderly, essentially the two ends of life's spectrum. I have witnessed positive changes in posture, alignment, weight, and body-mass distribution resulting from Pilates to a degree that has surprised even me. I have seen positive changes in self-image, athletic performance, and the ability to perform daily activities. My clients have shared heartwarming stories of improvement in their personal and sexual relations. I have witnessed—and personally experienced—postinjury and postsurgery rehabilitation programs incorporating Pilates that were successful beyond all expectations. It sounds too good to be true. Yet these transformations occur time and again throughout the world, and the international community is taking notice. Although more scientific research is needed, it is beginning to substantiate many of these anecdotal findings, bringing welcome credibility to the practice of Pilates.

Of course, Pilates is not a potion that cures all and brings about miraculous changes immediately. Change takes time, commitment, and discipline. If you are dedicated to regular Pilates sessions, three times a week for at least six weeks, some positive changes are inevitable. Although certain changes can and often do occur immediately—for instance, a change in body awareness, muscle activation, or alignment—it takes time for most changes and adaptations to become imprinted in the neuromuscular system, for muscles to transform, and for the transformation to be integrated into a person's life.

One of the most gratifying experiences I have had in my Pilates career was working with a woman named Stella, who came to me at age 76 with severe scoliosis and an array of muscular and structural imbalances. The medical literature would say that changes could not be made to this woman's alignment, posture, or even movement at this point in her life. In fact, it would probably say that without either surgery or bracing during her preteen years, no significant changes in her physical alignment could have been achieved at any point in her life. But Stella worked with a commitment and dedication that I had seldom seen. She inspired all those around her, people of all ages and fitness levels, including me. After my first session with Stella, I realized how unique she was, and she realized that she had found a system that could enhance her life greatly. Within the first few sessions her awareness improved

and she started recognizing the immense imbalances that had infiltrated her body. After 30 sessions she moved differently, her posture improved, her confidence was elevated—in fact, her whole life changed. She realized early on that these results were only the beginning; that remaining committed for the long haul—not for days, weeks, or months, but for years—was imperative. And remain committed she did!

Was it simply the method, the exercises, and the apparatus that brought about changes? I believe not. It was Stella. She had a positive outlook, determination, and a powerful drive. Pilates provided a vehicle and the tools for change. Did she suddenly have a straight spine? Absolutely not! Such a change to the skeletal structure could not take place at her age. Yet her alignment, muscular control, and efficiency in movement did change. Her level of pain decreased dramatically and she began to enjoy her daily activities, especially her beloved gardening, relatively pain free. I would not be exaggerating to say, it gave her a new lease on life!

I believe the body is the divine temple of all that lies within. It carries the nucleus of who we are and embodies our true potential. Although I have spent much of my life tuning my body as if it were a fine musical instrument, I knew viscerally from an early age (and later consciously) that physical activity—be it Pilates, yoga, dance, surfing, windsurfing, running, paragliding, biking, snowboarding, or skiing—ultimately serves my inner being. The physical benefits are undoubtedly important, but the effects on the inner being carry implications that are infinite. They influence how you function, how you feel, how you relate to yourself and those around you, and how successful you are in every respect. It simply makes you feel good. And if you feel good, you function well, you are fulfilled, and life seems more complete. The old adage that proclaims that within a healthy body lies a healthy mind could be taken one step further: A healthy mind guides a healthy body.

Benefits of Pilates

Develops many aspects of physical fitness: strength, flexibility, coordination, speed, agility, and endurance

Heightens body awareness

Enhances body control

Teaches correct muscle activation

Corrects posture and alignment

Facilitates optimal function of the internal organs

Improves balance and proprioception

Focuses on breathing and its related physical and psychological benefits

Offers a vehicle for concentration and focus

Promotes relaxation and the release of tension

Helps keep musculature and bone structure in an optimal state

Benefits pregnant women by providing a safe, effective, non-impact exercise activity

Serves as cross-training for athletic pursuits and daily activities

Distributes body mass aesthetically (people report looking and feeling slimmer)

Provides a path to inner harmony through a finely tuned body

Mind and Body As One

Discussion of the mind–body connection is as old as the ages; it rises up every now and again like a tidal wave. The 1970s and 1980s saw trends that focused on the physical being—hard-driving approaches with infamous mottos such as *No pain, no gain* or *Work till you drop*. More recently the fitness industry has returned to a mind–body focus—calmer, more introspective, refined and integrated systems of exercise and movement. We've seen a surge in the popularity of yoga and Pilates, an emphasis on nurturing the body rather than punishing it and a renewed focus on the power of the mind–body connection. Proof of this connection continues to accrue, especially in the form of research based on brain-scan imaging that reveals changes in the brain that occur as a result of changes in the body, and vice versa.

Joseph Pilates created his system of exercise with the intention that it should positively affect every aspect of a person's life—from movement to interpersonal relationships to heightened performance in daily tasks—leading the way to a state of total well-being. He believed that widespread practice of his system, based as it is on the mind–body connection, would eliminate many diseases and social ills. The Pilates method is more than a series of exercises; it is an approach to life, a philosophy. Time and again, the practice of Pilates reminds us that this system addresses the whole being. It dictates that we be aware of the changes that occur daily on every level of our being. These changes can be positive (such as rejuvenation and increased energy) or negative (such as rising stress and ailments). To reap the full potency of Pilates, you should make it an integrated part of your life; one that enriches every day. To practice Pilates is to strive to achieve balance and maximize the potential of the body, mind, and spirit.

The key to the positive effects of Pilates lies in its principles, not only in its exercises and equipment. It is a mind–body system that, unlike many other forms of physical fitness, addresses far more than the quantifiable aspects of human movement, such as strength, range of motion, and endurance. Pilates encompasses awareness, balance, control, efficiency, function, harmony, and the far reaching effects that these have on the body and the mind. Stabilization is developed, posture is refined, mechanics of movement are improved, muscle recruitment patterns are reeducated, and function and well-being are reinforced—the ultimate goal of any good conditioning program. Pilates can and will improve every facet of your life.

Three Higher Principles

Return to Life Through Contrology opens with these words: "Physical fitness is the first requisite of happiness." It is a bold statement and one that could seem judgmental, but the book quickly makes clear that Joseph Pilates recognized that each person has different capabilities. What his opening statement claims is that the mind and body are intricately linked and that the condition of the body influences the state of the mind, and vice versa. He continuously reinforces this premise in his writing and teachings, reiterating that physical condition relates not only to happiness but also to many other mental states (positive or negative, depending on the body's condition), such as relaxation and pleasure, anxiety, and depression. He claimed that by reawakening thousands of dormant muscle cells, we also awaken thousands of dormant brain cells. Stimulating the body enhances the functioning of the mind. It is essentially a case of the muscles building the brain.

Despite the vastness, complexity, and scope of the Pilates method, three themes remain constant. I call them the *higher principles*; guides that help us navigate the lifelong exploration of Pilates. The way we define certain elements of the work and describe the movements may change as new research is conducted and modern terminology is created. But these are only words, the glossary of the system. The philosophy encompassed in the higher principles never changes; it is the essence of the system itself.

1. **Completely coordinate the body, mind, and spirit.** This goal is the method's driving force—integrating into each exercise the balance of body, mind, and spirit. As Pilates wrote in *Return to Life Through Contrology*, achieving this balance "results in perfect posture." Without recognizing this principle and integrating it into your work, you will feel that your body lacks its life force. Although the relationship between the body, mind, and spirit is in a constant state of flux, these components are present throughout our lives. With the practice of Pilates we become aware of them. Finding the balance between them is a lifelong journey.

2. **Achieve the natural inner rhythm associated with all subconscious activities.** The highest level of motor learning we can attain is when an action is practiced to the point of becoming subconscious. This does not mean that we do it without concentration or awareness; instead, as the movement pattern becomes imprinted in the muscle memory, it becomes intuitive, and we can focus on fine-tuning, as opposed to being consumed with learning the action itself. Mastery cannot be achieved in a short time; it is the reward of consistent training over

a long period of time, sometimes years. In his book *The Outliers*, Malcolm Gladwell discusses the "10,000 hour principle," which states that a person needs that many hours of practice to master a skill—any skill. Such practice requires discipline and commitment on every level, as well as patience and endurance. This is the type of dedication to the practice of Pilates that leads to mastery of the system and ultimately to well-being. As Pilates wrote in *Return to Life Through Contrology*, "Correctly executed and mastered to the point of subconscious reaction, these exercises will reflect grace and balance in your routine activities" (page 63).

3. **Apply the natural laws of life to everyday living.** Pilates greatly admired nature and the animal kingdom. He often wrote about the graceful and efficient movements of animals, and he considered them far more evolved than humans in terms of movement and muscular development. Many of today's human ills and ailments are a result of people losing touch with the natural laws of living. Sitting at computers for many hours a day, watching television for many more, eating far in excess of our needs (often unhealthy food), driving and seldom walking are some of the lifestyle changes of the past few decades. Pilates wrote in *Your Health*, "Man has, in the race for material progress and perfection, entirely overlooked the most complex and marvelous of all Creations—Man himself!" We can learn a great deal from observing animals; their movements, their instincts and their habits. I have learned much from watching Shiloh, my little Jack Russell Terrier. He stretches his spine hundreds of times a day, usually doing what Pilates practitioners call an "Up Stretch" ("Down Dog" in yoga terms), and he definitely knows how to relax, despite his very spirited nature.

To achieve the highest accomplishments within the scope of our capabilities in all walks of life we must constantly strive to acquire strong, healthy bodies and develop our minds to the limit of our ability.

—Joseph H. Pilates, *Return to Life Through Contrology*

Ten Movement Principles

If the higher principles are the soul of the system, the ten movement principles I have identified through my personal experience in this work are its personality and character. They evolved from the three higher principles and are closely linked to their underlying philosophy. Pilates practitioners should be mindful of these movement principles at all times, during both the teaching of the movements and the execution of the exercises. Each movement principle applies to every exercise in this book and should be integrated into your practice. They are the foundation of this mind–body system, serving to guide teachers and students toward understanding, mastery, and well-being.

Principle 1: Become Aware

The first step into the wonderful world of Pilates, and every step that follows, should be filled with *awareness* and mindfulness. Be present in the movement with mind and body. In some forms of physical conditioning, everything about the environment seems designed to separate the mind from the body: loud music, television screens, computers mounted on exercise equipment, and a myriad of other distractions. Pilates is practiced in an environment that stimulates and fortifies the mind–body connection, beginning with an awareness of the body.

No one can address the process of realigning the body without awareness of its structure and how it moves. Often I will say to a client whose leg is not straight, "Please straighten your leg all the way." He will answer, "But it is straight" (when clearly it is not). At other times I will adjust a client's head so that it sits on the centerline of the body, and the response is, "That feels very lopsided." Over time we become accustomed to misalignments, and the less aware a person is, the more severe these misalignments become, until an off-center body part feels centered or a bent limb feels straight. Bringing awareness to the body and the intricacies of movement establishes a foundation for change. Without awareness, little can be achieved.

Principle 2: Achieve Balance

The term *balance* can mean many things. It can relate to components of fitness such as strength and flexibility, to the act of standing on one leg, or to the symmetry of the body. It can also describe a well-designed Pilates program, in which the exercises are proportionally distributed to work the different parts of the body in a session (an important consideration in Pilates). Due to the method's focus on the abdominal region, Pilates programs are often excessively weighted toward abdominal work, particularly in forward flexion. This is a mistake. There needs to be a balance in working the various muscle groups as well as the different planes of motion. The word balance may also refer to the well-being of the whole individual, a balance of body, mind, and spirit. You should strive to achieve balance, in every sense of the word and make it an integral part of your Pilates practice.

Joseph Pilates often mentioned the importance of a uniformly developed musculature, stating that only when the muscles are developed in such a way can the body function unhindered, true flexibility be present, and well-being be achieved. This idea touches on several issues, including muscular development, ease of function, and the mind–body relationship. Symmetrically and proportionately developed musculature allows the spine to perform its function to support the body and to assist in movement, ranging from fine, intervertebral articulation to large, powerful actions of the trunk.

Musculoskeletal conditions frequently show patterns of muscular imbalance for multiple reasons. Some patterns are associated with dominance on one side (referred to as *handedness*), some with postural deviations such as scoliosis and kyphosis, and others with lack of flexibility or excessive flexibility. Imbalances that affect body alignment or result from misalignment are important factors in many painful postural conditions.

The pursuit of awareness is endless—it is what makes Pilates so interesting, intriguing, and rewarding.

Balance is the internal scale of life, dynamic and ever-changing. Pilates offers the path to equilibrium.

At times muscles react to protect the body from harm or to reduce pain, with the result that certain muscles become overactive while others are inhibited. Muscle imbalance may result as well from occupational or recreational activities that involve movement habits in which certain muscles are used persistently while the opposing muscles are inadequately recruited. Examples include habitually holding the phone to the ear on the same side, resulting in a chronic tilt of the head; standing with the weight shifted onto one leg, resulting in a perpetual tilt of the pelvis; and playing a one-side-dominant sport such as tennis, resulting in asymmetric muscular development.

Each person has different needs in terms of imbalances and how to alleviate them. Identifying and addressing these needs is the first step on the path to achieving balance. As we practice and teach Pilates, we act as "movement detectives," constantly making observations about our own bodies and those of our students. I provide some basic tools later in the book, such as the Roll-Down exercise in chapter 2, that help assess alignment and identify imbalances. In fact, I view all the exercises in this book, and movement in general, as tools of analysis. They reveal a wealth of information about the intricacies of the body.

Principle 3: Breathe Correctly

At the root of the natural laws of life and natural inner rhythm is *breathing*. Pilates wrote in *Return to Life Through Contrology*, "Breathing is the first act of life, and the last . . . above all, learn how to breathe correctly." Breathing is synonymous with life and with movement. It is all-encompassing, the link between body, mind, and spirit. Breathing is immensely important and powerful, yet it is so often ignored. One deep breath can promote relaxation, release tension, and make you smile.

Everything, from the minutest movement to life itself, begins with breath. Breathing is the inner shower that cleanses the body, guides the mind, and rejuvenates the spirit; it promotes natural movement and is the first step to educating the neuromuscular system. Breathing is also a vehicle for the achievement of an inner focus and an inner rhythm, a path to relaxing the mind and calming the spirit. It is the engine that drives all movement, and it lies at the source of the Pilates method.

Certain muscle groups are recruited during the breath cycle to assist in respiration and therefore should be considered in determining a breathing pattern for a given exercise. For instance, we theorize that exhaling during abdominal work maximizes abdominal muscle recruitment because of the known participation of these muscles in exhalation. Conversely, we theorize that since the trunk extensors assist in inhalation, inhaling during trunk extension probably maximizes their recruitment. Note that both of these muscle groups can be recruited during inhalation and exhalation, but muscle contraction may be more prominent when it corresponds with the breath cycle. Although scientific proof for these assertions is lacking, my experience as a practitioner and a teacher has convinced me of their relevance. Saying that, although I teach a specific breathing pattern initially as a way of disciplining the mind and body, I do not promote being rigid and stuck with one pattern. Just as there is choreography for the movement, there is choreography for the breathing. This choreography can and should be changed around in the same fashion that we change the movement around to expand our movement vocabulary.

Normal breathing is a complex process that involves many joints and muscles and is responsive to both voluntary and involuntary control. Basic understanding of the breath cycle is important because it offers insight into exercise and movement in general. A crucial muscle to cite when discussing breathing is the diaphragm, a dome-shaped muscle that forms a canopy underlying the rib cage. The diaphragm plays an important role in breathing and in creating the "muscular corset," the internal support system that is addressed throughout this book.

Breathing

Oxygenates the blood and nourishes the body on a cellular level

Expels toxins from the body

Improves circulation

Improves skin tone

Calms the mind and the body

Encourages concentration

Provides a rhythm for movement

Assists in activating target muscles

During diaphragmatic breathing, 75 percent of the respiratory effort comes from the diaphragm. When this muscle contracts during inhalation, it flattens, increasing the vertical dimension of the thorax (figure 1.1a). In addition, the external intercostal muscles also contract, pulling the lower ribs upward. Because of the orientation of the ribs and their joints (the lower part of the rib cage is wider than the upper part), the lower region of the thorax expands laterally as the diaphragm contracts, increasing the lateral dimension of the rib cage. In contrast, as the upper ribs rise they increase the anterior-to-posterior dimension of the thorax, with the sternum moving forward (figure 1.1b). The overall effect is an increase in thoracic volume, a decrease in intrapulmonary pressure and air flowing into the lungs— in other words, inhalation.

When the diaphragm relaxes, the organs in the abdominal cavity and abdominal muscles push it upward into its dome shape, thus decreasing the vertical dimension of the thorax. Added to this, the elasticity (recoil) of the lungs and chest wall create decreased thoracic volume and increased intrapulmonary pressure, resulting in air flowing out of the lungs, or exhalation.

When practicing Pilates, abdominal muscle contraction typically accompanies most of the movements, which can be particularly challenging during inhalation. Therefore in Pilates, we emphasize the lateral and posterior expansion of the rib cage during inhalation (called *lateral* or *costal breathing*). Besides assisting in drawing air into the lungs, this mode of breathing facilitates maintaining abdominal muscle contraction throughout the exercise (during both inhalation and exhalation), which in turn assists in dynamic stabilization of the trunk.

This is not to say that the diaphragm does not contract or should be ignored. The diaphragm is a fundamental component of breathing and of the internal support system of the body. However the focus is placed on the expansion of the rib cage and contraction of the abdominal muscles as opposed to the relaxation of the abdominal muscles that often accompanies the contraction of the diaphragm.

This by no means implies that diaphragmatic breathing is undesirable; it is in fact the form of breathing that is primarily used in daily life. However, lateral breathing is the preferred mode of breathing during some forms of physical activity, including Pilates. An important point

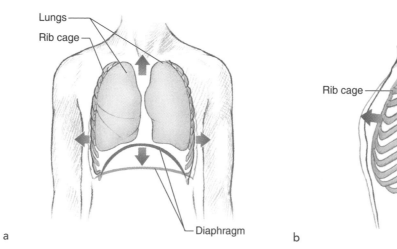

FIGURE 1.1 The diaphragm works with the abdominal muscles to deepen inhalation and expand the thorax.

Lungs

Rib cage

a

Rib cage

Diaphragm

b

to stress is that the process of practicing different types of breathing techniques should not cause tension; it should be viewed as expanding the breathing vocabulary so that the appropriate breathing technique can be employed for a given task. This can be equated to the different breathing techniques used to play the various wind instruments, from the trombone to the trumpet to the didgeridoo. None are wrong, just that each if these instruments requires a different breathing technique, and so it is with different physical activities.

During the exhalation phase of Pilates exercises, the abdominal muscles contract to assist the diaphragm and intercostals in expelling air. (Imagine a process of milking the lungs and wringing the air out.) This in turn promotes deeper inhalation on the part of the primary respiratory muscles and the auxiliary muscles (including the back extensors), bringing in a healthy quantity of oxygen-filled air to nourish and rejuvenate the body.

Many people have commented to me over the years that they have found learning lateral breathing and practicing this technique of breathing to be immensely beneficial. Those who have made such remarks have included singers, musicians, and yogis who are accustomed to using very specific breathing techniques. Focusing on the breath and training in various modes of breathing promotes breath control.

Breathing can be practiced anywhere and at any time. I find two exercises particularly helpful in mastering lateral breathing. The first is to wrap a three-foot length of rubber exercise band around your chest, holding the ends of the band in your hands, and expanding your chest against the resistance of the band amplifying the contraction of the intercostals. The other involves lying supine on a mat in a comfortable neutral spine position, knees bent, legs parallel, and arms by the sides of the body. Visualize that with each breath the chest expands and spreads laterally across the mat in both directions like two swells rising in the ocean and then gently falling back. This is an excellent form of meditation and good practice for breathing. Also imagine the breath

moving like a river of energy to either side of the chest, or any part of the body that may need to be activated or relaxed. This is particularly helpful if an imbalance is present and the musculature on one side of the thorax is not as active as the other, often the case when scoliosis is present and one side becomes relatively compressed.

Principle 4: Concentrate Deeply

I view *concentration* as the bridge between awareness and movement. As you establish the starting position for each movement, I encourage you to go through a checklist of important data: which muscles you need to recruit, how you should align your body, and what is your chosen breath pattern. Simply by concentrating on a particular muscle prior to the action, you can activate it more accurately and intensely than if you do not think about it. Concentrating on your body alignment will help you recruit the correct muscles and avoid unnecessary strain on the body. Concentrating on the breath pattern will help you maintain a good rhythm for the movement and keep your mind focused. However, keep in mind that concentration can be so intense that it becomes counterproductive. It can morph into tension, which leads to a tightening of the musculature, a restriction in breathing, and a halting rather than flowing movement. This is clearly not the intention and should be avoided.

Although awareness and concentration are closely related, I regard awareness as a state of mind—being mindful and feeling the movement. Concentration is a more cognitive process of understanding the movement. Concentration, combined with awareness, not only promises precise movement but also gives the work a meditative quality. Being meditative does not imply that the work will lack challenge, physical demand, or intensity; it means ensuring a deep focus to the work that allows you to block out unnecessary disturbances and perform each movement to the maximum of your ability, tapping into the full potential of Pilates.

Breath is the fuel for what Joseph Pilates called the powerhouse, the engine that drives the movement.

Pilates is meditation in motion—a physical, mental, and spiritual process.

Principle 5: Center Yourself

Centering yourself can be defined in purely physical terms—finding where your center of gravity lies. In women the center lies approximately anterior to the first and second sacral segments, floating in the middle of the pelvic bowl. In men it tends to be slightly higher, in the center of the body opposite the navel. Differences in anatomy result in different weight distribution—men tend to be top heavy and women carry their weight in the pelvic region. Discovering and experiencing your body's center of gravity is important, as it affects each exercise you do. This is also the region of the powerhouse. The concept of the powerhouse—that all movement emanates from this core—is a common thread in the practice of Pilates and is addressed in more detail in chapter 2 (see the section titled "Muscles of the Powerhouse"). In Pilates, centering yourself means more than finding your center of gravity; it means uniting body, mind, and spirit.

The concept of centering is not new. In Eastern practices we learn of *ki* in aikido, *chi* in tai chi, *tan tien* in chi gong, and *chakra* in yoga—all refer, in general terms, to the life force that lies within us like a bottomless well of energy. Interestingly, in all these practices this life force is located in approximately the same area of the body. Martha Graham focused on this area in her modern dance technique and altered the way dancers approached dance and movement; the *contraction* (flexion of the spine), involving deep abdominal activation, became the foundation of her technique. The feeling of being centered relates not only to the support provided by the area's strong, intrinsic muscles, but also to the energy emanating from this nucleus and a person's ability to make full use of this physical and metaphysical support system. It is not uncommon to hear a dancer speak of feeling centered or, conversely, lacking center. As you delve into Pilates and open yourself to finding and moving from your center, you will experience this most gratifying and elevating of sensations.

Principle 6: Gain Control

Gaining *control* is an amalgamation of all the preceding principles. When you watch people move, particularly during complex movements, it is immediately evident whether they have a high level of control. Few things are as beautiful and inspiring as viewing athletes, dancers, gymnasts, or figure skaters who have immaculate control over their movement. Similarly, watching a lion walk, a cheetah run, or a gazelle leap can evoke a feeling of awe. Kathy Stanford Grant, a student of Joseph Pilates who became a great teacher of his work, used to send me phenomenal pictures of animals in balance or in motion, pointing out their grace, their effortless power, and unencumbered movement. These qualities are lofty goals for us humans, but worthy of aspiring to nevertheless.

Initially, achieving control of movement is a conscious process. It occurs through practice, practice, and more practice. Ideally, a teacher who has achieved control should guide you in this process. As you continue to practice and integrate the work into your body, sometimes for years and many hundreds of repetitions, your own movement control becomes like that of an animal, intuitive—a part of your being.

Principle 7: Be Efficient

Who does not want to conserve energy? Waste has become a byproduct of our society in every way. Striving for *efficiency* teaches us to focus our energy. When performing Pilates, we do not grimace during effort or grunt as the movements become difficult and demanding. We focus the work where it is needed, exerting the required amount of energy, no more and no less. The rest of the body remains calm and relaxed. I have an internal agreement with myself when performing the work; the more difficult and demanding the movements are, the more consciously relaxed I become. I view efficiency of movement like a laser beam: focused and directed.

Achieving efficiency applies not only to athletic feats but also to everyday movements. An important phase in

A strong center enhances performance, be it in everyday activities or athletic pursuits.

When control becomes innate, you have reached the point of mastery.

the process of learning Pilates is transferal—the ability to transfer information that is learned and practiced in the Pilates session into everyday activities and to integrate it into all aspects of life. A session lasts approximately one hour and is often supervised by an instructor. What of the remaining 23 hours of the day? We must actively and consciously direct our attention to how we move. I recommend creating reminders to help you practice transferal. This is like placing notes on a bulletin board, except these notes are mental ones that remind you to keep your head centered and your spine aligned, to use your powerhouse, to relax, and ultimately to move effortlessly.

Principle 8: Create Flow

Like all the principles, *flow* manifests itself both physically and mentally. It is present within each movement as well as within the Pilates session as a whole. Flow can be described as the unobstructed channeling and translation of energy into movement. It is also the seamless connecting of one movement to the next, creating what appears to be a continuous stream of motion. Despite the fact that teachers offer correction and input to students and may need to stop the class periodically to do so, the overall sense of each individual movement and of the session as a whole should be one of a continuum.

If you observe people like inspirational golfer Tiger Woods, dynamic swimmer Michael Phelps, and brilliant dancer Mikhail Baryshnikov, you will note a common quality: an effortless flow in their movements. You can experience the same quality through the practice of Pilates.

Flow can be understood physiologically as the immaculate timing of muscle recruitment and movement through the joints. In each movement there is an optimum sequence in which the muscles should be activated, called a muscle-recruitment pattern or muscle-firing pattern. When muscle recruitment is not only correct but also timed down to the millisecond,

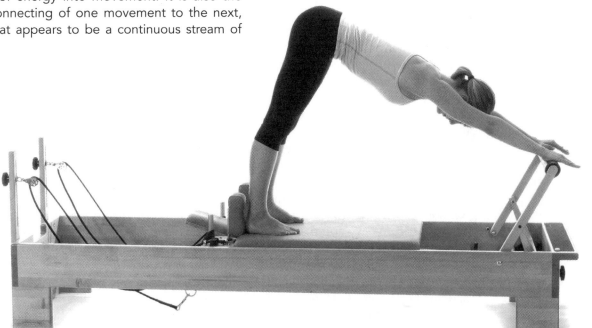

Precision is a fundamental ingredient in the practice of Pilates and a milestone on the path to mastery.

combined with the inner rhythm of unobstructed breath, the result is flow. Viewing two people performing an identical movement can be very interesting, as often they look quite different from one another. Flow, or lack thereof, is frequently the reason for this difference.

Principle 9: Be Precise

Without *precision*, Pilates work becomes almost meaningless. It is popular in the fitness industry to speak of isolating muscles during a particular movement. Isolation depends entirely on precision. Yet often those who claim to isolate muscles are doing anything but. Either they lack precision in isolating an area or they rely on external means, such as apparatus, to achieve this goal. For instance, someone who performs a biceps curl using a preacher curl bench is demonstrating nonfunctional isolation, because although he is using the biceps primarily, he is totally reliant on the bench. In life we cannot walk around with this type of support. Isolation is only meaningful when you can stabilize your body and support the isolated movement independently. This is a mindful process that takes us back to the first movement principle, awareness, followed by concentration and control. As you gain more insight into your body, you will be able to achieve increasingly fine muscle isolation. I strive for the day in which I am able to isolate and control every muscle fiber in my body; it is a dream that keeps me grounded and humble!

Precision requires complete integration of the body's musculature, which may then be followed by the isolation of certain muscles or muscle groups. You will feel the work more profoundly when you perform every movement with precision down to the finest detail. Precision is the basis of the "corrective approach" to working the body. We continuously strive to reach an ideal of balance and alignment. Students often comment that they feel an exercise more profoundly than ever, despite having done it many times before. Often it's a matter of adjusting the body one or two degrees this way or that—and suddenly the flame ignites. That

Moving through life in harmony with all around and within is the ultimate achievement of the practice of Pilates.

is precision. Pilates demands a great deal of precision, in the activation of each muscle, and in the execution of each movement.

Principle 10: Seek Harmony

Harmony is the whole, the culmination of all the preceding principles and all we strive to achieve it. It is the ultimate reward for commitment and hard work. Harmony means walking out of a session and feeling completely rejuvenated, being aware of each muscle and sensing the depth of each breath. It means being focused, centered and in control; efficient movement coupled with flow and precision. To feel all these qualities is to be in harmony with oneself and with the environment.

Few forms of conditioning can boast the profound outcomes that Pilates can, as millions are now experiencing. The greatness of human potential is realized when the infinite power of the mind is combined with the immaculate engineering of the human body. The principles I've described, individually and together, offer a path to harnessing the resources of the mind. The movements in Pilates, as beautiful and wonderful as they are, are only movements. The principles and philosophy of this system are what make it unique and able to transform lives. When correcting alignment and teaching positive movement patterns, you need to do more than only address physiological components, such as muscle strength and flexibility. You must also consider the principles behind the movements. They will guide you through the internal process of transformation that leads to well-being.

The practice of Pilates opens the path to new discovery each day. I can honestly say that I have never done a personal workout or taught a session without learning something new. Having done thousands of sessions and taught thousands of sessions, that statement in itself says much about the depth of the system. Of course your body, mind, and spirit must be open to such learning in order to benefit from it. If they are, the possibilities are never-ending.

2

Alignment, Posture, and Movement

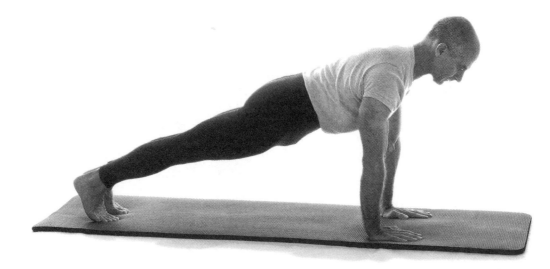

The previous chapter laid the foundation for understanding Pilates—its philosophy, principles, and ability to affect every facet of a person's being, as its creator intended. In the following chapters I discuss concepts that pertain to the science of human movement and their relationship to the Pilates method.

The human body is a complex instrument that can be likened, in its mechanical functioning, to a chain with multiple links—the *kinetic chain*. Exploring the kinetic chain is a fascinating study due to its infinite possibilities. Each body is different, even though all bodies share predictable patterns of movement and muscle development. As a movement occurs, the muscles are activated in a certain order, or pattern. If this pattern is faulty, the movement can often still be performed, but it will likely lack efficiency and could lead to injury. The Pilates method addresses the kinetic chain in its entirety, recognizing the influence that one region of the body can have on another. Through a process of refinement, Pilates can bring about profound changes, which enhance the body's performance and lay a path to well-being.

Musculoskeletal Structure

Let us view the body from the inside out. The skeleton is the body's infrastructure, on which all else is built (figure 2.1a). Onto this well-structured and balanced frame are layered the muscles, which provide support and movement (figure 2.1b). The bones act as levers and the muscles as cables that move the body part(s) in a desired direction. Because of this ingenious structure the musculature is able to work effectively. However, if the frame is out of alignment it affects the entire structure, resulting in inefficient muscle action, fatigue, and possible ailments.

The human body is the most masterful feat of mechanics, engineering, and physics imaginable. As a small example, consider the patella, the freely moving bone that sits above the knee (the largest sesamoid bone in the body). Besides protecting the knee joint, the patella creates a significant mechanical advantage for the quadriceps. If there were no patella, the quadriceps muscle would need to work approximately 30 percent harder and be much stronger (and larger) to create equivalent force. If the patella is out of alignment, knee function is affected and chronic ailments may

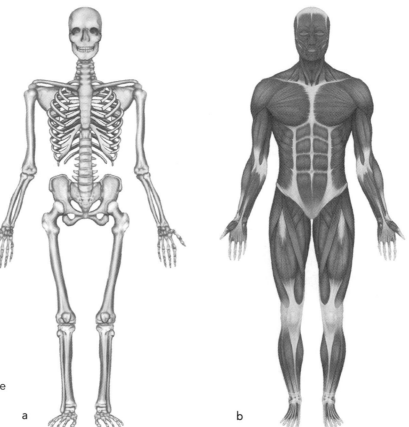

FIGURE 2.1 Proper skeletal alignment combines with good muscle mechanics to produce effortless and efficient movement.

a   b

result. How often do we give credit to this little bone for offering us such an enormous mechanical advantage in walking, running, and jumping? This is one tiny illustration of the body's wondrous mechanics.

The relationship between the skeletal structure and the muscular system is interesting and unique; it is the basis of all movement analysis. Often when exercising we place so much emphasis on the muscles that we ignore the skeletal structure. To achieve effective and efficient movement, we must consider both the skeletal and muscular systems (these categories are used in the broadest sense possible, including all bone and soft tissue—muscle, tendon, ligament, fascia, and cartilage). Joseph Pilates recognized and respected the marvel that is the structure of the human body. He invented a system that challenges this structure in every conceivable way, offering a path to discovering and utilizing its full potential.

Two well-known first-generation Pilates teachers, Eve Gentry and Bruce King, often described Pilates movements in terms of the *bones* (as opposed to the muscles) moving. Using this imagery can help facilitate effortless motion, devoid of tension or excessive force (and the inevitable grimacing and groaning!). It's as if the bones move as a result of an intangible internal force. Focusing on the skeletal structure also draws more attention to alignment. Correct alignment is the first step toward a positive outcome and success in achieving the desired goals.

Spine

One of the most fascinating parts of the skeleton is the spine (figure 2.2). Made up of 24 moving vertebrae and 9 that are fused (this number can vary slightly), the spine can be extremely mobile, allowing multidirectional movement of the trunk. At the same time, it can be very stable, serving as a solid platform to support movement of the limbs. In fact, each individual vertebral joint offers very little movement, yet combined they form a highly mobile mechanism. Distributing the work

through the spine and maximizing the movement of all the vertebral joints is preferable to stressing one or two vertebral joints, which can result in shearing forces and excessive load in a specific area. The pelvis and lower spine (the pelvic-lumbar region) is of particular interest in Pilates, because herein lies the *powerhouse*, the core, from which all movement emanates.

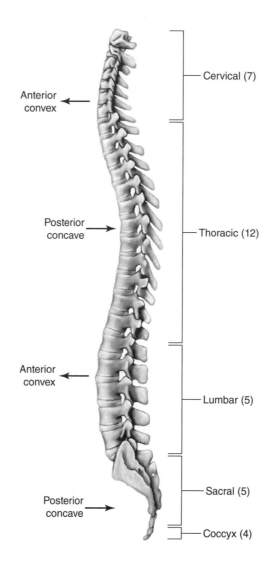

Anterior convex

Posterior concave

Anterior convex

Posterior concave

Cervical (7)

Thoracic (12)

Lumbar (5)

Sacral (5)

Coccyx (4)

FIGURE 2.2 This side view of the spine illustrates the natural curves of the spine and proper spinal alignment.

Pelvic Bowl

The pelvic bowl holds the essence of our being, the eternal spring of life. Here, where the body's center of gravity lies, is the meeting point of human anatomy with the metaphysical; the perfect merging of the musculoskeletal system with the life force. This concept forms the basis of Eastern and Western practices, such as yoga, tai chi, aikido, certain styles of dance and Pilates. The pelvis is indeed the powerhouse!

Dr. Arnold Kegel, innovator of the much-advocated exercises that bear his name (which involve contracting, holding, and releasing the muscles of the pelvic floor), recognized the importance of the pelvic floor muscles and their development, particularly for women before, during, and after pregnancy. He furthered the premise that training the pelvic floor muscles can help to prevent and cure urinary incontinence and improve sexual function and satisfaction. I am sure he would delight in the attention the pelvic floor is receiving today. A healthy pelvic floor—strong and flexible, able to adapt to changes in internal pressure—is one of the keys to well-being for both women and men.

Men are often surprised to learn that they even have a pelvic floor! Both genders need well conditioned pelvic floor muscles (coccygeus, iliococcygeus, and pubococcygeus) for optimum function, and recruitment of these muscles should be integrated into every comprehensive exercise program. Fortunately, because of the body's intricate neuromuscular patterning, when the transversus abdominis muscle is contracted (as it is throughout much of a Pilates session), the pelvic floor muscles also contract. A similar correlation seems to exist between contraction of the hip adductors, another muscle group that is activated frequently in Pilates, and the pelvic floor muscles. In addition, stopping the flow of urine activates the pelvic floor muscles, so, by nature's design; the pelvic floor is exercised throughout daily life, seemingly by default.

However, heightening awareness and control of this muscle group is extremely beneficial. A well-conditioned pelvic floor supports the internal organs and viscera and provides added support during pregnancy. In addition, it assists in preventing or overcoming urinary incontinence and contributes to heightened sexual function and satisfaction. Actively working the pelvic floor, particularly the coccygeus, influences positioning of the sacrum and may help relieve or prevent lower back pain. Much recent literature and research indicate that the pelvic floor is fundamental to healthy functioning of the core, in terms of strength, support, and stabilization, primarily due its role in enhancing intra-abdominal pressure.

Dr. Noelani Prietto, a specialist in gynecology based in Irvine, California, pointed out to me the uniqueness of the pelvic floor muscles: Like the diaphragm, they sit within a bony structure, in contrast to most of the skeletal muscles, which attach outside the bony structure. (In fact, the pelvic floor is sometimes referred to as the pelvic diaphragm.) The pelvic muscles work symbiotically; that is, they work cooperatively in order to adapt to the constant changes of internal abdominal and thoracic pressure. This mechanism of intra-abdominal pressure is thought to "un-weight" the spine and play a significant role in pelvic–lumbar stabilization (used in this context synonymously with the term core).

The pelvis is a fascinating structure, serving as a bridge between the upper and lower body. It is made up of three bones—the ischium, ilium, and pubis—bound together by cartilage (figure 2.3). Some people believe that these cartilaginous joints do not move at all; others (myself included) adhere to the belief that they do allow varying degrees of very subtle movement. I must stress that the movement is minute. I often hear people referring to the movement of the sacroiliac joint (SIJ) as if it glides around like the scapulae. That is clearly not the case. At the same time, if these joints become immobile, undue strain is likely to be placed on the pelvis and spine. The reasons for either hyper- or hypomobility vary (e.g., genetic, adaptive, or disease related), but for our purposes, simply being aware of the potential imbalances that can occur in the pelvis, addressing the imbalances, and seeking medical advice if a harmful condition prevails, will suffice.

I like to visualize the pelvis as being made up of two rotating discs sitting on their sides facing each other. The degree of rotation of each disc is quite limited in either direction, but a small amount of rotation is essential for healthy function of the pelvis and the body as a whole. This pattern of rotation of the two sides of the pelvis (innominate bones) is present during many basic activities, such as walking and running; as one innominate rotates in one direction, the other rotates in the opposite direction.

We need to consider the joints around, as well as within, the pelvis when discussing its function. The influence of the surrounding joints on the pelvis is profound and vice versa. In fact, the function of the pelvis can be best understood by viewing the movement of the surrounding joints. If the pelvis is misaligned, it adversely affects the function of body segments up and down the kinetic chain, resulting in inefficient movement, muscular imbalances, and stress on the structure of the body. Detecting the imbalances is the first step toward understanding the body's movement. Remedying them is the next step, and this is where Pilates can play a crucial role, in reeducating the neuromuscular system. Correct pelvic alignment is of paramount importance, whether you are performing daily activities, doing Pilates, or sitting at a desk. Balanced development of the muscles around the pelvis is fundamental in achieving a well-aligned pelvis and ideal posture.

One way to view the pelvis is as a suspension bridge with cables (the muscles) holding it from above, below, the sides and, very importantly, from the inside. As long as all the cables are tensioned correctly and proportionately, little strain is placed on any one cable and the bridge will be stable and level. However, the moment the balance of tension on the cables changes or the bridge is not level, excessive strain is placed on certain cables while others are underused. The result is that the entire bridge shows strain. Although the pelvis will not typically collapse under stress, as a bridge might, muscles that encounter excessive tension may become strained or even tear. Simply put, if the pelvis is out of alignment, the body is out of alignment.

We need only look at the list of some of the muscles that act on the pelvic complex—the pelvic floor muscles, spinal flexors and extensors, hip flexors and extensors, hip adductors and abductors, hip external and internal rotators—to understand the bridge analogy and the impact the pelvis has on the entire body. This list doesn't even include the tendons, ligaments, and joints that also add support and provide mobility to this intricate structure. The analogy can be taken beyond the structure to the location. The pelvis is the bridge between the lower and upper body, the all-powerful lower limbs and the trunk. It is no wonder that the source of much of our movement emanates from this region. Pilates provides a path to discovering the powerhouse and unleashing the power of the pelvis. Keep in mind that working with precision when exercising the pelvic–lumbar region is imperative, possibly more so than with any other area of the body.

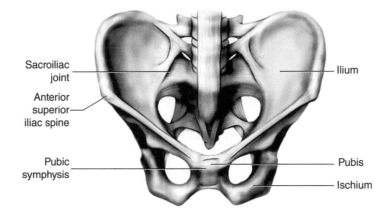

Sacroiliac joint

Anterior superior iliac spine

Pubic symphysis

Ilium

Pubis

Ischium

FIGURE 2.3 This front view of the pelvis clearly shows its structure and the joints that bind the parts together.

Muscles of the Powerhouse

In order to achieve good alignment and correct movement mechanics, the body must have the tools to do so; a well-balanced musculoskeletal system is the first step in this quest. Strength is obviously an important aspect of posture, yet other elements, such as habitual muscle activation patterns, genetics, and flexibility are also key components. In many instances, a lack of flexibility inhibits ideal alignment and recruitment of the correct muscles. Hypermobility, on the other hand, although not restrictive by nature, demands a great deal of body awareness and muscular control to maintain good alignment. In Pilates we strive to develop strong, flexible muscles that are effective in their function and adaptability.

Certain muscles play a crucial role in providing a stable and pliable core, without which good alignment and efficient function are not possible. These are the deep muscles of the pelvis and trunk. The superficial muscles are sometimes overdeveloped and overemphasized in comparison to the deep muscles, often at the expense of a strong, solid core. Being large does not necessarily translate into being functional. I regard muscle bulk that is not functional as extra baggage to carry around; ultimately, it can burden the body. As with a tree, the deeper layers, not the bark, provide the support for it to stand upright and the flexibility to bend with the wind.

The back extensors and abdominal muscles are key in providing the form and function of the trunk. They share a symbiotic relationship and there should be constant interplay between them. Both the abdominals and back extensors are made up of layers of muscle, and it is the deepest layers that are most prominent in providing stabilization and support to the spine. The abdominal group is made up of the rectus abdominis, external oblique, internal oblique, and transversus abdominis (figure 2.4). In back, the large superficial group (erector spinae) runs longitudinally along the spine, while the deep posterior spinal group (which includes the multifidus), the intervertebral muscles that connect between the vertebrae of the spine, lie deeper (figure 2.5). The back also serves as the attachment for many dual-purpose muscles, such as those connecting to the neck and head, the upper limbs and the pelvis. Within these two major muscle groups, the abdominals and back extensors, two muscles have been identified as having a particularly profound effect on stabilization and, in turn, function: the transversus abdominis (TA) and the multifidus.

The abdominals and back muscles, together with the diaphragm and the pelvic floor, create a cylinder of muscular support in the center of the body. I call this the *internal support system* (ISS). It is congruent with the powerhouse in Pilates, or the core in other forms of training. It is gratifying that scientific research is now substantiating much of what Joseph Pilates advocated so many years ago with regard to the importance of a strong, powerful, and functional core. During the practice of Pilates, you are encouraged to recruit the muscles of the ISS throughout. Movement is possible without activating the ISS; however, internal support, protection of the spine, and efficient function are likely to be diminished.

Another component that is important to consider in any discussion relating to the pelvis and the spine is the psoas. There are two psoas muscles, psoas minor and psoas major. Psoas major combines with the iliacus to form the iliopsoas (figure 2.6). Besides being powerful hip flexors, these muscles are believed to substantially influence spinal stabilization and alignment. Since the psoas is close to the axis of movement when performing flexion, lateral flexion, and extension of the lumbar spine, it compensates for imbalance between the anterior abdominal muscles

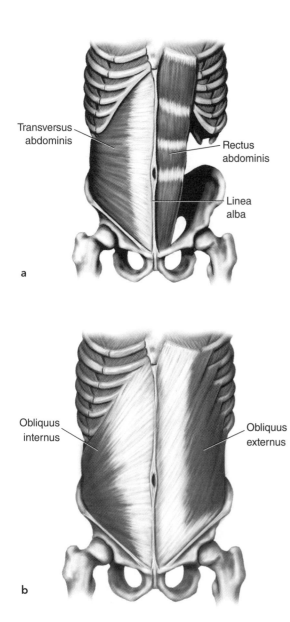

Transversus abdominis

Rectus abdominis

Linea alba

a

Obliquus internus

Obliquus externus

b

FIGURE 2.4 Major muscles of the abdominal muscle group.

and posterior spinal extensor muscles to stabilize the lumbar spine. Some practitioners believe that most dysfunction of the spine and the hip joint can and should be attributed to a disturbance of function of the psoas and iliopsoas. They postulate that tight or weak psoas muscles are associated with abnormal pelvic tilt, exaggerated lumbar lordosis, lower back pain, sacro-iliac dysfunction, degenerative disc disease, scoliosis, and misaligned posture, among other conditions. With extended sitting, a common byproduct of the modern lifestyle, the hip flexors become tight and weak. The psoas and iliopsoas in particular should be addressed in all exercise programs as they affect everyone, from the very active to the sedentary.

The psoas muscles and the abdominal muscles are agonists and antagonists as well as synergists—they can oppose one another's actions and work cooperatively; a dynamic interplay exists between the two muscle groups. The psoas plays an important role in much of the abdominal work in Pilates, particularly in the exercises in which the legs are held up off the ground. Typically, great emphasis is placed on recruitment of the abdominals, while the role of the hip flexors is often minimized or overlooked altogether. I believe that more focus should be placed on controlling and using the hip flexors correctly. They are vital to the successful execution of many Pilates exercises as well as to efficient function and general well-being.

Interestingly, all the muscles of the ISS are what I call *mind muscles*; activating them requires mental focus and a high degree of body awareness and concentration. Controlling the muscles of the ISS demands different skills than those used for controlling superficial skeletal muscles, such as the biceps or quadriceps, which are easily accessed and whose activation is readily apparent. It appears that nature intended that the journey toward mastery of movement and control, and the attainment of fitness, would incorporate mind-body exploration and, in turn would yield a multitude of rewards. As Joseph Pilates wrote in *Return to Life Through Contrology*, "exercises that produce a harmonious structure we

term 'physical fitness,' reflecting itself in a coordinated and balanced tri-part unity of body, mind, and spirit" (pages 32-33).

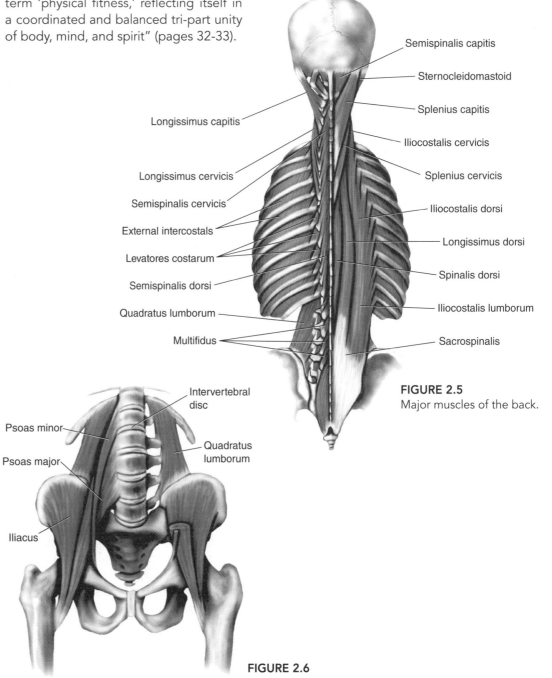

Semispinalis capitis

Sternocleidomastoid

Splenius capitis

Longissimus capitis

Iliocostalis cervicis

Splenius cervicis

Longissimus cervicis

Semispinalis cervicis

Iliocostalis dorsi

External intercostals

Longissimus dorsi

Levatores costarum

Semispinalis dorsi

Spinalis dorsi

Quadratus lumborum

Iliocostalis lumborum

Multifidus

Sacrospinalis

FIGURE 2.5
Major muscles of the back.

Intervertebral disc

Psoas minor

Quadratus lumborum

Psoas major

Iliacus

FIGURE 2.6

Ripple Effect

All movement emanates from the center, both anatomically and energetically. The path of movement is like the ripple effect that occurs when a pebble is dropped into still water. It creates a circular ripple that in turn creates many more ripples moving outward in progressively larger circles. So, each movement starts from the inner core (the first circle of energy) and moves outward; the trunk is the second circle of energy, followed by the limbs and finally the periphery, the hands and feet. But don't think of the energy stopping at the fourth circle; it should continue outward, as if the movement never ends. This is called the follow-through, and it has infinite value in terms of function and aesthetics. It is a concept promoted in all athletic activities, from jumping to throwing a ball to the elongated appearance of a ballerina.

Principles of Alignment and Posture

People often adopt a simplistic view when assessing posture and alignment; for example, they measure only strength and flexibility and ignore the complexity of the factors involved. Strengthening a certain muscle group or stretching another to improve posture and alignment is not enough. Correcting alignment is a process of neuromuscular reeducation that requires enormous commitment, patience, and, preferably, the scrutinizing eye and astute cueing of a good teacher.

Posture can be assessed in terms of the alignment of the joints and bony landmarks and understood in terms of muscle balance and function. Alignment is often described relative to a plumb line—a straight line that runs vertically through the body. Figure 2.7 shows ideal posture viewed from the side. By viewing the body from the side in relation to the plumb line, deviations in an anterior–posterior direction (in the sagittal plane) become apparent. When aligning a person up against a plumb line start by placing the plumb line slightly anterior to the lateral malleolus. The following landmarks of the body should then line up vertically on the plumb line: the lobe of the ear, center of the cervical vertebrae, shoulder joint, midpoint of the trunk, greater trochanter of the femur, and a point slightly anterior to the midline of the knee and slightly anterior to the lateral malleolus (ankle). Posture should also be viewed from the front and back as well as from the side, focusing on the symmetry of the body and deviations from the midline in a sideways (lateral) direction (in the coronal plane). The space between the arms and the trunk, which I call *windows of opportunity*, should also be observed as they offer much information regarding alignment of the pelvis, spine, and the upper girdle.

Please note that ideal posture is an *ideal*, a goal that one strives for but may never achieve. Each individual is different in body type, center of gravity, habitual movement patterns, mental state, and genes; it is inconceivable to think that one posture will fit all. However, the concept of an ideal posture serves as a guideline and a reference by which we can detect deviations and gauge changes.

Posture affects every movement, exercise, cue, and decision in an exercise program. Consider, for instance, a person who has *fatigue posture*, which is characterized by a rounded thoracic spine and the pelvis being forward of the plumb line in a posterior tilt. Although correction is complex, it generally involves strengthening the upper-back extensors, strengthening the iliopsoas, and stretching the external obliques of the abdomen. Bringing the shoulders into ideal alignment over the pelvis is also often helpful. On the other hand if a person has *lumbar hyperlordosis*, which involves an increased lumbar curve of the spine accompanied by an anterior tilt of the pelvis, correction generally focuses on strengthening the abdominals and stretching the hip flexors and lower back extensors. Clearly, these two people will receive different exercise programs, emphasizing different muscle groups, with the selection of exercises and the cueing being appropriate for their particular posture.

Alignment of the Spine

Good alignment translates into less stress on the spine and more economical muscular activity. When the spine is aligned with gravity, we are not fighting against gravity; in fact gravity is assisting us. The body is working in harmony with the laws of nature. The moment the body is unbalanced and out of alignment, certain muscles become overworked and others become weak, resulting in stress and inefficient movement. Maintaining the natural curves of the spine is important because they act as shock absorbers, protecting the body during impact, whether landing from a jump, running, or carrying a heavy load. We therefore always strive to attain ideal alignment and develop the musculature to support it.

Although much of our attention focuses on the musculature as it relates to posture and alignment, ideal alignment of the spine also facilitates efficient functioning of the internal organs. Deviations of posture over time can lead to malfunctioning of the inner organs. For instance, I have taught people who have scoliosis and who, with Pilates practice, begin to feel that they can finally breathe better. This is quite typical with scoliosis, because the muscles on one side of the thorax become tight, causing the rib cage to compress on that side and limit the function of the corresponding lung. Similarly, with kyphosis (increased thoracic curve of the spine) the rib cage becomes compressed and impairs respiration. Other systems can also be affected; for example, a posture with exaggerated forward flexion places constant pressure on the digestive system, hindering its function.

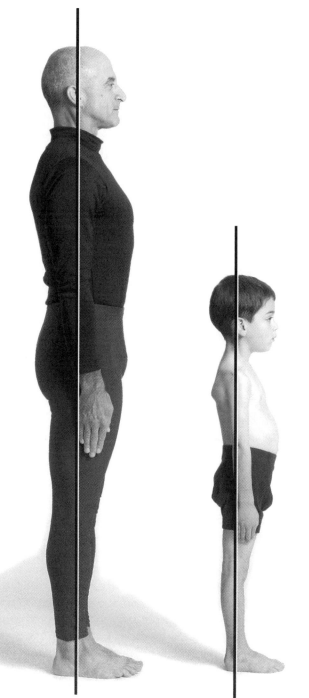

FIGURE 2.7 Good observation points and landmarks for assessing posture include the ears, shoulders, pelvis, knees, and ankles.

Placement of the Head

I like to think of the head as a ball balancing on a pin. None of the muscles should be strained; instead they should all act as cables that keep the ball balanced, in harmony with the forces of nature. Adjusting the position of the head is one of the most common and important corrections I give when I teach. I view the head as simply a large vertebra (or a large ball encompassing the first vertebra), an integral part of the spine, and as such it should follow the line of the spine. Deviations from this alignment, particularly because of the head's relatively heavy weight, inevitably result in neck tension and strain and can be aesthetically unpleasing. This situation tends to progressively deteriorate with time and age. It is even more pronounced when a person has a long neck, which essentially acts as an extended lever arm. For instance, if someone has forward head posture (the head is carried anterior to the plumb line), the neck extensors will become tight and overworked and the flexors relatively weak and inactive. The head weighs 12 to 14 pounds (approximately 5 kilograms), so shifting it away from the base of support has a significant effect on the musculature, an effect that grows exponentially as the head moves further away from the plumb line with a longer lever (neck).

During forward-flexion abdominal exercises such as the Mat Work: Chest Lift exercise, the trunk lifts up and forward, and the spine, including the head, must follow the natural curve. When forward flexion is inadequate, the head lies further from the body's center of gravity creating a longer lever. The result is often neck strain and tension. This inevitably happens when weak abdominals, tight lower back muscles, or both restrict the forward flexion of the trunk, and is often exacerbated by attempts to maintain a neutral pelvis when the body is not adequately prepared or able to do so (discussed in the next section). To understand proper positioning, visualize the body in forward flexion with the sun shining directly overhead. The shoulder girdle would cast a shadow on the ground below slightly larger than the actual size of the shoulder girdle. This shadow marks the base of support of the upper girdle; the head should be held within this area. Establishing a good C-curve position of the spine in this exercise is extremely beneficial, as it lays the foundation for many of the abdominal exercises that follow, both on the mat and on the apparatus (figure 2.8a).

The Mat Work: Roll-Up exercise offers a good illustration of spine and head alignment and a perfect example of how the art and science of human movement merge. In the sitting phase of this exercise, many people place the head down between the arms. I prefer that the head follow the natural C curve of the spine and be held above the arms, with the arms remaining parallel to the floor (figure 2.8b). Not only does this present a longer, more continuous line, which is visually pleasing, but it also encourages better placement of the head, shoulders, and scapulae, and a balanced interplay between the spinal flexors and extensors—leaving the body devoid of tension.

Neutral Pelvis and Neutral Spine

Neutral pelvis is defined as a position in which the anterior superior iliac spines (ASIS) and the pubic symphysis (PS) are in the same coronal plane (horizontal plane when supine) and the two ASIS are in the same transverse plane. The term *neutral spine* indicates that the natural curves of the spine are present. If the PS is higher than the ASIS, the pelvis is in a posterior tilt; if the ASIS are higher than the PS, the pelvis is in an anterior tilt (see figure 2.9).

The neutral position of the pelvis and spine is a reference against which to compare and describe all other positions of your body during your Pilates practice and other activities. This is not to say that we never deviate from it, we do quite frequently. However neutral is the foundation, and from this neutral alignment infinite positions and movements emanate. When the spine is in a neutral position, the pelvis by definition must also be neutral; however, instances do occur in which the pelvis is in neutral and the spine is not, such as during the Mat

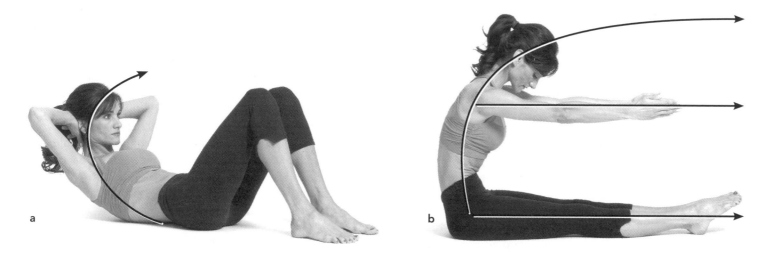

FIGURE 2.8 The head and spine align in a natural, elegant C curve in the *(a)* Chest Lift and *(b)* Roll-Up exercises.

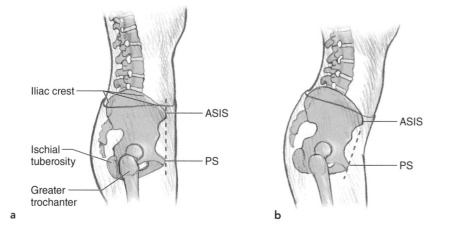

Iliac crest

ASIS

Ischial tuberosity

PS

Greater trochanter

a

ASIS

PS

b

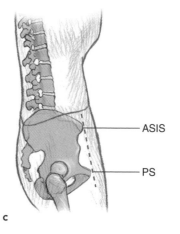

ASIS

PS

c

FIGURE 2.9 *(a)* Neutral pelvis, *(b)* anterior tilt, and *(c)* posterior tilt.

Work: Single-Leg Stretch (figure 2.10) and many other abdominal exercises.

Performing exercises in the neutral pelvic position yields several benefits. It encourages balanced muscular development of the pelvic complex and correct muscle recruitment. It teaches and reinforces efficient posture and ideal alignment, which is particularly important when upright. It can also assist in unloading the pelvis of undue stresses. However, keep in mind that the pelvis is dynamic and constantly adjusts to the body's movements and its ability, or inability, to perform a movement. At times, maintaining a neutral pelvis could prove counterproductive and lead to negative results. Therefore appropriate positioning of the spine and pelvis should be assessed on a case-by-case basis. This is particularly pertinent during abdominal exercises. A neutral pelvis is the ideal, but it may be necessary at first to work with a slight posterior pelvic tilt in order to elongate (and at times relax) the back muscles of the lumbar region and strengthen the abdominals. Once both flexibility of the lower back and strength of the abdominals have been achieved, the position of the pelvis can be adjusted from posterior to neutral.

It is important to recognize, as stated previously, that neutral pelvis and neutral spine do not always occur simultaneously, and they have different implications. I sometimes encounter students who claim to be working in a neutral spine position during abdominal exercises in forward flexion. Clearly they are not (nor should they be). Once the head and trunk lift into forward flexion, the spine is no longer in a neutral position. When in a neutral position the natural curves of the spine must be present; in forward flexion the natural curves cannot be present. So to say that you do abdominal work with a neutral *spine* while in forward flexion is a contradiction in terms. However, maintaining a neutral *pelvis* during abdominal work in forward flexion is quite possible and in many instances desirable.

When teaching the chest lift I instruct students to lift into forward flexion. Some lift only their heads off the mat, and not the entire upper girdle, in a misguided attempt to maintain a neutral spine. By performing neck flexion, and not trunk flexion, they are missing the point of the exercise, which is abdominal work. As a result they are not working the abdominals effectively, and are probably acquiring more neck tension and excessive lower back tension than abdominal strength. I have witnessed similar scenarios with oblique abdominal work entailing rotation of the trunk, such as in the Mat Work: Criss-Cross. In an attempt to maintain a neutral spine in such exercises, students exhibit a great deal of neck flexion but little or no trunk flexion and rotation. The lumbar spine is sometimes lifted off the mat, placing excessive strain on the back.

I do advocate maintaining a neutral pelvic position during many of the abdominal exercises, but not at all costs. For example, if you have hyperlordosis and a tight lower back, performing abdominal exercises while maintaining a neutral pelvis could result in excessive contracture of the lower back muscles. This translates into insufficient forward flexion of the trunk, ineffective abdominal recruitment, possible excessive hip flexor activation (particularly when the legs are held off the mat), plus stress on the lower back and probably the neck. In an endeavor to work with neutral pelvis, people sometimes compromise the outcome of the exercise and reinforce negative movement patterns, coming away with neck pain, back pain, and, to make it worse, weak abdominals.

A series of actions allow the lumbar spine to imprint into the mat during forward flexion in a supine position: the abdominal muscles contract, intra-abdominal pressure is increased, the back extensors elongate, and the lumbar vertebrae flatten out. This does not mean that the pelvis should be forcefully thrust into a posterior tilt (commonly called a *tuck*) in order to imprint the back into the mat. Rather, the trunk is lifted into forward flexion while maintaining a neutral pelvis, and if the pelvis must tilt posteriorly at the end range of the forward flexion in order to achieve maximum abdominal activation, elongate the tight lower back extensors, and imprint the lower back into the mat, then so be it! Continue modifying the position of the pelvis until you have addressed and overcome the limiting factors. Ultimately, as the strength of the abdominals increases, you will be able to perform the abdominal exercises with integrity and a positive outcome, free from excessive tension and hopefully in a neutral pelvic position.

Assessing Alignment

Over the years I have found it important to develop convenient methods of assessing posture. Very sophisticated systems of assessment are available, yet most are impractical to use at home or during a Pilates session.

I recommend the Mat Work: Roll-Down as a simple but useful tool for assessing posture and alignment. It offers valuable information regarding structure, muscular development, and compensations. At the same time it allows one to gently mobilize the spine and coordinate the breathing with the movement. Teachers who are assessing a student's alignment should observe the roll-down from the back, front, and side, since certain postural deviations are more apparent from a coronal (front/back) view and others from a sagittal (side) view. When using this exercise as a self-assessment tool, stand on a firm, level surface in front of a mirror if possible. Self-assessment demands heightened inner awareness and observation skills that should be honed constantly.

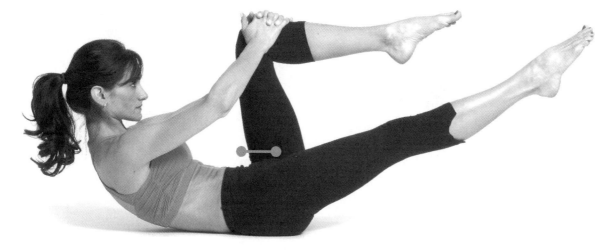

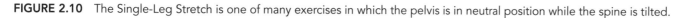

FIGURE 2.10   The Single-Leg Stretch is one of many exercises in which the pelvis is in neutral position while the spine is tilted.

Muscle Focus

- Abdominals and back extensors

Objectives

- Develop articulation of the spine
- Stretch the back extensors
- Improve control of the abdominals and back extensors
- Align the body and focus the mind

Roll-Down

I encourage the use of the roll-down at the beginning and end of a session; however, the exercise is *not* appropriate for everyone and should not be performed in certain instances, such as when lower back problems are present. If you have any reservations about yourself or a student doing this movement, substitute with a modified roll-down by leaning the back against a wall, placing the feet hip-width apart, one to two feet (30 to 60 centimeters) from the wall, and bending the knees. Doing the exercise in this position allows the wall to bear the weight of the body and provides tactile feedback.

During the roll-down, become internally aware of weight shifts within the body. Notice asymmetries and imbalances, and take note of deviations from the plumb line. Use the roll-down not only as a tool for assessment but also as a means of focusing the mind and tuning the body, just as you would tune a musical instrument before playing it.

Imagery

Imagine your back pressing against a pole that is keeping you upright and aligned. The head fills with water and becomes very heavy. It rolls forward, pulling the body away from the pole one tiny segment at a time. At the bottom the water runs out the top of the head and the body becomes light so that the spine rolls back up the pole, one segment at time.

☐ Establish ideal alignment in relation to the plumb line from the outset.

☐ Keep the movement relaxed and avoid forcing a stretch of the hamstrings at the end range.

☐ Relax the arms and hands, with the palms facing the sides of the body.

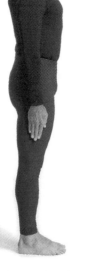

Inhale. Stand upright in ideal alignment with the feet hip-width apart and parallel. Prepare for the movement by going through a mental checklist of ideal alignment.

Exhale. Roll down through the spine, beginning with the head and articulating through each vertebra. Allow the knees to bend as you roll down, alleviating any pressure on the lower back. This is particularly important if you have tight back extensors and hamstrings. While in this position, inhale, holding a relaxed (but not slumped) position at the bottom. Relax the neck and allow the head to follow the line of the spine. Expand the chest laterally when inhaling, feeling the back expand and the vertebral joints releasing all tension.

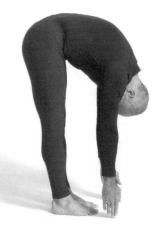

Exhale. Roll back up, articulating through the spine and placing each vertebra back on the plumb line like building blocks until you have established ideal alignment, returning to the starting position.

Effects of Center of Gravity

The body's center of gravity (COG) is important for both alignment and understanding the mechanics of exercises. Weight distribution can make exercises easier or more difficult, depending on the person's body type. Sometimes, difficulty executing an exercise successfully has little to do with lack of strength and much to do with physical build—specifically the weight distribution of the body. For instance, a man with broad shoulders, a well-developed upper body, and short legs may find the roll-up extremely challenging, while a woman with a petite torso, substantial hips, and long legs will find the exercise relatively easy. The man is not weaker; in fact he may well have far stronger abdominal muscles, but he is top-heavy, while the woman has a lower COG. In other exercises, such as the Wunda Chair: Full Pike and the Reformer: Long Stretch, this man would have an advantage.

Given that each person's COG is slightly different, the way each person performs an exercise is also different. Understanding this fact is important in order to cue effectively, make exercises easier or more difficult and, most importantly, make them safe. Joseph Pilates had a very muscular build, like that of a gymnast. Add to that a male's naturally strong upper body and propensity to develop it as well as his innate desire to create exercises that feel good (and look good), and it is not surprising that many of the exercises Joseph Pilates created require a strong, well-developed upper girdle. (This in no way implies that women cannot perform the repertoire very beautifully and successfully.) Understanding the mechanics of the body and the exercises will allow you to overcome obstacles for yourself and your students.

Let's take, for example, the Mat Work: Roll-Up. If a person is struggling with this exercise and the reason appears to be body type rather than weak abdominals or tight lower back and hamstrings, an excellent solution is to drape a light (2.2 pounds/1 kilogram) ankle weight over the ankles. This does not allow the person to rely on the ankle weight to pull the body up, as would be the case if the feet were placed under a secure foot strap; it simply changes the weight distribution, adding weight (or, in effect, length) to the legs and lowering the COG toward the pelvis. The individual became *taller* for the sake of the exercise. (If only it were so easy to become tall!) At other times, being top-heavy or shorter may prove an advantage. Regardless of body type, everyone faces challenges and obstacles that can be overcome . . . so enjoy your body and relish the journey!

Foot Alignment

The feet are the foundation of the body when upright: standing, walking, running, and jumping. Any misalignment of the feet, in a static position or in motion, results in postural deviations and compensations all the way up the kinetic chain. The foot is a complex structure, made up of many joints, and citing any one joint or aspect of the foot as particularly vulnerable is difficult. However, I will single out the subtalar joint (often mistaken for the ankle joint) due to its importance in relation to foot alignment. The subtalar joint controls the inward and outward motion (supination and pronation) of the foot and is vital to achieving correct foot alignment. A good guide, when assisting someone to achieve neutral alignment of the foot when standing, is to observe the Achilles tendon from the back (see figure 2.11). The tendon should be perpendicular to the ground, and fine adjustments of the subtalar joint can be made to achieve this alignment. Becoming acquainted with neutral alignment is particularly helpful during the foot work on the Pilates apparatus.

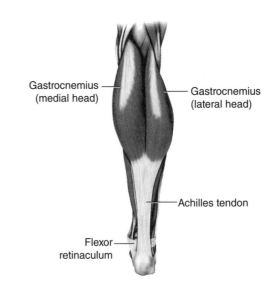

Gastrocnemius (medial head)

Gastrocnemius (lateral head)

Achilles tendon

Flexor retinaculum

FIGURE 2.11 Alignment of the Achilles tendon.

3

Powerful Pilates Practice

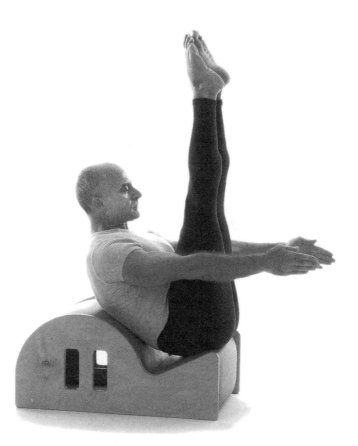

The foundation of the Pilates method as Joseph Pilates intended it, and as I approach it, is working with the *whole* in mind. The body is the most intricate of instruments, and imbalance in one area will inevitably cause imbalances in other areas. Therefore, all Pilates programs should be comprehensive, regardless of a person's age, fitness level, or ability. In some cases, you may certainly direct more attention toward a particular area of the body, but you should always keep in mind the intricate patterning of human movement. An injury, compensation, or any other restriction that adversely affects the integrity of the body's ability to function can be regarded as a weak link in a chain. For the chain to function as a complete unit, you must address the weak link without losing sight of the fact that the goal is the efficient functioning of the chain as a whole.

Structure and creativity may seem to be diametrically opposed, yet one cannot exist without the other. Both are essential components of an effective Pilates program. Having a structure allows you to be creative and to adapt to personal and specific needs without compromising the concept of the whole. If you view Pilates as *only* exercise, and, furthermore, as exercise for only one part of the body, you risk sacrificing the essence of the system. Adhering to a structure allows you to compile an efficient, comprehensive program. It also allows teachers to maintain the flow in a studio when teaching several people at the same time, while offering each person an individualized program and personal attention. I liken the process to a conductor leading an orchestra or a chess master playing several games of chess at one time—the conductor always knows where he is in the composition and what each section of the orchestra is doing, just as the chess master has in mind the strategy for not only the next move, but the next several moves in each match. Maintaining flow within all the individual sessions simultaneously can only be achieved with a clear and well-learned structure.

Over the years I have witnessed Pilates classes that lack structure, direction, and the concept of the *whole*.

I have always come away feeling that these sessions are missing the point; without a logical progression, they lack the elements that make Pilates so valuable and its effects so profound. I sometimes see this happening in clinical environments, where Pilates is used as a treatment modality. A therapist might take a patient through a few exercises on the reformer and then move on to another method of treatment. Using a Pilates exercise here and there is not Pilates. The exercise happens to be done on Pilates equipment and it may or may not be a Pilates movement, but it is not Pilates because it does not embody the system's philosophy and approach. I cannot say this is wrong; I can only say it is not the system that Joseph Pilates created. Therefore, it is unlikely to achieve the outcome that Joseph Pilates described in *Return to Life Through Contrology* as "the highest accomplishments within the scope of our capabilities." (Of course many therapists have studied Pilates in depth and have integrated it very successfully into their practices as a complete system.) The method's creator was explicit in his belief that you must address both the mind and body, concurrently and comprehensively. This belief has been proven to be a powerful approach to wellness and is now receiving the widespread recognition it deserves.

Structuring Your Practice: The Block System

My quest to find a useful structure for the practice of Pilates led me to develop the BASI (Body Arts and Science International) Block System. Derived from many years of practicing and teaching the method and directing programs around the world, the block system is the nucleus of my approach to Pilates. It is solidly grounded in the Pilates method while, at the same time, it adheres to the principles of exercise physiology and contemporary knowledge. The structure of the BASI Block System ensures that practitioners address the whole body, providing a framework and clear guidelines for individual development while allowing for adaptability and creativity.

The block system organizes the vast Pilates repertoire in such a way that each exercise has a home, a block that it belongs to. It can be likened to a family tree; all the exercises emanate from the same roots and are related to each other, some more closely than others. Familiarity with the intricacies of the whole tree is essential in order to implement the block system successfully, and this knowledge can be used to compile programs that are individualized according to level, personal needs, restrictions, and goals.

Without such a system, the hundreds of Pilates exercises become just that—exercises, like words without context or meaning. They are valuable in and of themselves, but they convey a message only when put together in sentences. The more finely crafted the sentences, the more profound the message. So it is with Pilates. The teacher compiles the session with the blocks, which are like chapters in a book; together, they create the whole story. Each movement takes on more meaning when it is placed within a well-conceived structure and sequence of movements—like poetry in motion. This is where the art and the science of human movement unite. At this level, mind and body work as one and all the principles of Pilates are in effect; the work becomes deeper, yet more effortless. This is the level we strive for, where the greatest and most profound changes take place.

Fully grasping the many levels of the block system can take years. However, even in its most simple form, the system provides a way to categorize the vast repertoire, maximize work time and use the session to its full potential. Because it is a standardized system, it allows practitioners who are trained in it to communicate and collaborate in a seamless and meaningful fashion, wherever they may be in the world. The BASI Block System is now used in studios around the world, and I am always filled with pride when I see how successfully it has been implemented in different cultures.

All exercises in this book are laid out according to the block system, which means that you can learn each exercise and its place in the overall structure concurrently. For example, the exercises on the reformer that focus on the upper girdle fall into the *arm work block*, a pool of upper-body exercises of varying levels of difficulty from which to choose. Each block comprises individual exercises or series of exercises. A series is a compilation of several exercises that complement each other to create a complete, integrated *exercise unit* for a particular area of the body. The exercises within a series are all performed together. There is one other term that is used regularly. I use the term *group* of exercises to refer to multiple exercises that share a common denominator, such as being performed with the long box placed atop the reformer. In contrast with a series, the exercises in a group are not typically performed together in one session. It would be very unusual for someone to perform all the long box exercises together in a session, yet we refer to them collectively as the long box group.

Two different block systems have evolved over the years. The first is used for a typical Pilates session that utilizes the full complement of apparatus. It is called the *comprehensive block system*. The blocks that make up this system are as follows:

Warm-up. This block prepares the body for the work, both physically and mentally. It is typically a selection of mat work exercises.

Foot work. Devoted to the lower limbs, foot work is performed on the reformer, cadillac, and wunda chair. The focus is on the entire leg: foot, ankle, knee, and hip. This block is regarded as part warm-up and part specific training for the lower limbs. (Use of the name *foot work* is to differentiate from *leg work* later on)

Abdominal work. This selection of exercises is focused on developing the abdominal muscles. Although the abdominals are engaged throughout the Pilates session, these exercises are specifically aimed at this region and address all the abdominal muscles.

Hip work. This section demands work and control of the hip joint and is typically performed with the feet in the straps on the reformer, or using the leg springs on the cadillac or other apparatus, such as the Avalon chair and Avalon barrel. Focus on control of the pelvic–lumbar region is key because of the close relationship of the pelvis to the hip joint.

Spinal articulation. This block is devoted to spinal mobility and developing control of the trunk muscles, particularly the deeper lying muscles. Spinal articulation exercises can be found on almost all the apparatus, including the mat.

Stretching. Selections from this block can be performed on or off the apparatus and typically include stretches for the hip flexors and hamstrings. The selection of exercises depends on the needs and ability of each individual.

Full-body integration (FBI). Although all Pilates exercises work the entire body, these exercises defy categorization by muscle group or area of the body and are specifically geared to full-body motion. There are two levels: FBI fundamental/intermediate (FBI F/I) and FBI advanced/master (FBI A/M).

Arm work. This block is devoted to the upper girdle of the body. I have compiled several series, consisting of exercises that work the various muscle groups of the arms and shoulders. Typically a complete series is practiced to ensure comprehensive work of the upper body.

Leg work. These are exercises for the lower body to supplement the foot work. They typically emphasize the hip abductors and hip adductors. However, the system accommodates flexibility, so that this section may be utilized for specific skill training, such as when working with dancers, skiers, and runners, or for corrective and therapeutic work of the lower limbs.

Lateral flexion and rotation. This block refers to exercises that work the rotators and lateral flexors of the trunk, with an emphasis on the oblique abdominal muscles. These muscles are vital to healthy functional movement and support of the spine. Often imbalances exist between the muscles on either side of the body, for reasons ranging from scoliosis to one-side–dominance (handedness), due to the practice of certain athletic or occupation-related activities. I recommend always working toward balance and symmetry.

Back extension. This block is devoted to exercises for the trunk extensors. These muscles lie along the spine and span the back in layers. The superficial muscles are long, large muscles that are responsible for gross movement. The deeper intrinsic muscles are intervertebral muscles that control fine intricate movement of the spine. As with the abdominals, it is the deeper layers that are largely responsible for stabilization. This block should *not* be compromised.

The mat exercises focus predominantly on the powerhouse—the spinal flexors (abdominals), lateral flexors and rotators, and back extensors. Therefore, a specific block system has been created for the mat work and is presented here in this second edition. The blocks that make up the *mat system* are as follows:

Foundation

Abdominal work

Spinal articulation

Bridging

Lateral flexion and rotation

Back extension

Because of their versatility and transitional qualities, the mat exercises lend themselves more naturally to arrangement according to progression and flow. The mat work block system is described in further detail in the introductory section of chapter 4.

I sometimes hear an unjustified criticism of Pilates as having inadequate rotation and extension exercises. My standard answer is simple: "I am sorry, but either you or your teacher do not know the full extent of Pilates, or, at the very least, you are not utilizing it." There are myriad options in the Pilates repertoire for both spinal rotation and extension, which are important components of any comprehensive exercise program.

Spinal extension becomes all the more important in an exercise program as we age. Over time gravity tends to pull us forward into flexion. This tendency is exacerbated by the ravages of our modern lifestyle—hours spent sitting in front of computers, driving cars, checking smartphones, and taking part in recreational pursuits that demand forward flexion. The result is bleak, with a high incidence of round-shoulder syndrome and other shoulder problems, lower back pain, and neck tension. If Pilates or another fitness regimen is performed in a way that focuses excessively on working the abdominals, with the majority of exercises performed in trunk flexion, the picture gets even bleaker. Effective abdominal work is important, but it must be complemented proportionally with working other areas of the body, specifically the lateral flexors, rotators, and extensors of the spine. Proportional muscle development is a key component in achieving good alignment, balance, efficient movement, and general well-being.

I often look to babies and young children for guidance. Seldom do you see toddlers with bad alignment; they have strong backs and straight spines. I recall a wonderful incident when Lolita San Miguel, one of the Pilates "elders" and a first generation teacher, was visiting my family in our home. My son Elan, who was about two years of age, was taking a bath and Lolita and I were standing in the bathroom looking on. Together we marveled at the amazing musculature and posture of this little rambunctious ball of energy as he stood, sat, jumped, splashed, and showed off his athletic skills to his guest. This is the type of spine nature intended us to have, not only as infants, but also throughout our lives.

Yes, toddlers have little potbellies, and as children reach their early teens emphasis on developing the abdominals is important. However, we should not lose sight of the tendency toward deterioration of certain muscle groups—notably the hip extensors, hip abductors, and back extensors—as we age and the importance of keeping them strong and flexible.

Exercise Descriptions

In order to fully understand an exercise or movement (for the purposes of this book these two words are used interchangeably), you must first analyze it. You will then be able to apply the movement at the right opportunity and in the most appropriate manner to achieve the desired outcome. I have formulated a clear and succinct form of movement analysis. This analysis opens the door to understanding, as well as learning and teaching the movement. It is also invaluable in compiling exercise programs. In the following sections I explain the categories used for each of the exercises presented in chapters 4 through 11. These categories not only describe the exercise, but also serve as a means of analysis.

I present each exercise by name, apparatus, block, level of difficulty, and the amount of resistance to use (if applicable). This information is followed by a discussion about the exercise, its muscle focus, its objectives, and the imagery that I suggest using to achieve optimum results. Imagery is a very powerful and personal teaching tool. Specific imagery may work in a given situation and with certain people, while in a different situation and with different people it will not. At the very least, I hope the imagery I offer sparks your imagination to create your own imagery and cues for teaching. I also include a checklist of key points you should observe to ensure a successful outcome for each exercise. Finally, photographs illustrate the movement, accompanied by a description of the movement according to the breath pattern.

Classifying the Movement

The blocks are used to classify the exercises into categories. Each is also defined by its level of difficulty—fundamental, intermediate, advanced, and master level. (Master-level exercises, as the name implies, take years to study and master. I offer only a few, as that realm of the repertoire exceeds the scope of this book.) Classifying movements by level is a subjective process, since what is difficult for one person may be relatively easy for another. Contrary, for example, to weight training, where progression may be based solely on increasing resistance, progression in Pilates is far more intricate. Therefore I allocate levels according to the complexity of the movement—the more complex the movement, the higher the level of difficulty.

I must emphasize that this system is not one in which, once you have learned an advanced movement, you no longer practice the fundamental or intermediate movements that prepared you for it. Each exercise becomes part of your movement vocabulary, to be used and enjoyed. Ultimately, the goal of each movement is to assist in the pursuit of well-being. When I construct programs for advanced students, I select exercises from all levels, not only the advanced repertoire. Including a wide range of exercises in a program is important, both physically and mentally. The level should not be a goal in and of itself, but a milestone in the lifelong process of learning and practicing Pilates.

I have spent much of my career mastering the most difficult moves in this method, and I certainly enjoy the exhilaration of performing the master-level work. Yet it is only part of the picture. With commitment, people can reap similar benefits from Pilates at any level of practice. The benefits depend not only on the movements per-

formed, but also on their quality and the integration of the Pilates principles into one's practice and one's life. Too often, I see the master-level repertoire becoming the sole focus, at times being performed by people who have little experience in this work. A talented gymnast or dancer could probably perform all the master-level work almost immediately. Does this mean they know Pilates? No. It means that they can learn choreography and perform it.

I see as much value in the Mat Work: Pelvic Curl, one of the most fundamental exercises, as I do in the high bridge single leg (not included in this book), one of the most advanced movements in the repertoire. In this example, the two exercises are actually closely related, and the relationship between fundamental and advanced work should be established early on in the practice of Pilates. Acknowledging and utilizing these relationships allows you to prepare methodically for the next level, growing and maturing within the system. The process of working through the levels and understanding each building block is the path to mastery and well-being, not the performance of an advanced exercise. You can do an exercise thousands of times and always find new meaning in it. I do not believe that any movement is *easy or simple, nor should it become boring*. Besides the enormous complexity in terms of neuromuscular and biomechanical activity, each movement embodies an entire philosophy. The work manifests itself on so many different levels. Fundamental? Possibly. Less complex than another exercise? Yes. Easy or simple? Never.

Some people try to learn the repertoire as quickly as possible, steering away from the fundamental exercises, preferring to move on to the more difficult work. But every movement has infinite complexity, regardless of the level. I encourage you to delight in the process of becoming intimately familiar with each exercise rather than rushing. The development of familiarity and understanding, not the ability to perform an advanced exercise, reflects true learning.

Pilates is not the performance of choreography; it is the never-ending process of learning about the body, controlling movement, and striving for well-being.

34

Resistance

Pilates is unique in its ingenious use of both gravity and springs for resistance. The pull of gravity will always be consistent, although its relative effect on the body depends on a variety of intrinsic factors such as body type and center of gravity, therefore the impact of gravity has not been noted specifically for each exercise in this book. However, for exercises using springs for resistance (as in the majority of exercises on the apparatus), the appropriate amount of resistance is noted. In some instances, there is an effect from both the springs and gravity, and an understanding of the mechanics of the apparatus and the exercise is essential. Springs provide *progressive resistance*, meaning that the resistance increases as the spring is tensioned. This differs from *constant (non-variable) resistance,* in which the resistance does not change, for example, when using weights. Take into account that when working with resistance, whether constant or progressive, the effect on the muscle changes through the range of motion because of the mechanical advantage or disadvantage at certain angles of the joint.

Much debate surrounds the question of which type of resistance is preferable. This cannot be resolved simply, and I think the points made in favor of each are valid. Ultimately, it comes down to personal preference. I personally favor working with springs because they can be easily adapted to simulate other activities and skills, and can be more functional in their effect. They also feel alive with energy, a sensation that I enjoy.

The spring settings on the equipment are a complex issue. Settings vary from one piece of apparatus to another, and even the same piece of apparatus can vary depending on the manufacturer. Unfortunately, no universal standard exists. Adding to the complexity is the fact that the spring setting for an exercise will depend on a person's fitness level, Pilates level, body type, gender, experience, and restrictions. In addition, you can dramatically change the intensity and outcome of an exercise by increasing or decreasing the tension.

Even the age of the springs can become a factor when choosing a setting.

Let me also distinguish between absolute and relative resistance. *Absolute resistance* means, for instance, that two springs are always two springs. *Relative resistance*, on the other hand, refers to how heavy or light the tension feels for a particular exercise. For example, two springs would typically be regarded as light for foot work, but would be heavy for arm work.

Pilates professionals must become familiar with the resistance settings for every exercise on each piece of apparatus, as they are unique to that apparatus. As an example, when doing foot work on the reformer, heavy might mean four springs; on the cadillac the equivalent might be two heavy springs; and on the wunda chair two heavy springs on the top setting. The only way to learn how to determine spring settings and their effect on an exercise is through practice—doing each movement many times, experimenting with different spring settings. There will always be a logical range within which to execute an exercise, yet determining your place within that range requires practice, knowledge, and experience.

Because of the variables mentioned previously, I have not included an actual spring setting for each exercise. Instead I offer an absolute weight range, which translates to a limited number of spring setting options. You must then make micro-adjustments according to your individual needs.

The following are Body Arts and Science International guidelines for resistance and spring settings on the reformer. The same concept can be applied to the other apparatus; although the number of springs will change. Through experience you can establish the setting for each resistance category on the respective piece of apparatus.

Extra-light	→	0.5 spring (light spring)
Light	→	1 to 1.5 springs
Medium	→	2 to 3 springs
Heavy	→	3.5 to 4 springs
Extra-heavy	→	4.5 to 5 springs

Muscle Focus

The muscle focus identifies which muscle or group of muscles are targeted by the exercise. Although it is usually one muscle or muscle group, there may be more depending on the complexity of the exercise and positional changes. Identifying the muscle focus assists you in achieving the desired goal of the exercise. Note that in many instances, increasing or decreasing the resistance or adjusting the body position even slightly will change the muscle focus. Therefore, precision is all-important.

You are encouraged to recruit the internal support system (ISS)—the transversus abdominis, pelvic floor, diaphragm, and the multifidus—throughout the session. Therefore, these muscles are not mentioned in each exercise as target muscles. The muscle focus refers to muscles other than the ISS unless the exercise is specifically for one or more of these core muscles.

Objectives

Objectives relate to the broader context of an exercise or action. In contrast to the muscle focus, which is very specific, the objectives describe the action of all the muscles involved. An exercise may have only one muscle focus, but it can have several objectives—and those objectives may not necessarily relate only to the area of the muscle focus. For example, in the case of the Mat Work: Hundred (chapter 4), a signature Pilates abdominal exercise, the muscle focus is the abdominals, while the objectives are to strengthen the abdominal muscles, develop trunk stabilization, and stimulate the cardiovascular system. The objectives for many Pilates exercises relate to increasing control or strength, stabilization, disassociation, and isolation.

Strength Versus Control

In describing the objective and effect of an exercise, I use the words *strength* and *control* in a very specific and separate manner. The term *strength* is often used too liberally and broadly in Pilates. In order to strengthen a muscle, certain criteria need to be met, one being *overload*. If insufficient load is placed on a muscle, it will not increase significantly in strength. That is not to say the muscle is not being activated, which in itself has value in terms of neuromuscular patterning and body awareness. However, the muscle is not being strengthened significantly. So I use the term *control* when a muscle is being recruited but not overloaded sufficiently for significant strength gains to be realized.

Stabilization

Developing stabilization in a particular area of the body is a common objective in Pilates. Each exercise can be broken down into muscles that stabilize movement (stabilizers) and muscles that produce movement (movers). Both are important in maintaining the integrity of the exercise. There is also a third category, the synergists, which are recruited to neutralize undesired muscle actions and assist in achieving the correct movement. For instance, in the Reformer: Chest Expansion (chapter 5), a shoulder extensor exercise, the following sequence of events should occur.

The stabilizers are recruited first; initially the stabilizers of the trunk (local stabilizers) are activated, then those of the scapula and elbow (global stabilizers). The movers, in this case the shoulder extensors, come next. Prominent among these is the latissimus dorsi, a shoulder extensor, shoulder adductor, and shoulder internal rotator. In this exercise, we encourage the first two actions but do not want shoulder internal rotation. Therefore, we must recruit the shoulder *external* rotators to neutralize the *internal* rotation component of the latissimus dorsi and prevent the shoulder from internally rotating. The shoulder external rotators function as synergists to keep the shoulder in the desired neutral position and assist the prime mover in maintaining the integrity of the exercise.

In any exercise, I encourage first focusing on the stabilizers, since without correct stabilization efficient movement cannot occur. Once you have achieved correct stabilization, focus on the initiator, which can be described as the primary focus or initial cue of the movement. This is a crucial link in any movement. Finally, focus on the movers. I call this the *SIM (stabilize-initiate-move) formula*. After this process has been learned and practiced many times it becomes second nature; an instinctive response to movement.

Most traditional forms of movement analysis address the stabilizers and movers but not the initiator. This is understandable, because the initiator is in fact either a stabilizer or a mover and therefore falls into one of these categories. However, using the concept of the initiator encourages mental focus, concentration, body awareness, and control, all of which in turn contribute to deriving maximum effect from the exercise.

Besides highlighting the importance of stabilization, Pilates also focuses on ranges of motion of the joints and different types of muscle contraction. The stabilizers work to a large extent isometrically, meaning that the muscles contract with no change in their length or in the angle of the joint(s) on which they are acting. Note that this is a dynamic process of agonist and antagonist muscles working in a symbiotic and dynamic relationship, adjusting constantly to the changes occurring in the body. The movers work isotonically (dynamically), both concentrically (decrease in muscle length and the angle of the joints on which they are acting) and eccentrically (increase in muscle length and the angle of the joints on which they are acting.)

Pilates encourages the development of both agonist and antagonist muscles and highlights the relationship that exists between them; as one muscle or group contracts concentrically the other contracts eccentrically. In certain instances they both contract isometrically to stabilize a joint or area (co-contraction). It is important to strive for a good balance between agonist and antagonist muscle groups in terms of strength, flexibility, and control.

Stabilizing the Trunk and Pelvis The term *trunk stabilization* describes a stable position of the spine and in this context is synonymous with *spinal stabilization, core stabilization, torso stabilization,* and *pelvic-lumbar stabilization*. It is important to recognize that stabilization is dynamic and that the stabilizers are continuously adapting to a changing environment.

I typically use the term *trunk stabilization* when the trunk is stable and the upper girdle is being mobilized, because of the close relationship between the two regions. The movement of the arms has a direct influence on the thoracic spine and, conversely, certain muscles of the thoracic region play an important role in correct mechanics of the shoulder girdle. Furthermore, achieving good head alignment and shoulder function is impossible without correct alignment of the trunk. Similarly, I use the term *pelvic-lumbar stabilization* when the lower limbs are being mobilized due to the close relationship between the lower limbs and the pelvis. If the pelvis is out of alignment or not stable, it will directly affect the function of the limbs as well as the alignment and function of the spine. Essentially, the pelvis acts as a bridge between the lower limbs and the spine. The position of the spine and the direction of the pull of gravity determine which muscles are recruited and to what extent.

Maintaining a stable position of the trunk and pelvis is fundamental to the success of many Pilates exercises. In order to achieve trunk stabilization, the ISS must be recruited. Depending on the position of the trunk, certain muscles are activated more than others. For instance in the Mat Work: Front Support, the abdominals play a vital role in stabilizing the trunk and avoiding collapse through the center. In the Mat Work: Back Support, on the other hand, while the abdominals are recruited to add support to the structure, it is primarily the back extensors, together with the hip extensors and shoulder extensors, that hold the structure up.

In the Mat Work: Rolling Like a Ball, stability of the trunk needs to be sustained in forward flexion. In this case, the abdominals contract concentrically and play a greater role than the back extensors, which contract eccentrically; the agonist (abdominals) and antagonist (back extensors) work in tandem to create the desired curve of the trunk, which is necessary to achieve the smooth, rolling motion. By contrast, the Mat Work: Swan Dive demands a great deal of back extensor work to achieve the desired position. Yet, the coordinated contraction of the abdominals is crucial in maintaining stability, helping create the desired shape of the body, distributing the load through the spine, and protecting the lower back from excessive pressure.

In each of the preceding examples, of course, once the desired position has been established, both the flexors and extensors of the trunk contract isometrically to maintain the position.

In a standing position, the gravitational pull is equal in the front and back of the body (ideally). In this case the abdominals and back extensors work in a state of co-contraction to stabilize the trunk. The back extensors hold the body upright and prevent it from folding forward. At the same time, the abdominals play an important role in creating a girdle of support around the midsection, preventing excessive stress on the lower spine. In effect, they function as a second spine.

Note that the abdominals tend to decondition more rapidly than the back extensors, and the back extensors tend to respond to conditioning more readily than do the abdominals. Add to this the fact that the back extensors are used most of the time to keep us upright, and the result is that they are typically better conditioned than the abdominals. However, the almost constant use of the large back extensors, particularly the erector spinae, can in itself create a problem. These superficial muscles may become hypertonic (overused) and very tight. "Switching them off" (inhibiting them) or at least "dimming" them to allow the abdominals and deep posterior spinal extensors, such as the multifidus, to fully engage is a first crucial step in creating balance in the trunk and achieving healthy trunk and pelvic stabilization.

To stay well-conditioned, the muscles of the trunk should be worked in all ranges of motion: flexion, extension, lateral flexion, and rotation. Individual needs vary, but a safe guideline is to allocate 50 percent of the time spent working muscles of the core to the spinal flexors, 25 percent to the lateral flexors of the spine, and 25 percent to the spinal extensors. Of course, Pilates exercises often include the combined activity of many muscle groups in various ranges of motion. It is interesting to note that exercises geared toward endurance, as opposed to strength, appear to have a more prominent effect on enhancing spinal stability. The block system helps ensure that all these factors are addressed in a well-rounded Pilates session.

Stabilizing the Scapulae   We tend to think of the shoulder as only the glenohumeral joint, the ball-and-socket joint that facilitates arm movement in every direction. But the shoulder is in fact an intricate structure that involves precise interplay between various bones, joints, and muscles. The humerus, scapula, and clavicle form the shoulder complex, which is connected to the axial skeleton (the central "axis" of the body) only at the tiny sternoclavicular joint. The scapulae articulate with the ribs, connected only by muscles. Because of the lack of bony and ligamentous support, the shoulder is *muscle dependent*—it relies heavily on the musculature for its function and stability. Although the terms *shoulder stabilization* and *scapular stabilization* are often used interchangeably, *scapular stabilization* may be a more precise term because the stabilization mechanism of the shoulder typically emanates from the scapulae (in the same way pelvic-lumbar stabilization relates to the movement of the hip). Scapular stabilization does not necessarily mean keeping the scapulae still, but rather preventing them from moving excessively in an undesired direction. For instance, in many exercises the scapulae tend to elevate and adduct, requiring that they be depressed and abducted to maintain the integrity of the movement. In this book I use scapular stabilization to refer to keeping the scapulae in the correct, desired position—most often a neutral position.

The shoulder complex is of great personal interest to me, having been born with a hooked acromion process. Throughout my life I have participated in activities with a high level of shoulder activity (swimming, dancing, yoga, gymnastics, surfing, windsurfing, and Pilates) and my supraspinatus eventually tore and retracted, on both sides. After extensive open (as opposed to arthroscopic) rotator cuff surgery, I began a personal journey of exploration to find solutions within Pilates that would help bring me back to 100 percent functionality. I learned a tremendous amount, including how difficult and painful rehabilitation can be. In the process my awareness of the power of Pilates and its limitless possibilities was reaffirmed. But probably the most important lessons I learned were how intricate the mechanics of the shoulder are, how few people use their shoulders correctly, and how far-reaching the implications of incorrect use are. The most common corrections in any Pilates studio around the world relate to the shoulders. Clearly there is a universal need to address the shoulder complex.

The back extensors, particularly those of the mid-back, play an important role in correct shoulder mechanics, not only because of their direct participation in the positioning of the scapulae, but also because of their importance in alignment and posture of the body (figure 3.1). As mentioned previously, certain postural deviations, such as round-shoulder syndrome, are encouraged by the dominance of forward-oriented activities in the modern lifestyle. We tether ourselves to electronic devices, drive for hours, and sit for much of the workday—and then for recreation we watch movies, ride bikes, play golf, or go to the gym and do push-ups, crunches, and bench presses! All these activities are forward-oriented and typically lead to problems—weak back extensors and shoulder external rotators; tight pectorals, hip flexors, hamstrings, and shoulder internal rotators; and, often, overactive levator scapulae and upper trapezius. Throw in some mental tension and you have a recipe for the type of neck, shoulder, and lower back problems that are so prevalent in our society.

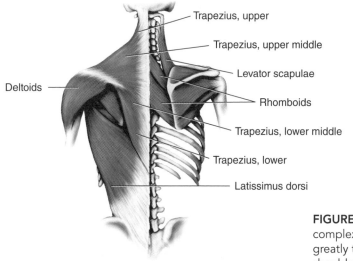

FIGURE 3.1 The muscles of the shoulder complex and the mid-back contribute greatly to the mechanical function of the shoulder joint and to shoulder stabilization.

So where do we start? We start with the muscles that hold us up, the back extensors, supported by the ISS. As long as the body is in good alignment, as close to the plumb line as possible, achieving good shoulder mechanics is possible. Conversely, without proper alignment and posture, good shoulder function is impossible—and faulty shoulder mechanics will probably result in shoulder problems. Rounded shoulders can lead to impingement; impingement can lead to rotator cuff inflammation; inflammation to tearing and, potentially, incapacitation and surgery. This downward spiral begins with habitual movement patterns that in turn cause incorrect posture and muscular imbalance.

Disassociation

Disassociation is when one area of the body remains stable while a connecting part moves freely. The more stable the foundation, the more precise and efficient the movement. Disassociation requires the synthesis of two of the pillars of human motion: stabilization and mobilization. The value of disassociation can be described thus: *Effective stabilization equates to efficient movement, and efficient movement equates to safer movement.* Conversely, ineffective stabilization translates to an unstable base of support, wear and tear on the body, and possible injury. Ineffective movement lacks efficiency and fluidity, and typically relies on muscle-substitution patterns (compensations) to perform the motion.

Muscle Isolation

Achieving muscle isolation, which is a goal of many exercise disciplines, requires the integration of many muscle groups in order to maintain a stable body while moving only one region. Therefore while muscle isolation and muscle integration may appear to be diametrically opposed concepts, attaining *functional* muscle isolation relies heavily on muscle integration. It's true to say that *Effective integration equates to heightened isolation,* and Pilates offers a roadmap to mastering both integration and isolation. Much of the conventional fitness equipment found in gyms is designed to support the body from every angle, thus facilitating the isolation of a muscle group without requiring integration. I do not consider this functional isolation, however, because the support is provided by extrinsic rather than intrinsic means; the equipment provides the stabilization. Intrinsic stabilization, provided by the body itself, involves heightened body awareness and control.

Imagery

One of the tools commonly used when practicing or teaching Pilates is imagery. This effective and artful means of understanding an exercise is a key category in the exercise chapters that follow (chapters 4-11). An image can convey a large amount of information instantaneously, whereas explanations involving large amounts of technical information and in-depth description can at times be confusing and counter-productive. In fact, describing a directive anatomically is often almost impossible. For example, if you want the movement to flow, how would you describe it anatomically?

Yet, simply saying, "Flow," accompanied by an illustrative gesture or calming tone will most likely produce the desired effect.

Imagery should be used with insight to avoid misunderstandings and breakdowns in communication. The image should be suited to the client's life experience and *image vocabulary* so that he or she can relate to the image and inferred meaning. If not, the image may seem meaningless or even ludicrous. Common expressions such as "inner pillar of support," "internal reinforcement," and "bracing the center" are examples of imagery that refer to the action of engaging the ISS. Teaching the recruitment of the ISS (and use of the powerhouse) is challenging because of the high level of awareness, concentration, and control required. Appropriate imagery is often the key.

Effectively cueing an exercise (for yourself or others) by means of imagery requires good understanding of the movement, of human science, and of the person being cued. Cueing is an art that comes in different forms—tactile, verbal, and visual—and you can deliver each type in different ways. Through cueing, information can be conveyed, received, and integrated almost instantaneously. Succinct cueing is equivalent to good communication, in this case between teacher and student. Good communication leads to better understanding and positive outcomes, as in every relationship. Deeper understanding is the basis of quality practice. *Consistent, high-quality practice is the path to mastery and success.*

A key component in developing and improving cueing skills is experience, there is simply no short cut, and this process takes time. Just as a student cannot learn all the nuances of an exercise in one session, so a teacher cannot learn all the cues from the pages of a book. Knowledge, practice, experience, intuition, compassion, understanding, and life experience are all ingredients that make for good cueing and effective teaching. It is also the reason cueing is such a personal realm. Cues for an exercise may change from person to person and day to day, illustrating the reason cueing is truly an ever-changing, lifelong exploration and the essence of teaching itself.

Following are brief explanations of some of the terms that I often use in my imagery when teaching and therefore often appear in the imagery descriptions in this book.

Lengthening

The term *lengthen* is frequently used in Pilates. This is a complex directive that can mean different things to different people. Working full ranges of motion can encourage lengthening. It is also helpful to think of the co-contraction of the muscles of all the joints along a kinetic chain (such as a limb) working symbiotically to create the desired shape. This can give the appearance and feeling that the whole kinetic chain is functioning as one long segment (reaching out in space) rather than as short individual links.

When using imagery, it is important to stress the difference between concept and physiological fact and to not confuse the two. For example, commands such as "Lift the leg from the back [the hamstrings]," "Lengthening out of the hip joint," and "Reach up from under the arm" utilize imagery to achieve a physical result but are anatomically imprecise. This is not to say these images cannot and should not be used—they can often be used very effectively—but teachers and students should always be aware of the line between fact and poetic license.

A related point of discussion is the question of how straight is straight? Because of the often-heard instruction to avoid locking the knees or elbows, many people no longer straighten their limbs completely. This results in inefficient movement, incomplete use of the joint, an unstable joint, inadequate muscle recruitment, and even the possible onset of problems such as patella-femoral syndrome (caused by misaligned tracking of the patella). *Locking* refers to hyperextension of the joint, which should be avoided when doing Pilates. However, it does

not mean that you should never completely straighten the joint; it means reaching the straightest line possible without going beyond the straight line. This is achieved by becoming aware of what *straight* is. First, create an imaginary straight line across the joint. Then activate both the agonist and antagonist muscles groups (co-contraction). In the case of the knee, the hamstrings and quadriceps should be in a state of co-contraction with the knee joint fully extended. In this position the joint is well supported, the correct muscles are perfectly activated, and a long line is achieved.

Remember, a straight limb is longer than a hyperextended or slightly bent one. This is easy to feel on the reformer when doing the foot work (chapter 5). As long as the carriage is traveling away from the foot bar, the leg is still straightening. Once the leg is completely straight, the carriage will no longer move in that direction, and it is time to bend the knee and return. If the knee continues extending past the straight line into hyperextension, the carriage will actually start returning toward the foot bar. It is a slight but distinct movement, illustrating that hyperextension is shorter than full extension.

Ultimately, creating length is both anatomical and an inner quality and is conveyed better through relaxed, rather than tension-filled, movement. A wonderful dance teacher once showed me how a straight arm can look short, or by contrast, appear infinite in length. It was difficult to identify exactly what the difference was, but it was clearly apparent and I have never forgotten that lesson. I try to re-create that quality in every move I do.

Relaxing the Ribs

In discussing imagery, we need to pay particular attention to the lower rib cage, which tends to thrust forward when in an upright position or lift off the mat in a supine position. This is typically a result of overusing the back extensors, particularly those of the lower back. I like to think of the lower ribs being connected to the pubic symphysis with two rubber bands, one from each side of the rib cage, which allow the ribs to glide up and down the front of the body, but remain controlled and not thrust forward. This image encourages the muscles of the lower back to elongate and the abdominals to activate. You will often hear Pilates teachers say, "Drop your ribs" or "Relax your ribs." What is being implied in physiological terms is to engage the abdominal muscles (without going into spinal flexion) and decrease the intensity of contraction of the spinal extensors, resulting in ideal alignment with appropriate co-contraction of the abdominals and back extensors. Breathing can play a valuable role in this process. Often one deep exhalation achieves the desired result. Try it right now—inhale and exhale fully!

Imprinting

Credit for the concept of *imprinting* must be given to Eve Gentry, one of the great first-generation Pilates teachers. It was a central motif of her teaching and the powerful imagery she used with great success. I had the pleasure of experiencing Eve's teaching firsthand, and a tremendous honor it was.

Lying on a mat, visualize the body sinking into soft sand, making an imprint. Note that the spine still maintains its natural curves; the very reason the image of soft sand works well is that it conforms to the shape of the body. The bones are then moved out of, and back into, the imprint. In this form of work, the focus on the individual muscles is minimized while attention is shifted to the motion of the body part, as if moving only the bones. Ideally, this results in movement that is fluid and void of tension. For example, when performing the pelvic curl you may imagine an imprint of the spine in the sand. The pelvis and each vertebra is first lifted out of its imprint and then returned to the same place. The result is sequential articulation of the spine without excess muscle activity (or at least without the tension associated with trying too hard). You can apply this concept to any part of the body in any position. It allows the body to move with graceful correctness without being bogged down with information.

In conclusion, effective learning and teaching strategies may vary according to the movement, the student and the instructor. Some people learn better when presented with a picture or a demonstration of the movement, which they then emulate and practice. Others learn better by breaking the exercise down into small movements. Still others prefer a verbal explanation, an image or the use of touch. In most cases, a combination of approaches is best, using every angle to improve performance and increase understanding.

The following general guidelines will prove helpful in achieving a positive outcome:

- Precede the movement with the breath.
- Set up the exercise before moving (engage the ISS).
- Go through a full body scan, to make sure the positioning is correct and to eliminate excessive tension.
- Concentrate on the muscle focus (initiator).
- Keep the head aligned with the spine.
- Direct the eyes forward, in line with the head.
- Breathe throughout the exercise (even if it is not the recommended breathing pattern).
- Keep the shoulders and neck relaxed.
- Create long lines with the movements.
- Move with efficiency, flow, precision, and harmony.

Movement Description

Each exercise in the following chapters includes a description of the movement, with step-by-step instructions for correct execution. Although the words *exercise* and *movement* can be, and are, used interchangeably, I often refer to *movement* rather than *exercise*, in an endeavor to differentiate the Pilates approach from the notion that an exercise is a merely a physical action. Even the most basic movement has many layers of

Repetition in Pilates

Joseph Pilates spoke of *mindless repetition*; I like that term because I believe that a high rate of repetition invariably becomes mindless and produces diminished returns. You can practice an exercise routine that is based on a high number of repetitions, with no real focus or control, and it becomes mindless as opposed to mindful. Being mindful in each exercise and each repetition is the goal. In order to achieve this, both physically and mentally, I recommend a limited number of repetitions, usually 5 to 10, depending on the intensity and complexity of the movement. The more complex the movement, the fewer the repetitions required. Use the low end of the scale for the very difficult and complex repertoire, and the high end (10 repetitions, still relatively low compared to many typical endurance-based workouts) for the fundamental work.

One reason profound effects are achieved from so few repetitions is the precision with which Pilates movements are executed and the resulting recruitment of the appropriate muscles. When many repetitions are done, compensations often creep in; other muscles (usually the larger, superficial ones) take over and the effect on the desired muscles is minimal at best. Other negative effects of doing excessive repetitions are fatigue, wear and tear on the joints, boredom and, in some instances, injury. Pilates encapsulates the concept of *less is more* (quality versus quantity), which holds the key to deeper work, enhanced performance and in many cases better results.

information, with the physical motion being only one of them (and the most superficial one at that). This is not meant to devalue the physicality of an exercise but to bring attention to the underlying approach, in which the movements are a means to an end: a vehicle for reaching a higher purpose—well-being.

Before starting an exercise, it is important to set up the body to perform the movement correctly. I often say to students that the *setup* is 90 percent of the exercise and the movement is 10 percent, because without a good, precise setup, the movement has little chance of being correct and producing the desired results. The setup allows the mind and body to work together to achieve optimum alignment and muscle recruitment.

The setup may take 5 seconds or 30 seconds—take the time you need to engage the ISS and establish a connection with the muscle focus of the exercise. Review the breath pattern and do a body scan to make sure that every body part is aligned and in place. Go through a checklist of the nuances of the movement. If

you are working alone, cue yourself and make corrections to the movement before the mistakes or deviations ever occur. The better you know your body and recognize your own habits and compensations, the more refined this process becomes. In essence the exercise begins long before movement is apparent. The process of setting up gives each exercise, and the session as a whole, a deep focus and a meditative quality.

Achieving Symmetry

Is symmetry attainable? Is it desirable? My wife, Adelle, likes to remind me that in nature there is no absolute symmetry—close, but not absolute. So should we strive for symmetry in our bodies? This question leads to the interesting issue of symmetrical versus asymmetrical training. I have worked with athletes who questioned whether it was worth tampering with the physical asymmetries that had resulted from their many years and thousands of hours of practice in sports such as tennis and volleyball. It is certainly legitimate for them to strive for core strength and enhanced performance, without altering the balance (or imbalance) in their bodies that is serving them well. Personally, I like to promote symmetry as an ideal, a reference point for which we strive and against which improvement can be measured. Symmetry can also serve as a guideline for cueing. I believe that training toward symmetry ultimately enhances performance and function, in both everyday and skill-specific activities; it prevents undue stresses on particular areas of the body and possibly the eventual deterioration of the body as a whole.

Furthermore, when practicing movement on one side of the body, a transferal of information to the other side occurs. That means that if one side is injured, exercising the non-injured side has a positive effect on the injured side through information transfer. This transferal applies not only to injuries but also to all motor skills, including athletic activities.

Training toward symmetry is complex; therefore a conservative approach is the most prudent one. Do not rush to make drastic changes. I use the following steps when dealing with imbalances. Note that I use the first and second steps in a well-rounded session for several months before proceeding (only if necessary) to steps three and four.

1. Work bilaterally, raising awareness to asymmetrical muscular activity and development.
2. Work unilaterally, using the same number of repetitions and resistance on both sides.
3. Work unilaterally, loading the weaker, less-dominant side more than the other.
4. Work unilaterally, working only the weaker, less-dominant side.

Moving With the Energy Lines

As a dancer I was taught to think of movement in terms of energy lines or energy paths; this is a concept that adapts well to Pilates. Energy paths can be straight, circular, or spiral shaped. Fundamental movements such as the Mat Work: Pelvic Curl or Mat Work: Chest Lift have only one or two energy lines (see figure 3.2a). More complex movements have more energy lines, since various parts of the body reach in different and often opposing directions. For example, the Mat Work: Spine Twist has longitudinal, horizontal, and spiral energy lines (see figure 3.2b). The longitudinal line, which travels up and down the spine and continues into space, keeps the trunk upright. The horizontal line, running across the shoulders and traveling outward in both directions, keeps the arms, shoulders, and back as broad as possible and on one plane. We add to this a spiral, which travels up the trunk, illustrating the rotation that occurs. The energy moves in all these directions at the same time, making this movement relatively complex.

Think of the energy lines as a form of notating the energy of the exercises. Understanding these lines will bring clarity and simplicity to the exercises and result in precise movement. You can utilize this principle in every exercise. Once you understand the energy lines of an exercise, the choreography becomes clear and the correct muscles will likely be activated in the most effective manner.

Adapting Exercises

There is no need to reinvent the wheel. I've seen people create variations of Pilates exercises simply to be different or to avoid boredom. Others choreograph variations because they are unfamiliar with the original exercises, or possibly cannot do them as prescribed. I do not support changing an exercise for any of these reasons. I believe the essence of the exercise is often lost in a mass of choreography, at times ceasing to have any resemblance to the original exercise or its intention. Yes, we must evolve. But evolution does not mean throwing out this vast, ingenious body of work. It means refining it according to advances in scientific knowledge and the needs of the individual—but always building on the foundation of the original work. The goal is to promote

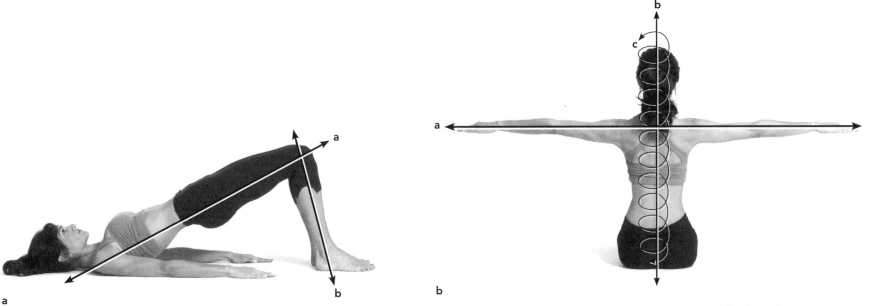

FIGURE 3.2 Focusing on the energy lines of exercises will guide you along the correct movement path(s). The energy in the *(a)* Mat Work: Pelvic Curl moves along two simple lines, while the energy in the more complex *(b)* Mat Work: Spine Twist moves in multiple directions simultaneously

growth, keep the system alive and contemporary, and to adapt the work to individual and societal needs, while still preserving the legacy of Pilates.

The original body of work must be seen in the context of the time and place it was created, the early part of the 20th century in Europe and New York. That world was very different from the 21st century in terms of people's habits, occupations, and lifestyles. Computers were nonexistent, cars were scarce, air travel was a dream, the Internet was decades away, and recreational activities were simple and low-tech. Surely the evolution of this system and its adaptation to the needs of people today is justified and should be celebrated. But as we progress, we must not lose sight of the value of Joseph Pilates' work.

Modifying exercises is necessary at times in order to avoid negative movement patterns, compensations, and contraindications and to achieve the desired objectives. When I say *modification*, I mean changing the choreography of an exercise to meet certain goals.

However, maintaining the essence of the exercise is critical, which means that one must understand the intention and mechanics of the exercise and its possible contraindications. Creating modifications is an integral part of being a creative, innovative, and interactive teacher.

This approach to modifications applies also to *assists*. Assists are external aids such as springs, rubber bands, cushions, balls, or adjustments to the apparatus that help achieve the goal. Again, complete understanding of the exercise and the exerciser is essential. Also important is being well informed about the many choices of apparatus and, which would be best suited for each scenario. In short, intimate familiarity with the Pilates repertoire, the human body and its movement, as well as the myriad choreographic directions and apparatus available make this work an evolutionary process.

In the first edition of *Pilates* I intentionally abstained from offering modifications and assists. Too much information and too many variations can lead to confusion. I wanted people to gain knowledge, understanding, and experience in the original repertoire. I also wanted to encourage individual creativity, which is a multiphase process. The first phase is learning the original exercises—their form, function, and intent. The second is gaining knowledge of the equipment as well as an understanding of anatomy, physiology, and kinesiology. and the final and most important is acknowledging the body you are working with—the possibilities for developing variations become infinite.

Following many requests from students and readers that I offer variations of exercises, I have included modification options for many of the exercises in this second edition of *Pilates*. My intention is to spark ideas. I stress that each person is an individual with particular needs, restrictions, and personal goals that must be taken into account when selecting or choreographing a variation of an exercise. Body type, suitability of apparatus, and desired outcome must also be considered. Finally, safety is always an underlying concern. Choose or create movements that will allow you and your student to perform the work safely and to enjoy years of Pilates practice.

4

Mat Work

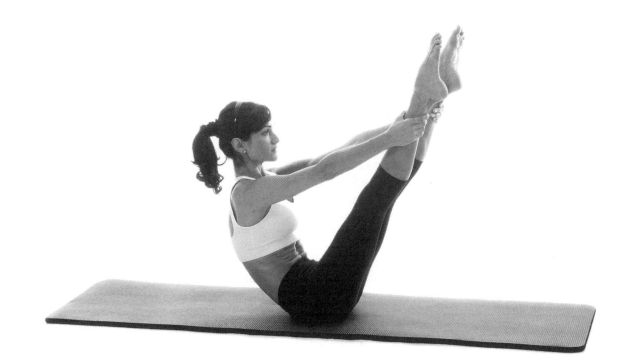

Pilates mat work is the essence of the Pilates system. It is the source of all that follows, the root of most exercises in the Pilates repertoire, and it never ceases to challenge. Without an intricate familiarity with the mat work, you will lack a fundamental component in your Pilates practice.

Mat work can be practiced anywhere and everywhere, with no special apparatus other than a mat. You can practice it at any time of the day and at any level of challenge. You can structure it to meet different goals: as a warm-up for a Pilates class on the apparatus or for other athletic activities, as part of a daily conditioning program, as a means of improving general body awareness, or as a pre- and postnatal fitness routine.

The block designations provided in this chapter will assist you in structuring workouts. As noted in chapter 3, the *mat block system* differs from the *comprehensive block system* used to structure a session that utilizes all the apparatus. Most mat exercises focus on developing the core, and therefore the mat work blocks relate primarily to the movements and position of the pelvis and spine.

The exercises in this chapter are presented with both progression and flow in mind. Mat work embodies the principle of flow more fully than the work on any of the other Pilates apparatus. I have created what I call flow sequences, which offer a unique way to practice traditional mat work. These sequences incorporate the original movements, arranging them according to level of challenge and duration and in such a manner that each exercise flows seamlessly into the next.

I typically conclude a mat work session with a few minutes of relaxation and focusing. Whether it involves performing slow, guided movements, sitting still in a comfortable position and listening to calming words or music, or going through a short, guided meditation, this relaxation period serves as a cool-down for the body and a chance to mentally and spiritually integrate the work that you have just done. This is possibly the most valuable part of the session.

Don't view the mat work as the underdog in the Pilates system; it is the crown jewel. Enjoy!

Foundation

The foundation block focuses on exercises that are typically performed at the beginning of the mat session and serve as an introduction to the session or a warm up for other activities. These exercises lay the foundation to all that follows, on the mat and on the apparatus. They place great emphasis on the *powerhouse*, and they increase physical and mental awareness of the core.

Although these exercises are not as complex as some of the movements that follow later in the book, they should be performed with concentration, control, and precision. Foundation exercises are performed slowly, providing a perfect opportunity to pay attention to the internal aspects of the work and the finer details of proper execution.

The essential muscle actions of this block are the recruitment of the pelvic floor muscles, the abdominal muscles, in particular activation of the transversus abdominis, the co-contraction of the abdominals, back extensors, the hip flexors and hamstrings that help position the pelvis and hip flexors. The hip flexors, unobstructed articulation of the spine is pivotal. Also important is the establishment of certain body shapes, including the neutral spine position, the C curve of the trunk, and the tabletop position of the legs, which will be applied later to more complex and demanding movements.

Pelvic Curl

The pelvic curl exercise has myriad benefits. Not only does it mobilize the spine and prepare it for exercise, but it also teaches recruitment of the internal support system (ISS). The pelvic curl develops body awareness and brings focus to the powerhouse. This exercise promotes mobility and stability in the pelvic region and spine, releasing both physical and mental tension in the process.

Imagery

The image I like to use is that of a banana peel being peeled off the fruit slowly and deliberately. Allow the feeling of gentle resistance and fine movement to prevail throughout.

☐ Begin and complete the movement in a neutral spine position.

☐ Tilt the pelvis slightly posteriorly and stretch the hip flexors when at the top.

☐ Keep the shoulders and neck relaxed and uninvolved.

VARIATION

Perform this same exercise with a single leg lifted from the mat. Hold the lifted leg in a tabletop position (right angles at the knee and hip joints) from the outset. The angle in the hip joint will change as the body is lifted, but keep the right angle in the knee, with the shin parallel to the mat, constant throughout. Although most of the variations offered in this book make the exercises less challenging, this particular variation adds exponential challenge in terms of pelvic stabilization and hip extensor control.

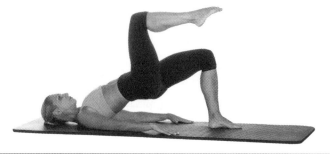

Muscle Focus
- Abdominal muscles
- Hamstrings

Objectives
- To improve spinal articulation
- To establish pelvic–lumbar stabilization
- To develop abdominal and hamstring control

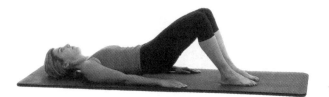

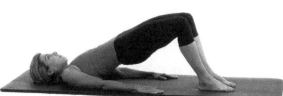

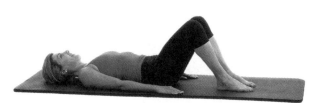

Inhale. Lie supine with the spine in a neutral position, keeping the entire body relaxed. Bend the knees and place the feet hip-width apart. Sense the elongation through the spine while keeping the scapulae in a neutral position, the arms straight by the sides, and the fingers reaching toward the feet. Make sure the neck is relaxed and the chin is tilted slightly toward the chest.

Exhale. Draw in the abdominal muscles. Begin to curl the pelvis, lifting the lower back vertebra by vertebra off the mat. Midway through the motion, recruit the hamstrings to lift the pelvis and trunk higher, continuing to articulate the spine one vertebra at a time.

Inhale. Keep the body still and the legs parallel, maximizing the hip flexor stretch. Engage the shoulder extensors to accentuate the extension of the upper back.

Exhale. Articulate the spine in reverse order from the top of the spine, vertebra by vertebra, accentuating the flexion through the lumbar region. Return to the start position.

Spine Twist—Supine

Muscle Focus

- Oblique abdominal muscles

Objectives

- To improve flexibility for spinal rotation
- To increase abdominal control
- To encourage pelvic–lumbar stabilization

This exercise prepares the body (specifically the spine) for rotational movements. It also activates and brings awareness to the oblique abdominal muscles. The degree of rotation should be dictated by your flexibility and abdominal control. Maintain strong pelvic–lumbar support, avoiding hyperlordosis throughout the movement. This is particularly pertinent when in rotation, because the tendency to exceed the controllable range of motion often results in the back arching excessively.

Imagery

Imagine the pelvis turning like a doorknob, with the pelvis, legs, and feet rotating fluidly, as one unit, from side to side.

- ☐ Keep the shoulder girdle and neck relaxed and still.

- ☐ Focus the movement in the waist area (although anatomically the majority of the rotation occurs in the thoracic spine).

Perform the same movement pattern, but instead of placing the legs in a tabletop position to begin, bend the knees and place the feet on the mat. The legs again move as one unit; as the pelvis and legs move to the right, the left foot rises slightly off the mat, and vice versa.

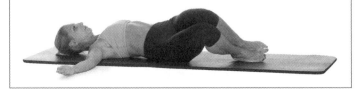

- ☐ Keep the knees and feet together, avoiding any gliding back and forth.

- ☐ Maintain a long line across the chest, from the fingertips of one hand to the fingertips of the other.

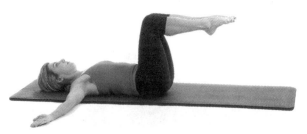

Exhale. Lie supine with the arms in the T position, palms facing upward. Draw the lumbar spine into the mat, maintaining a slight posterior pelvic tilt. (You can begin this exercise from a neutral pelvic position, although greater control is required to avoid hyperlordosis and excessive stress on the lower back). The legs are in a tabletop position (legs together, right angles at the knee and hip joints).

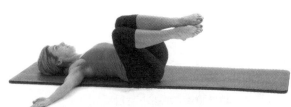

Inhale. Rotate the spine; moving the pelvis and the legs as one unit to one side, keeping the knees together. The movement is in the transverse plane, with the shoulder girdle providing a stable base around which the movement occurs.

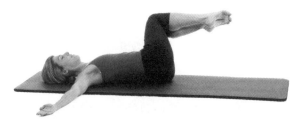

Exhale. Draw the pelvis and legs as one unit back to the center.

Inhale. Rotate to the opposite side.

Chest Lift

This exercise strengthens the abdominal muscles, teaches correct recruitment of the internal support system, and lays the foundation for much of the abdominal work that follows. Although it resembles the infamous crunch, it is a completely different exercise. Most notably, the pace is much slower, which eliminates momentum and allows the abdominal muscles to drive the movement. The positioning of the spine and pelvis are also different in that the crunch is typically done with the pelvis in posterior tilt and the spine pressing into the mat, while the chest lift begins in a neutral spine and neutral pelvic position and the neutral pelvis is maintained throughout. The chest lift should be challenging, regardless of your fitness level. Remember: Exercises do not get easier as we get stronger, they get better (more intense)!

Imagery

Imagine the spine being a strip of spring metal, flexible and strong. The lower part is riveted down onto a stable surface. The mid and upper part is free to be lifted. As you begin to lift the mid and upper part of the metal strip, it curves; as you continue, the curve is distributed evenly throughout the movable portion, while the lower part of the strip remains absolutely stable.

VARIATION

After lifting the upper spine, vertebra by vertebra, bringing the bases of the scapulae off the mat, inhale while placing the hands behind the thighs. Exhale; lift the trunk slightly higher, using the arms for support. Inhale; place the hands back behind the head and maintain the same height of the trunk. Exhale and slowly lower the spine. Return to the start position.

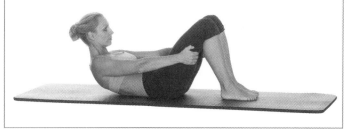

☐ Avoid pulling on the neck.

☐ Lift the head, shoulders, and upper trunk as one unit.

☐ Maintain a neutral pelvis, keeping the hip flexors as uninvolved as possible.

Muscle Focus

- Abdominal muscles

Objectives

- To strengthen the abdominal muscles

- To develop pelvic stability and control

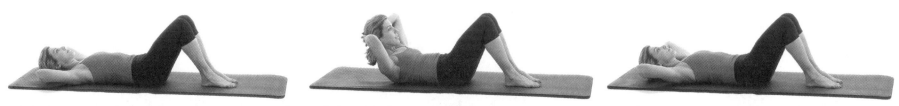

Inhale. Lie supine with the pelvis and spine in a neutral position, the knees bent, and the feet hip-width apart. Feel a sense of elongation through the spine. Interlace the fingers and cradle the head in the hands. Make sure the neck is relaxed, with the chin tilted slightly toward the chest. Engage the internal support system, highlighting awareness of the abdominal region.

Exhale. While drawing in the abdominal muscles, lift the upper spine, beginning with the top of the head, and allow the lumbar spine to sink into the mat. Sense a hinging action just under the sternum, and maintain absolute stability of the body below this point. Continue lifting the upper spine, vertebra by vertebra, until the bases of the scapulae have risen off the mat.

Inhale. Maintain the maximum height you can achieve with the upper trunk. Contract the abdominals further and focus on the neutral position of the pelvis.

Exhale. Lower the spine without releasing the contraction of the abdominal muscles. Return to the start position.

Muscle Focus

• Oblique abdominal muscles

Objectives

• To strengthen the abdominals, emphasizing the obliques

• To develop pelvic stability while performing spinal rotation

Chest Lift With Rotation

This exercise is an extension of the Mat Work: Chest Lift. It adds the element of rotation and further challenges the abdominals by loading the oblique muscles in a bilateral pattern. This lays the foundation for much of the rotational abdominal work, such as the Mat Work: Criss-Cross, and prepares the body for the many rotational activities that everyday life and athletic activities demand.

Imagery

A good image for this exercise is a combination of the door-knob turning described in the spine twist supine, and the spring metal strip described in the chest lift. Together these images describe the type of movement used in this exercise.

☐ Move the head, arms, and upper trunk as one unit.

☐ Avoid pulling on the neck and moving the elbows forward.

☐ Maintain consistent forward flexion as you transition from side to side.

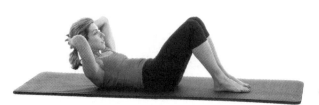 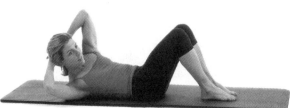 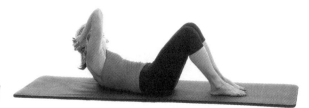

Inhale. Lie supine with the pelvis and spine in a neutral position, the knees bent, and the feet hip-width apart. Interlace the fingers and cradle the head in the hands. Engage the internal support system, draw in the abdominal muscles, and lift the upper spine, vertebra by vertebra, until the bases of the scapulae have risen off the mat.

Exhale. Rotate the upper girdle to one side. Focus on drawing in the abdominal muscles and moving from above the pelvis without any lateral flexion of the trunk. Maintain stability of the pelvis throughout.

Inhale. Rotate the upper girdle through the center to the opposite side without lowering the trunk.

Continue moving from side to side. On the final repetition rotate back to the center, contracting the abdominal muscles further, before returning to a supine position.

Leg Lift

This exercise uses the abdominal muscles as stabilizers rather than as movers. It is particularly useful when pelvic stability is lacking or abdominal strength is insufficient to lift the trunk into forward flexion. By keeping the entire body still, particularly the pelvic–lumbar region, and moving only one leg up and down, you learn to bring awareness to the powerhouse and stability to the pelvis.

Imagery

The pelvis should be as stable as a rock and the leg as light as a feather, floating up and down without affecting the pelvis. These opposing images help create the correct sensation in the body.

- ☐ Avoid tension in the lower back and possible hyperlordosis when lifting the leg.

- ☐ Move the leg as one unit, maintaining a right angle at the knee.

- ☐ Minimize the weight shift onto the supporting leg when lifting the opposite side.

Muscle Focus
- Abdominal muscles

Objectives
- To develop pelvic–lumbar stabilization
- To develop hip-joint disassociation
- To improve abdominal and hip flexor control

VARIATION

To raise the level of difficulty and challenge, work both legs at the same time: Lift one leg into tabletop position. As you lower that leg to touch the mat with the tip of the toes, lift the other leg into tabletop position. Continue changing legs simultaneously, performing the same number of repetitions on each side. This version of exercise is appropriately called Leg Change.

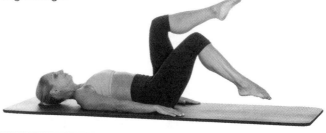

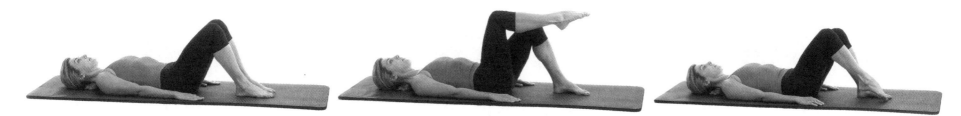

Inhale. Lie supine with the spine in a neutral position, bend the knees, and place the feet hip-width apart. The arms are straight by the sides, the fingers reach toward the feet, the neck is relaxed, and the chin is tilted slightly toward the chest. Emphasize pelvic–lumbar stability and an even distribution of weight on the feet.

Exhale. Lift one leg, focusing the movement in the hip joint only and maintaining a perfect right angle in the knee throughout the full range of motion. Continue the movement until your hip joint reaches a right angle and the thigh is perpendicular with the floor (tabletop position).

Inhale. Keep the knee at a right angle and lower the leg gently, touching the floor with the tip of the toes without placing any pressure on the foot. Repeat several times before switching to the other leg.

Leg Circle

Muscle Focus

- Abdominal muscles
- Hip flexors

Objectives

- To develop pelvic–lumbar stabilization
- To improve hip disassociation
- To develop control of the hip flexors
- To relax the muscles around the hip joint

This exercise is an excellent example of coordinated stabilization (of the trunk) and mobilization (of the leg) producing disassociation of the hip joint. While the pelvis remains anchored and the spine remains still, the hip joint fluidly rotates and the leg circles effortlessly. Hip mobilization and disassociation, a pattern often found in Pilates exercises, is a requisite for many activities, such as cycling, running, and certain dance and gymnastic movements. When executed correctly, it may also help release lower back tension and assist in remedying sacroiliac dysfunction.

Imagery

Imagine the leg as a big spoon that is stirring thick syrup in a large pot. The motion should be gentle and smooth, with a continuous flow. Thinking of a fall-and-retrieve action, like a yo-yo rolling down and then up, may also be helpful.

☐ Maintain a neutral pelvis and spine throughout the exercise.

☐ Keep the movement in the hip joint unrestricted and fluid.

VARIATION

This exercise can be performed with a rubber exercise band draped over the foot of the lifted leg, with an end of the band held in each hand and the elbows firmly planted on the mat by the sides of the body. This version allows the hip flexors to relax and assists in achieving the desired fluidity of movement in the joint as the leg rotates—it is a very helpful option when the hamstrings are tight.

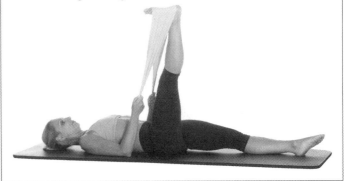

☐ Keep the neck, shoulders, and chest relaxed.

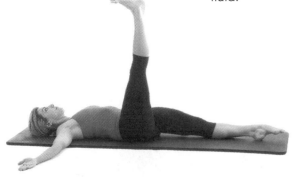

Exhale. Lie supine and place the arms by the sides of the body or in a T position palms facing up. Keep the legs straight and together, with the feet gently pointed. Bend one leg toward the chest.

Straighten the leg upward, to form an angle of 90 degrees (perpendicular) to the floor and dorsiflex the foot. Keep the other leg straight and actively engaged, with the foot plantarflexed.

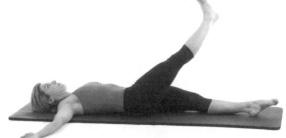

Inhale. Circle the raised leg inward, bringing it slightly across the centerline of the body then down and around. The circle should be only as big as you can make it while maintaining a stable pelvis.

Exhale. Repeat the movement, alternating the breathing on each circle and pausing slightly (suspending the movement) each time the foot reaches the 12 o'clock position (leg perpendicular to the floor), 5 to 10 times.

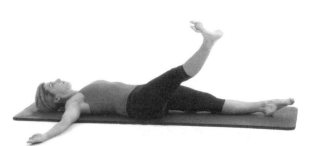

Inhale. Reverse the circle and repeat the breath pattern, one circle of the leg on each breath. Start by taking the leg away from the centerline and circling it outward and downward. Emphasize pelvic–lumbar stability and the free-flowing movement of the hip joint. Repeat 5 to 10 times, returning to the 12 o'clock position after the final repetition. Bend the leg to the chest and straighten it on the mat. Return to the start position.

Abdominal Work

Despite the fact that the abdominals are engaged to some extent in nearly every exercise in Pilates because they are integral to the concept of the *powerhouse*, this block is devoted specifically to their development. The abdominals are also a key element in the concept of core strength and spinal stability, which is increasingly popular in the areas of general fitness, rehabilitation, and athletic performance. In addition well-conditioned abdominals play a vital role in ensuring healthy functioning of the back and protecting the back from injury.

The exercises in this block focus particularly on strengthening the abdominals in their action of spinal flexion and on recruiting the abdominals for trunk stabilization. As always, precision in activating the muscles and executing the movement is crucial to achieving a positive outcome. If done poorly, not only will the exercise fall short of its goal, but it may actually result in injury or compound an existing problem.

With all its emphasis on precision, Pilates is not a one-size-fits-all method of conditioning. Often, particularly when working the abdominals, modifications need to be made in order to achieve the desired objectives. It is imperative to work at an appropriate level and increase the challenge incrementally. Ultimately, well-conditioned abdominals contribute positively to the many activities of daily living and to athletic pursuits.

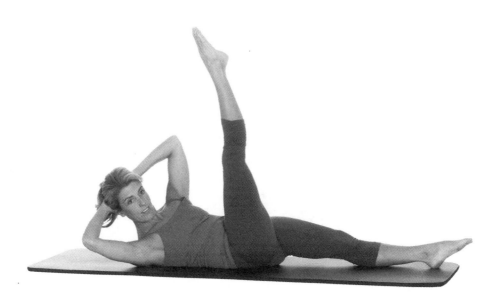

Muscle Focus
- Abdominal muscles

Objectives
- To strengthen the abdominal muscles
- To develop trunk stabilization
- To stimulate circulation and elevate body temperature

Hundred

This exercise is one of the signature abdominal exercises of the Pilates method, highlighting the powerhouse. The name of the exercise is derived from the breathing pattern—each inhalation and exhalation in a single breath cycle should last for 10 counts (5 counts for the inhalation and 5 counts for the exhalation). This breath pattern is repeated 10 times, totaling 100 counts. This does not mean taking 100 breaths!

I often use *active breathing* during this exercise, in which the work of respiratory muscles is accentuated by dynamically contracting the muscles involved in exhalation and inhalation. Ron Fletcher, a wonderful first-generation teacher, and pioneer, whom I am honored to have called a friend, coined the term percussive breathing. The percussive quality does make the breath more active and dynamic—this is a good if done well, but not if it induces tension.

The hundred can be counterproductive if certain elements are not in place, including strong abdominals and the ability to lift the trunk into adequate spinal flexion. I encourage you to practice preparation exercises to build up to the hundred (see Variation). When doing the hundred, keep the legs at a height that your abdominal strength and control can support. (Legs perpendicular to the floor is less challenging; legs lower toward the floor is more challenging. The lower back must not lift off the mat.) The classic version of the hundred, as Joseph Pilates performed it, is with the feet at eye level. However, keeping the legs at this height demands a great deal of strength, control, and practice.

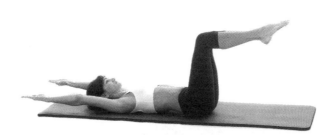

Inhale. Lie supine with the legs in a tabletop position (right angles at the knee and hip joints). Hold the arms straight, directly overhead and shoulder-width apart, with the palms facing up.

Exhale. Lift the trunk into the Mat Work: Chest Lift position by drawing in the abdominal muscles, lifting the upper spine, and allowing the lumbar spine to sink into the mat. Continue lifting the upper spine, vertebra by vertebra, until the bases of the scapulae have risen off the mat.

Inhale. Maintain the maximum height you can achieve with the upper trunk while straightening the legs to the appropriate height for you. Lower the arms toward the sides of the body until they are parallel to the floor.

Inhale. Prepare for the movement by focusing on the contraction of the abdominal muscles.

Imagery

Visualize the movement of the arms generating energy like a generator; this energy helps keep the body stabilized, the abdominal muscles active and the legs supported.

☐ Contract the abdominal muscles throughout the exercise, imprinting the lower back into the mat.

☐ Relax the neck and shoulders throughout.

☐ Keep the pumping motion smooth, small, and free of tension.

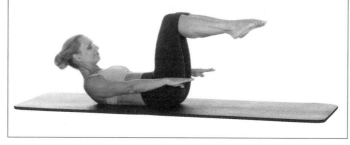

VARIATION

To make this exercise easier while building up the required skills, keep the feet on the floor or keep the legs bent in table-top position, thereby decreasing the load on the hip flexors and, in turn, the demand on the abdominals. If you have tight hamstrings, I recommend bending the knees during this exercise to reduce the load on the hip flexors.

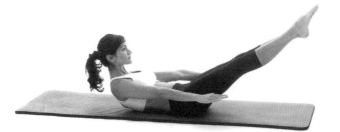

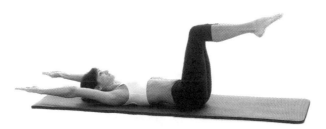

Exhale. Pump the arms up and down with a small pulsing movement for the duration of five counts. The lower the legs are held, the more challenging the exercise becomes.

Inhale. Continue to pump the arms for the duration of five counts. Keep the arms close to the sides of the body throughout. Repeat this cycle 10 times. Return to the start position.

Exhale. Lower the spine without releasing the contraction of the abdominal muscles. Return to the start position. Repeat this cycle 10 times.

Roll-Up

Muscle Focus

- Abdominal muscles

Objectives

- To strengthen the abdominal muscles
- To develop spinal mobility and stability
- To stretch the muscles of the back

The roll-up activates the abdominal muscles, both as movers and as stabilizers. In the initial phase, the abdominals are recruited to move the body into spinal flexion. Next, the hip flexors are introduced to lift the trunk and pelvis off the mat, flexing the body at the hip joint as the abdominals (with assistance from the back extensors) stabilize the trunk and maintain the C curve of the spine. In the top position, with the shoulders directly above the hip joints, concentrate on further engaging the abdominals, remaining in the C curve and elongating the muscles of the back.

I have made several choreographic changes to this exercise from the classic form. The first is that I advocate pausing in the position described above, with the shoulders above the hips, rather than reaching all the way forward with the trunk over the legs. The reason for this change is to avoid stretching the hamstrings excessively too early in the session, when they may not yet be ready to be stretched. The objective is to gently warm up the back muscles and the abdominal muscles while providing a very light stretch for the hamstrings.

The second change is the positioning of the head. In the classic form, the head is lowered and placed between the arms when in the sitting phase of the exercise. I prefer that the head follow the natural line of the spine, in which case it is held higher up so that the neck and face can be clearly observed from the side, with the arms parallel to the floor.

Finally, in the classic form the feet are dorsiflexed. I prefer the feet to be in moderate plantar flexion, with the knees soft (very slightly bent). The reason is that when the feet are dorsiflexed, there is a strong tendency to overuse the quadriceps, including the rectus femoris (a two-joint hip flexor). I prefer to downplay the activity of the hip flexors in this exercise. The hip flexors have a tendency to overshadow the work of the abdominals, making it difficult to maintain the C curve when lifting off the mat. However, the hip flexors clearly play an important role, particularly at that point when the pelvis, together with the trunk, is lifted off the mat. This version of the roll-up accentuates the long lines of the arms, legs, and spine and is aesthetically very appealing, in my opinion.

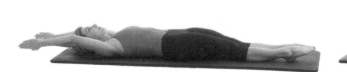

Exhale. Lie in a supine position with the arms overhead, palms facing each other, legs straight and together, and feet moderately plantarflexed. Draw the ribs down and together while accentuating the overhead reach of the arms. Keep the arms shoulder-width apart.

Inhale. Engage the abdominal muscles and begin the movement with the arms, following with the head and upper spine. Pause in this position, further engaging abdominal muscles and imprinting the lower back into the mat. Prepare to lift forward off the mat to a sitting position by activating the hip flexors.

Exhale. Maintain stability of the trunk with the abdominal muscles as you peel the spine off the mat, vertebra by vertebra, keeping the C curve of the trunk. Pause when the shoulders are above the hips. The curve should extend from the top of the head and the fingertips through the spine to the tips of the toes—hollow and deep.

Imagery

As you roll up, visualize holding the reins of a horse and being gently raised off the mat and then lowered back down. The movement should appear effortless and the gentle C curve of the body should remain constant when lifting and lowering the trunk.

☐ When supine, do not allow the ribs to thrust upward as the arms reach overhead.

☐ Maintain a C curve of the trunk when lifting off the mat and lowering back down and in the sitting position.

☐ Keep the head aligned with the spine throughout the exercise.

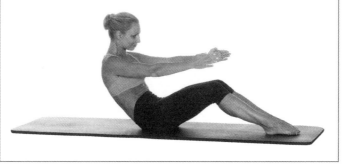

VARIATION

If the regular roll-up proves difficult because of tight lower back muscles, tight hamstrings, or insufficient abdominal strength, start the exercise with the knees bent. Inhale; lift the arms, head, and upper trunk. Exhale; roll up, simultaneously straightening the legs. Inhale while maintaining the C curve in the sitting position. Exhale, and roll down, simultaneously bending the knees. Return to the start position.

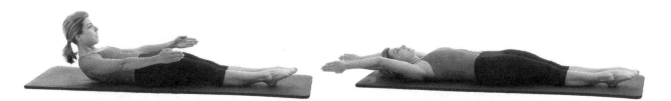

Inhale. Maintain this stable position with the trunk, emphasizing the stretch in the lumbar spine. Hold the arms at shoulder height (parallel to the floor) to accentuate the long neck position, keeping the neck and shoulders relaxed.

Exhale. Roll down, vertebra by vertebra, through the spine. Avoid burying the head between the arms.

Establish a stable core with the abdominal muscles, controlling the tendency to thrust the ribs forward. Lower the head and take the arms back overhead.

Neck Pull

Muscle Focus

- Abdominal muscles

Objectives

- To strengthen the abdominal muscles
- To improve spinal mobility
- To increase hamstring flexibility
- To develop back extensor control

Ironically, contrary to what the name implies, pulling on the neck is the one thing to avoid in this exercise. Tackle this exercise only after having achieved proficiency in the Mat Work: Roll-Up. Placing the hands behind the head (as opposed to the arm movement in the Roll-Up) alters the center of gravity and the levers of the movement, making the neck pull more difficult than its "cousin." In addition, reaching forward over the legs with the trunk requires more flexibility than is called for in the Roll-Up. Extending the spine in a sitting position and establishing upright alignment of the trunk demands core strength and well-conditioned trunk stabilizers, particularly back extensors, as well as adequate hamstring flexibility.

From the sitting position, hinge the trunk backward as one unit, keeping the back straight, before rolling down. Due to the demands of this exercise, it should be performed later in a session and not as part of a warm-up.

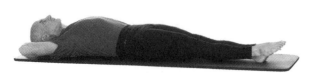

Exhale. Lie supine with the legs straight and together, feet gently plantarflexed. Interlace the fingers behind the head and keep the elbows wide.

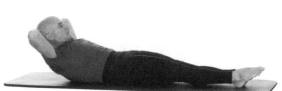

Inhale. Lift the head and shoulder girdle, sinking the lower back into the mat.

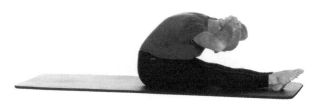

Exhale. Roll up, continuing the movement forward until the trunk is over the legs.

Imagery

The smooth, rolling motion that is desired in this exercise is similar to that of a carpet rolling up. The second phase, the move from forward flexion into the upright sitting position, can be likened to pulling over a young tree and then allowing it to slowly spring back.

☐ Keep the elbows wide throughout the exercise.

☐ Avoid pulling on the neck and thrusting the head forward during the roll-up phase.

☐ Hinge back with a straight trunk before rolling down through the spine.

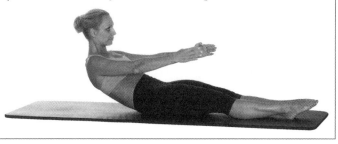
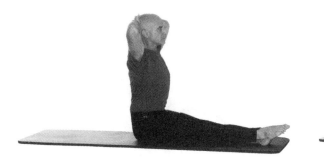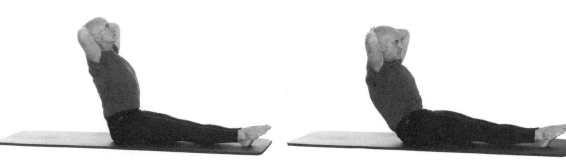

Inhale. Roll the spine up to a sitting upright position, articulating each vertebra on the longitudinal axis.

Exhale. Hinge back, keeping the trunk straight.

Roll down to the supine position, articulating through each vertebra. Return to the start position.

Muscle Focus

- Abdominal muscles

Objectives

- To strengthen the abdominal muscles
- To develop pelvic–lumbar stabilization

Single-Leg Stretch

This exercise belongs to a relatively large group of abdominal exercises that develops abdominal strength in a stabilizing mode (isometric contraction), holding the trunk and the pelvis absolutely still as the limbs move. It is important to pay attention to the positioning of the head, which should be aligned with the spine, supported, and absolutely still. The pumping action of the legs, which amplifies the abdominal work, should not affect the stability of the pelvis. With each repetition, press firmly into the shin just below the knee and bear down as if driving the hip into the mat. This helps to accentuate the contraction of the abdominal muscles.

The single-leg stretch is an excellent preparation for the double-leg stretch in which both arms reach overhead as both legs straighten forward, making stabilization of the pelvis and trunk much more challenging. In the case of the single-leg stretch, only one leg straightens at a time while the other offers support as the hands hold onto it.

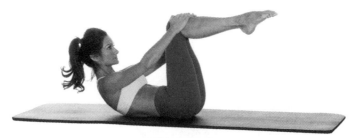

Inhale. Lie supine and draw the knees toward the chest. Lift the trunk into forward flexion with the scapulae off the mat, flex the hips, and lift the shins into a position parallel to the floor. Place the hands on the shins just below the knees.

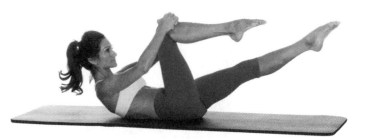

Exhale. Straighten one leg and place the hands firmly on the shin of the opposite leg just below the knee. The bent knee is slightly closer to the chest than in a typical tabletop position; however, the shin remains parallel to the floor.

Imagery

The in and out movement of the legs conjures up the image of the pistons of a machine as they fire, moving in and out with absolute precision. The powerhouse serves as the engine that drives the pistons.

☐ Keep the trunk still throughout the movement.

☐ Keep both feet at approximately eye level as they alternate in and out.

☐ Make sure the shin of the bent leg is parallel to the floor and do not bring the knee in too close to the chest (the angle of the thigh should be approximately 10 degrees beyond the perpendicular).

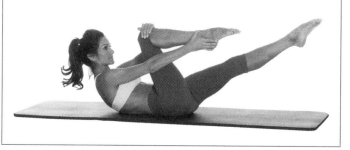

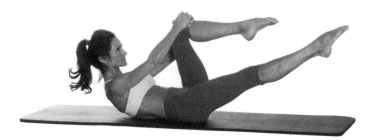

Inhale. Let go of the shin and simultaneously change legs, keeping the feet on the same horizontal plane and the legs close to the centerline of the body as you do so.

Exhale. Straighten the opposite leg fully, and transfer the hands to the bent knee.

Muscle Focus

- Abdominal muscles

Objectives

- To strengthen the abdominal muscles
- To develop trunk stabilization

Double-Leg Stretch

The double-leg stretch is a very challenging abdominal exercise that emphasizes pelvic and trunk stabilization. The lower back remains firmly anchored on the mat as the arms and legs stretch away from the center of the body and then are drawn back toward the center. Keep the eyes focused forward, head stable, and the neck and shoulders relaxed. The abdominal muscles provide support and stability for the structure as the hip flexors draw the legs in toward the chest. As the hips reach approximately 100 degrees of hip flexion and the shins are parallel to the floor, place the hands on the shins firmly below the knees, press down and deepen the abdominal contraction. The hip extensors and knee extensors then straighten the legs as the shoulder flexors take the arms overhead.

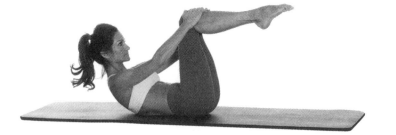

Exhale. Lie supine and draw the knees toward the chest. Lift the trunk into forward flexion with the scapulae off the mat, the thighs at approximately 100 degrees of hip flexion, and the shins parallel to the floor. Place the hands on the shins just below the knees.

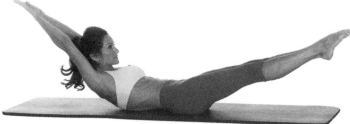

Inhale. Move the arms overhead and simultaneously straighten the legs in the opposite direction, keeping the trunk stable and the feet at eye level. Recruiting the abdominal muscles and imprinting the back into the mat is vital at this point.

Imagery

I use the image of a rubber band being stretched from both sides and then rebounding, just as the arms and legs are stretched out in opposite directions and are then pulled back to center. This recoiling quality provides the dynamic essence of the exercise.

- ☐ Maintain a stable spine from the tip of the head to the tailbone, imprinting the lower back into the mat.

- ☐ Reach the arms as far back overhead as possible without lowering the trunk or elevating the shoulders.

- ☐ Keep the feet at eye level (if abdominal strength allows), or raise them if the back starts lifting from the mat.

- ☐ Keep the eyes focused forward throughout the movement.

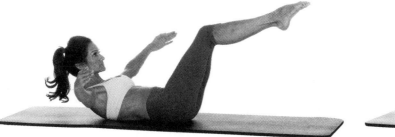

Exhale. Circle the arms out and around while still maintaining a stable spine. Begin drawing the knees toward the chest.

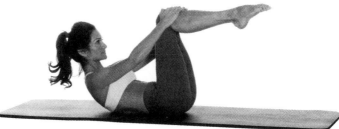

Draw the knees in toward the chest. Then firmly place the hands on the shins, returning to the start position.

Muscle Focus

- Abdominal muscles

Objectives

- To strengthen the abdominal muscles
- To develop pelvic–lumbar stabilization
- To increase hamstring and hip flexor flexibility

Hamstring Pull

The hamstring pull prepares you for the high level of pelvic–lumbar stabilization and abdominal work needed for other intermediate exercises and for advanced and master-level exercises. With each pulse of the leg, you should focus on deepening the abdominal contraction as well as that of the hip flexors, specifically the psoas and iliopsoas, rather than pulling on the hamstrings as the name implies. The support for the position emanates from the abdominal muscles, not from holding onto the leg. Although this exercise is often performed with the lower leg floating about 6 inches (15 centimeters) above the mat, anchoring the lower leg on the mat creates a stable base for stretching both the hamstrings of the lifted leg and the hip flexors of the lower leg. The movement of the legs should be independent of the pelvis and not affect its stability. Lift the leg only as high as your flexibility and pelvic control allow.

Imagery

A wonderful image for this movement is a handheld fan opening and swishing closed, then opening in the other direction. The legs move so swiftly that they create a blur of movement.

☐ Maintain pelvic–lumbar and trunk stability as you change legs.

☐ Maintain consistent trunk flexion throughout the exercise.

☐ Cradle the lifted leg with the hands behind the calf (if flexibility allows).

☐ Keep the shoulders and neck relaxed.

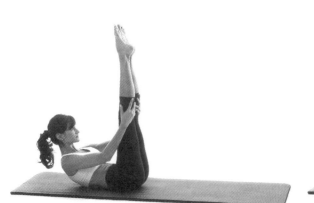

Inhale. Lie supine and lift the head and chest forward into the Mat Work: Chest Lift position. Bend the knees toward the chest, and then straighten the legs so they are toward the ceiling and perpendicular to the floor.

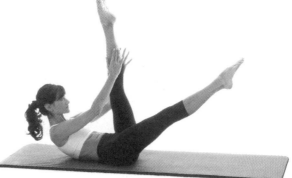

Still inhaling, place the hands behind the calf of one leg, and lower the other leg to the mat and anchor it.

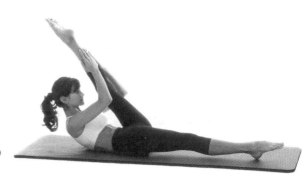

Exhale. Draw the lifted leg slightly closer to the chest, deepening the abdominal contraction, and do two small pulses with the leg. Use percussive breathing, exhaling a puff of air with each pulse.

For additional challenge, place the hands behind the head with the fingers interlaced. To add even more challenge, rotate the trunk toward the lifted leg. The regular, hands behind the head and trunk rotation versions can be done in a sequence, performing 10 repetitions of each. People with tight hamstrings or hip flexors can bend the knees slightly to assist in achieving proper alignment and positioning of the pelvis. Those with weak abdominal muscles can switch the legs one at a time, bringing the anchored leg back to the start position before lowering the other; then, as they gain more strength, they can perform the switch of the legs simultaneously.

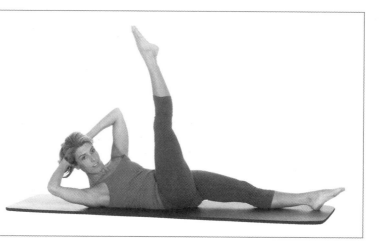

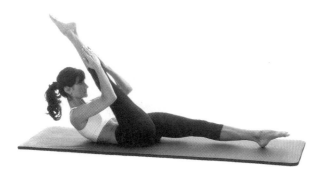

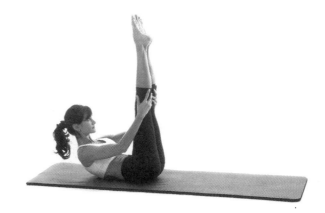

Inhale. Change the legs simultaneously—lowering the lifted leg to the mat and lifting the other toward the chest. The switch should be swift, with absolute stability in the pelvis and trunk. Continue the exercise, alternating legs with each repetition.

Finish the exercise in the start position, with both legs perpendicular to the floor.

Teaser Prep

Muscle Focus

- Abdominal muscles
- Back extensors

Objectives

- To strengthen the abdominal muscles and back extensors
- To develop control of the hip flexors
- To prepare for the Mat Work: Teaser

This exercise prepares you for advanced abdominal work and full body integration movements. Here you incorporate the principles of several more basic mat work exercises, such as the Roll-Up, Rolling Like a Ball, and the Open-Leg Rocker. However, this exercise is more difficult because it requires a high level of control and eliminates the support of the hands and the use of momentum. Find the point of equilibrium, using the back extensors supported by the abdominals and the hip flexors, to create a stable structure. Note that the legs should be still and the shins parallel to the floor. As with the earlier exercises, focus on articulation of the spine when transitioning from extension to flexion and vice versa.

Imagery

The image of a fishing line, unwinding as the body rolls down and then being reeled in as the body rolls back up, helps to give the feeling of continuous, seamless and effortless movement, as if being controlled by an external force.

- ☐ Use the back extensors to complete the movement.
- ☐ Articulate the spine when lowering and lifting the trunk.
- ☐ Initiate the roll-down and roll-up with deep lumbar flexion.

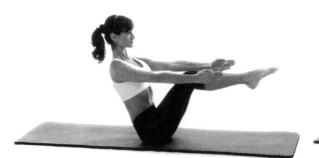

Inhale. Sit upright, balancing on the base of the pelvis (sit bones), arms reaching forward in front of the shoulders. Bend the knees with the shins parallel to the floor.

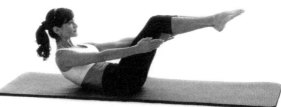

Exhale. Round the lower back and lower the spine to the floor. Go down only to the point where you can maintain complete control, no further than the base of the scapulae.

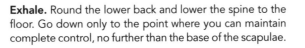

Inhale. Roll back up, maximizing the articulation of the spine.

Complete the movement by extending the back. Return to the start position

Teaser

This is a combination of the abdominal exercises, particularly the Mat Work: Teaser Prep and Mat Work: Roll-Up, and the balancing exercises, specifically the Mat Work: Open-Leg Rocker. The start position is identical to that of the open-leg rocker except that the arms are overhead and the legs are held together. Roll down the spine without moving the legs. After a complete roll-down with the arms reaching overhead, roll up as you would in the roll-up exercise, except that in this exercise the legs are in the air. Maintaining this leg position demands hip flexor strength and control, which in turn demands strong abdominal engagement to prevent pressure on the back, hyperlordosis and an anterior tilt of the pelvis. Although this full-body exercise places great emphasis on the abdominal muscles, the strength of the back extensors and hip flexors plays a large part in the success of the movement and should not be overlooked.

Imagery

Visualize holding the reins of a horse and being gently raised up off the mat and gently lowered back down. The image of an inflated tire rolling smoothly applies here too, as does the image of fishing line being reeled in and then let out.

☐ Articulate the spine when rolling down and up.

☐ Initiate the roll-down and roll-up with deep lumbar flexion.

☐ Keep the legs at the same angle throughout the exercise; avoid moving them up and down.

Muscle Focus
- Abdominal muscles
- Back extensors
- Hip flexors

Objectives
- To strengthen the abdominals and back extensors
- To develop hip flexor control
- To develop trunk stabilization
- To develop balance

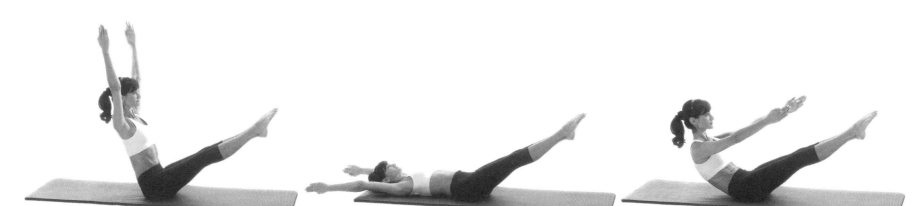

Inhale. Sit upright, balancing on the base of the pelvis (sit bones), straighten the legs at approximately 60 degrees to the floor, creating a V-position with the body. Lift the arms overhead.

Exhale. Roll down, lowering the arms to shoulder height as you begin to articulate down through the spine, and then reaching them overhead after rolling out the spine onto the mat. Keep the legs still throughout the movement.

Inhale. Roll up, emphasizing the articulation through the spine.

Complete the movement with back extension and arms overhead. Return to the start position.

Spinal Articulation

The spine is an awe-inspiring structure that, when functioning as a coordinated and integrated unit, can move in many directions and ranges of motion with great flexibility. Yet each vertebral joint alone actually offers very little motion.

Spinal articulation refers to the fine, precise, sequential movement of each vertebra of the spine relative to the next vertebra, as opposed to movement of the spine in stiff sections. This concept of sequential spinal mobility was one that Joseph Pilates promoted tirelessly. In fact, he went as far as to say that when a person's spine is mobile and articulate, the person is young, no matter their chronological age, and conversely that if the spine is immobile, the person is old.

The focus of this block is fine articulation of the spine during spinal flexion. It is common for people to be very inflexible in their lower backs, particularly during spinal flexion, because of the lower back's natural orientation toward an arched shape (the very opposite of flexion). The motions of spinal flexion and spinal articulation tend to stretch this area and can be very helpful in restoring healthy flexibility to the lower back. Even when individuals have adequate flexibility, they often lack the fine control of the spine required to perform spinal articulation.

Since the abdominal muscles are the flexors of the spine, they are pivotal in the action of spinal articulation. Yet the back extensors should not be ignored. Spinal articulation is a delicate interplay of the flexors and extensors of the spine.

It should be noted that extreme flexion of the spine and exercises that demand bearing weight on the shoulders and neck are controversial because of the risks involved. This chapter contains exercises that involve both extreme flexion and weight bearing on the neck and shoulders, therefore extra caution should be adopted and decisions made on a case-by-case basis. Seek medical advice when in doubt.

Spine Stretch

This exercise teaches articulation of the spine in a sitting rather than supine position. Emphasize rolling or peeling the spine, as if off a wall, vertebra by vertebra as the trunk moves into forward flexion. Then articulate through the vertebrae in reverse as the trunk moves back into the upright position, along the plumb line. The prominent interplay between the spinal flexors and extensors in this exercise helps develop spinal mobility and stability and enhances core control. This exercise can improve seated posture enormously.

As the upper body rolls forward and then back to the seated position, focus on keeping the legs shoulder-width apart, the pelvis stable and the feet dorsiflexed. Keep the toes facing the ceiling; this ensures that the legs remain in a neutral position.

Imagery

Visualize the motion of a young tree being pulled over by its top branches and then slowly being released to find its stable, upright position.

☐ Maximize articulation of the spine when moving from sitting to spinal flexion and when moving back through spinal extension to sitting.

VARIATION

This more challenging variation should only be done once you have mastered the standard version. When in the forward flexion position over the legs, extend the spine to create a diagonal line reaching forward and upward from the lower back through the trunk and head, completing the movement with the arms in line with the ears before returning to forward flexion and restacking the spine.

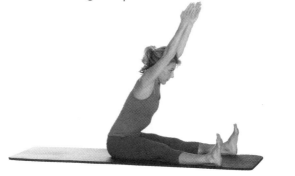

☐ Keep the feet dorsiflexed, with the toes reaching toward the ceiling.

☐ Keep the shoulders relaxed.

Muscle Focus

- Abdominal muscles
- Back extensors

Objectives

- To develop spinal articulation
- To develop core control and trunk stabilization
- To improve hamstring flexibility

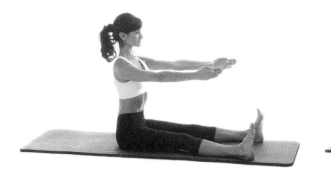

Inhale. Sit with the trunk upright and the legs straight, shoulder-width apart. Dorsiflex the feet and reach the arms forward, shoulder-width apart and parallel to the floor, with palms facing each other.

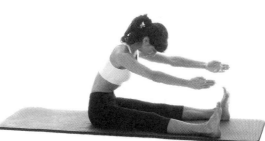

Exhale. Roll down and forward through the spine, starting from the head.

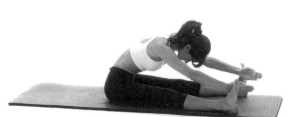

Inhale. Deepen the abdominal work, drawing the spine further into forward flexion and stretching the back muscles. The shoulders remain relaxed and the neck elongated.

Exhale. Restack the spine back to return to the start position.

71

Muscle Focus
- Abdominal muscles

Objectives
- To improve trunk stabilization
- To learn to use energy efficiently
- To elongate the lower back muscles and deepen the abdominal work

Rolling Like a Ball

This exercise embodies the concepts of stabilization and internal flow of energy. The more stable the position is, the smoother the movement will be. It illustrates well the controlled elongation of the back muscles (in particular those of the lower back), deep engagement of the abdominals, and the gentle and consistent rounding of the spine, which is so necessary for the successful execution of much of the abdominal work in Pilates. It is worth noting that although the focus is placed on the abdominal muscles, it is in fact a coordinated contraction of the back extensors together with the abdominal muscles that creates the desired elongated C curve of the trunk. This exercise also introduces balancing on the sit bones, a position that repeats itself in several increasingly challenging exercises. The key to the success of the exercise is keeping the ball shape of the body as contained and stable as possible.

Imagery

Visualize an inflated wheel that rolls effortlessly and without obstruction. The more inflated it is, the more smoothly it rolls. When it is deflated, the rolling is interrupted and halting, just as this exercise appears when a consistent, smooth spinal curve is not maintained, usually due to a tight lower back or a lack of abdominal control.

- ☐ Keep the trunk as still and stable as possible throughout the movement.

- ☐ Maintain a consistent curve in the spine from the head to the tailbone.

- ☐ Pause momentarily on the sit bones and on the shoulders in each repetition.

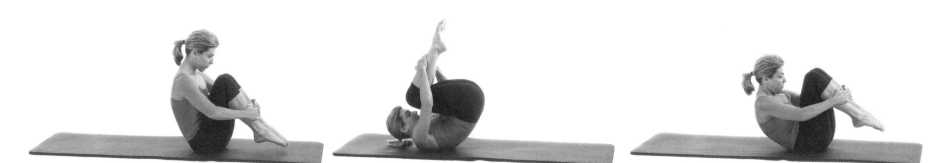

Exhale. Sit on the mat with the legs pressed together, holding each leg just above the ankles. Draw the spine into an elongated C curve and lift the feet slightly off the mat. Balancing on your sit bones, keep the head aligned with the natural curve of spine. (Do not bury the head between the knees.) Deepen the C curve and solidify the position, holding onto the legs for support. Keep the heels as close to the back of the thighs as possible.

Inhale. Allow the weight to shift within the body and roll back, visualizing a further hollowing and rounding of the lower back region. Roll only as far as the shoulder girdle, avoiding pressure on the cervical spine.

Exhale. Pausing (but not stopping), reverse the internal energy and the direction of the roll. Continue holding the trunk in a firm C-curve position, slightly increasing the pull on the legs with the hands. Roll forward through the thoracic and lumbar vertebrae. Return to the start position.

Inhale. Focus on the internal work occurring in the body to maintain this dynamic balanced position, and keep the internal energy flowing as you prepare to repeat the movement.

Seal Puppy

The seal puppy is often done at the end, or near the end, of a mat work routine as a form of stretching and relaxation. I encourage using this exercise to focus on the many movements that have been performed in the session and to allow the effort to culminate in this moment of flow and balance.

This exercise stretches the back (the trunk is held in deep flexion) and the upper trapezius (the shoulders are drawn down by the legs). As with the Mat Work: Rolling Like a Ball and Open-Leg Rocker, you should focus on the internal flow of energy and on the balance. The clap of the legs when balanced on the sit bones, and when the legs are overhead, require you to pause without stopping the flow of the energy within the body.

Imagery

The image for this exercise is the same as that of several of the rolling exercises, such as rolling like a ball—keeping the feeling of an inflated tire rolling back and forth without obstructions or jarring movements. In the balance position, I like to imagine I am balancing on a precipice or floating on a cloud without any tension. This is the position in which I often do some relaxation, inner focusing, and meditation.

☐ Maintain a constant C curve of the spine.

☐ Keep the head aligned with the spine, and relax the shoulders.

☐ Place the inside of the legs as high up on the arms (as close to the shoulders) as possible.

Muscle Focus
- Abdominal muscles

Objectives
- To stabilize and develop control of the trunk
- To improve hip-joint flexibility
- To focus and relax

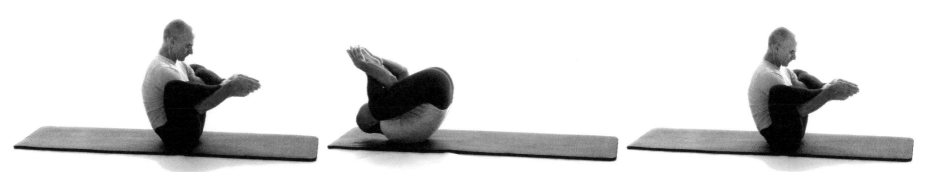

Exhale. Sit with the knees open and feet together. Lift one leg and place it over the arm on the same side, as close to the shoulder as possible. Reach the arm under the leg and wrap it around the lower leg, placing the palm on top of the foot. While balancing, do the same with the other arm and leg. Balance in this position, with the back rounded, the arms wrapped around the legs, and the hands resting on the feet.

Inhale. Roll back onto the shoulders (avoid reaching the neck and head) and clap the feet together three times by moving the legs slightly in and out from the hip joints. The feet remain relaxed.

Exhale. Roll up to the balance position and again clap the feet together three times while balancing.

After 5-10 repetitions, unwrap the legs and arms, place the feet on the mat and roll the spine up to an upright position, hands resting on the legs and arms providing support for the trunk. This is a perfect way to complete a mat routine, if you so choose.

Muscle Focus

- Abdominal muscles
- Back extensors

Objectives

- To develop trunk stabilization
- To improve balance
- To increase spinal mobility

Open-Leg Rocker

This exercise demonstrates the movement principles of Pilates clearly and profoundly. Not only does it integrate awareness, balance, breath, and control, but it also demands concentration, centering, efficient use of energy, precision, flow of movement, and harmony. It demonstrates coordinated activation of the abdominal muscles and the back extensors. Mastering the open-leg rocker is exceptional preparation for more advanced, full-body exercises, such as the Mat Work: Teaser series as well as the teasers on other apparatus.

Imagery

Visualize an inflated wheel that rolls effortlessly and without obstruction. Maintaining a smooth spinal curve keeps the wheel moving smoothly; conversely a tight lower back or a lack of abdominal control deflates the wheel, causing the rolling to be interrupted and halting. Sitting on the sit bones in the V-shape, at the point of balance, should be effortless. This pinnacle is where body, mind, and spirit unite; it is the culmination of every Pilates principle—the point of harmony.

VARIATION

Perform the exercise with the legs bent and the hands holding the back of the thighs. This version is particularly suited for people with tight hamstrings.

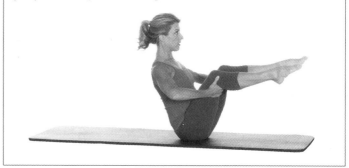

☐ Use the back extensors to complete the movement.

☐ Keep the arms straight throughout the exercise.

☐ Hold the legs firmly without pulling on them.

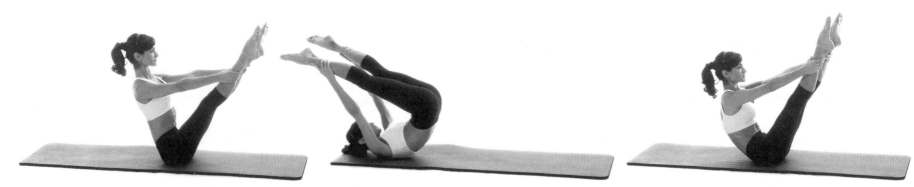

Exhale. Sit balanced on the sit bones in a V-position with the back and legs straight. Hold the ankles firmly with the hands, keeping the legs shoulder-width apart and focusing the eyes straight ahead.

Inhale. Round the back, initiating the movement from the lumbar spine, and roll back to the shoulders. (The head should barely touch the mat, if at all.)

Exhale. Roll up, first keeping the spine round and then extending it as you return to the start position. Balance momentarily in the sits bones before rolling back again.

Control Balance

In addition to requiring a great deal of core strength, this exercise relies greatly on hip flexor flexibility and hip extensor strength. The extensors, primarily those of the hip and back, facilitate the lifting of the leg perpendicular to the floor, essentially creating a straight line through the trunk and up through the leg.

This exercise serves as an excellent preparation for the Mat Work: Jackknife, in that it is a one-legged version of that exercise. Both this exercise and the jackknife place greater pressure on the cervical spine than does the Mat Work: Roll-Over, so I advise erring on the side of caution when performing them. They are absolutely contraindicated for anyone with neck problems, particularly those related to disc dysfunction.

Imagery

I like to visualize two energy lines in this exercise: one that runs from the shoulders through the trunk and the upright leg to the ceiling, and the other creating a stabilizing force by stretching from the hip joint down through the lower leg and foot into the ground.

☐ Keep the focal point of your weight on the shoulder girdle.

Muscle Focus
- Hip extensors

Objectives
- To strengthen the hip extensors
- To improve hip flexor flexibility
- To strengthen the core

VARIATION

An alternative version, which places less weight on the cervical spine, is to do exactly the same movement pattern but roll onto the upper back and shoulders, as opposed to the shoulders and neck. In this version, which in fact is the classical version, the leg switch will remain the same, but due to the position of the trunk the lifting leg will not reach as high toward the ceiling. The work of the hip extensors and the stretch of the hip flexors is not quite as profound but it is certainly a wonderful exercise and does bypass the issue of weight of the cervical spine.

☐ Keep the pelvis and trunk still as the legs change.

☐ Minimize bearing weight on the cervical spine.

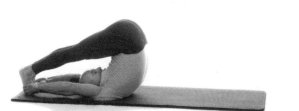

Exhale. Lie supine with the arms by the sides and the legs straight. Bend the knees toward the chest and then straighten them at a 60-degree angle to the mat.

Inhale. Lift the legs to a 90-degree angle in the hip joint, so they are perpendicular to the floor.

Exhale. Round the lower back and roll over. Rest the weight on the shoulder girdle. Anchor the feet on the floor and circle the arms overhead to hold onto the feet.

Exhale. Extend one leg up toward the ceiling. Perform two pulses with this leg when reaching maximum height (aiming to increase the hip extension with each pulse). Use percussive breathing, exhaling a puff of air with each pulse.

Inhale. Switch the legs simultaneously, keeping the pelvis and trunk as stable as possible.

After the final repetition, bring the extended leg back to a dorsiflexed position on the floor overhead, and then roll down, keeping the thighs close to the chest. When the legs reach a 60-degree angle to the floor, bend the knees toward the chest, place the feet on the mat and straighten the legs, returning to the start position.

Roll-Over

Muscle Focus
- Abdominal muscles

Objectives
- To develop spinal articulation
- To stretch the lower back and hamstrings
- To improve control of the abdominal muscles

You must follow certain guidelines to make this exercise effective and meet its desired objectives. The roll-over motion should be facilitated by flexion of the spine, particularly the lower spine, which is achieved through deep abdominal contraction. Avoid the tendency to use the momentum and long lever of the legs to roll over. Instead, when the legs are lifted in the initial phase to a 90-degree angle of hip flexion, maintain this angle during the roll-over phase, which helps to maximize the abdominal work. On the return, however, you can enhance the stretch of the hamstrings and the lower back by drawing the thighs close to the chest, creating a tight pike position.

People who have neck problems should be extremely cautious when doing this exercise; some individuals may need to avoid it completely (as with all other Pilates exercises that place weight on the cervical spine), even though most of the weight should be borne on the shoulder girdle rather than the neck.

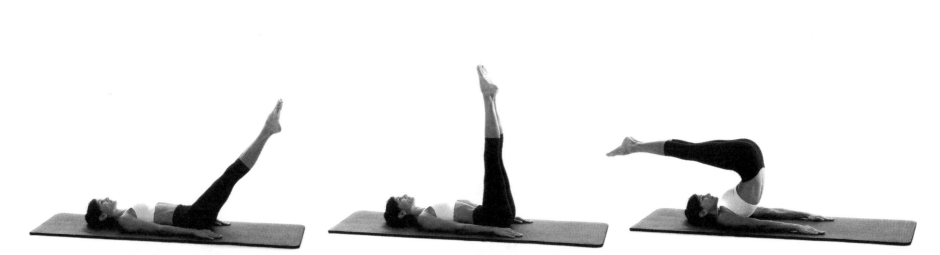

Exhale. Lie supine with the arms by the sides and the legs straight. Bend the knees toward the chest and then straighten them at a 60-degree angle to the mat, legs held together.

Inhale. Lift the legs to a 90-degree angle in the hip joint, so they are perpendicular to the floor.

Exhale. Round the trunk and roll over, peeling the spine off the mat and bringing the legs up and over. Rest the weight on the shoulder girdle, keeping the legs parallel to the mat.

Imagery

In the roll-over phase, when rolling back, visualize creating a ball out of the lower back (see also Mat Work: Rolling Like a Ball). The feeling should be like spring metal being bent in half and then opening out to the start position.

☐ Do not use momentum to roll over.

☐ Keep the hip joint at a consistent 90-degree angle during the roll-over phase.

☐ Deepen the abdominal contraction to achieve maximum lumbar flexion.

☐ Keep the thighs close to the chest in the roll-back phase.

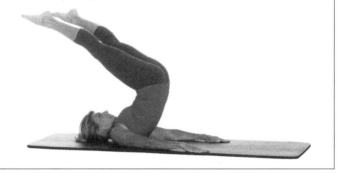
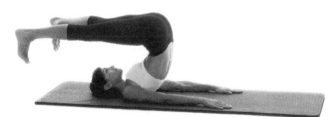

Inhale. Dorsiflex the feet and separate the legs to shoulder-width.

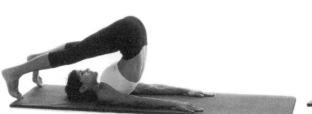

Continue inhaling as you lower the feet toward the floor above the head (touch the floor if flexibility allows).

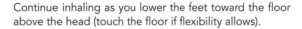

Exhale. Keeping the legs close to the chest, articulate the spine down to the mat. Anchor the pelvis on the mat, and lower the legs to the 60-degree angle as you bring them together. Return to the start position.

Jackknife

Muscle Focus
- Hip, back, and shoulder extensors
- Abdominal muscles

Objectives
- To develop spinal articulation
- To improve trunk stabilization
- To strengthen the hip and shoulder extensors

The jackknife is an extension of the Mat Work: Roll-Over and should not be attempted until you have mastered that exercise. Initially the feet reach overhead and are parallel to the floor, before being lowered to the floor as in the roll over. At this point, however, rather than roll down again, you recruit the hip extensors and spinal extensors to reach the legs in a swooping action up toward the ceiling, creating a perpendicular line from the floor up through the shoulders, trunk, hips, legs and feet. In this position, it is legitimate to use the shoulder extensors to assist in keeping the structure stable and upright and in alleviating pressure on the cervical spine. When rolling the spine down, vertebra by vertebra, keep the feet above the face until the pelvis reaches the floor, and then return to the start position.

Because of the weight that this exercise places on the cervical spine, people with neck problems should avoid it. Although the weight is distributed between the shoulders and the arms, and the pressure on the cervical spine is minimized, the neck still bears significant pressure.

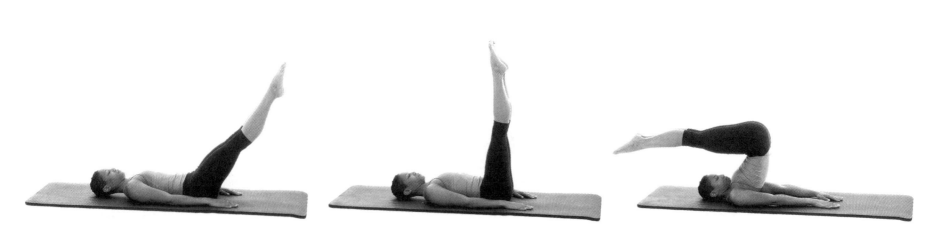

Exhale. Lie supine with the arms by the sides of the body and the legs straight at approximately 60 degrees to the floor as with the roll-over. Brace the trunk and prepare for the Mat Work: Roll-over. Imprint the lower back into the mat.

Inhale. Raise the legs to 90 degrees, anchoring the pelvis and continuing to sink the lower back into the mat.

Exhale. Roll over, maximizing the flexion of the lumbar region and maintaining a 90-degree angle in the hip joint. Complete this phase with the legs parallel to the floor and the weight on the shoulders.

Imagery

As the name implies, the jackknife should feel like a spring-loaded hinge or knife closing and opening (at the hip joint), with a swooping movement of the legs into the air.

☐ Maximize flexion of the lumbar spine during the roll-over phase.

☐ Use the hip, shoulder, and back extensors to achieve maximum height of the legs and trunk.

☐ Roll down with the feet opposite the face (but held as high as possible rather than close to the face).

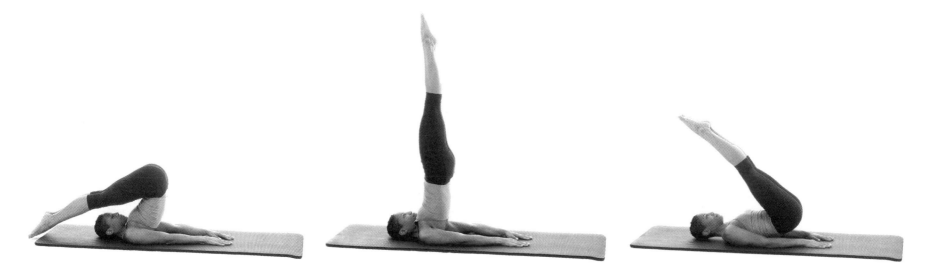

Inhale. Lower the legs toward the floor.

Still inhaling, lift the legs toward the ceiling. Move the pelvis forward and press the arms into the mat.

Exhale. Slowly roll down, articulating the spine and keeping the feet opposite the face. As the pelvis reaches the mat, anchor it with the legs at 90 degrees, and then lower the legs to return to the start position.

Muscle Focus

- Abdominal muscles
- Back extensors
- Hip flexors

Objectives

- To strengthen the abdominal muscles and back extensors
- To develop hip flexor control
- To stretch the muscles of the chest
- To develop balance

Boomerang

This is a high-level exercise because of its complexity. It also demonstrates the progression of exercises in Pilates, the logical methodology of one exercise building on another. The boomerang requires strength, flexibility and, most important, coordination. It draws from the Mat Work: Roll-Over and Teaser, which should be mastered before embarking on the boomerang. It resembles the Reformer: Rowing Back 1 in its movement pattern.

Imagery

It takes a while to understand why this exercise is called the boomerang, but once you achieve a flow, it becomes apparent. At the point where the body rolls down to the lumbar region, before the legs are taken overhead, the shape resembles a boomerang. In this position the body should feel firm, and the legs and trunk should be integrated so that you can rock back and forth like the base of a rocking chair.

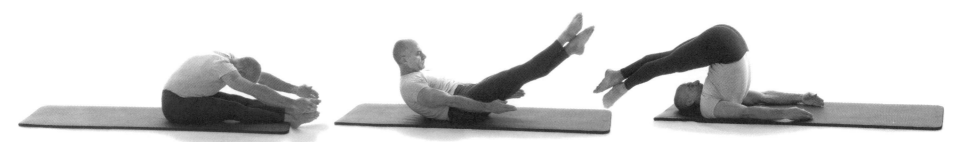

Exhale. Sit with the legs straight and crossed in front, and the feet plantar-flexed. Round the trunk over the legs and reach the arms forward.

Inhale. Roll down while lifting the legs, feet opposite the eyes, and pause when you reach the lumbar region. Hold the trunk and legs stable in this boomerang position.

Exhale. Lower the chest and head and lift the legs so they are perpendicular to the floor. Round the lower back further and roll over. Lower the crossed legs toward the mat, keeping the feet plantarflexed.

In fact I often use the rocking in this difficult position as an exercise unto itself. It demands tremendous core strength and control. I call it the "BASI rock"! I believe I created it during a huge mat class in Turkey where I was trying to explain the name and the feeling of rocking in this exercise. It worked! After the legs change position overhead, the body rolls back momentarily to the boomerang position before lifting into the teaser position. This is the point where exceptional balance is needed, as the arms reach back and are then circled around to the front returning to the start position—and there we have the boomerang!

☐ Keep the movement fluid.

☐ Open and stretch the muscles of chest as the arms reach back.

☐ Use trunk stabilization during the balance phase, keeping the legs as high as possible.

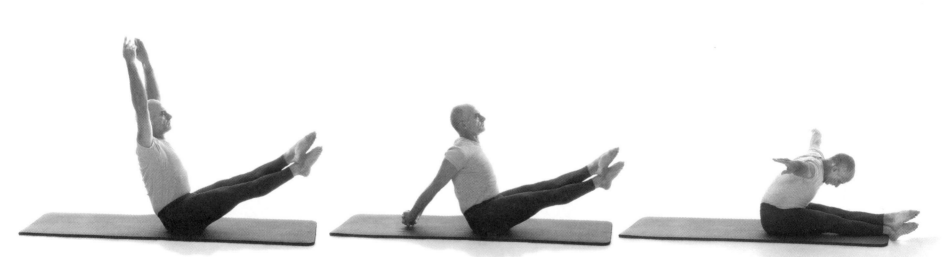

Inhale. Switch the crossed legs.

Exhale. Take the legs back over to return toward the boomerang position, and then roll up into a teaser position.

Inhale. Circle the arms around and interlace the fingers behind the back as you lift the chest and extend the trunk further.

Exhale. Lower the legs and release the hands. Circle the arms around to the front, bringing the body forward over the legs. Return to the start position.

Muscle Focus
- Abdominal muscles

Objectives
- To stretch the neck and lower back
- To develop trunk stabilization

Crab

Although this exercise appears uncomfortable and even dangerous because it involves leaning forward onto the head and seemingly transferring weight onto the neck, it is enjoyable and beneficial if done correctly. The key point is that the body's full weight should never be placed on the neck. Instead, transfer the weight cautiously and with control onto the head, with most of the weight remaining on the legs. Other than the rolling onto the head, the rest of the exercise is very similar to Mat Work: Rolling Like a Ball and the Mat Work: Seal Puppy, with an element of coordination added. In addition, because the legs are held close to the body by the arms in the cross-legged position, the possibility of compensating by opening the legs and using them for momentum is diminished.

Imagery

I have never been able to relate this exercise to a crab, despite spending hours observing crabs run across many a beach. I suppose the cross-legged position itself does have some remote resemblance to the underside of a crab. I find using the image of a rolling wheel, keeping a smooth back and forth flow of energy, more beneficial.

☐ Transfer weight cautiously onto the head.

☐ Maximize lumbar flexion when rolling.

☐ Keep the legs close to the body.

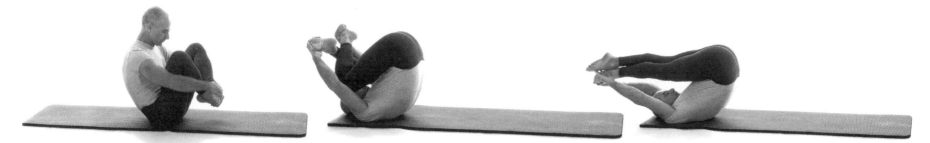

Inhale. Sit in a balanced position on the sit bones with the body in a ball shape. Cross the legs, reach the arms around the legs from the outside, and hold the feet. The left hand holds the right foot, and the right hand holds the left foot.

Exhale. Roll over onto the shoulders.

Inhale. Straighten the legs overhead and switch them, as in the boomerang. Bend the knees and take hold of the feet again, tucking back into a ball shape.

I have choreographed an alternative for those who cannot or do not wish to place any pressure on the head and neck. Instead of rolling over the legs and forward onto the head, roll over the legs but lift into an upright position, kneeling with the legs still crossed and arms overhead. The upright position is a welcome change after the deep spinal flexion that is maintained in this exercise. This position demands good balance and core strength. Use great control as you lower the pelvis back down, and return to the sitting start position.

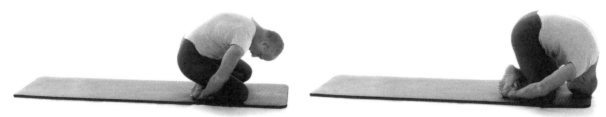

Exhale. Roll forward, transferring the weight over the legs. Use the arms to assist rolling over the legs by pressing into the hands.

Inhale. Place the head on the floor and roll slowly over onto the head, cautiously transferring the weight toward the neck and stretching the neck extensors. Return to the start position.

Bridging

This block is unique to the mat block system. Its name is derived from the bridge shape formed by the trunk of the body in all the exercises, with the pelvis lifted off the mat and the limbs supporting the structure. The term *bridging* can have different connotations depending on the context in which it is used. Here it relates primarily to the shape of the body and not to muscle function.

The importance of abdominal strength and control in achieving spinal stabilization has been discussed in connection with other blocks. In contrast with the exercises in the abdominal block and the spinal articulation block, which are performed in spinal flexion, the bridging exercises are performed with the pelvis and spine in a neutral, or very close to neutral, position. Developing the muscles in this position is thought to be more functional than developing them in spinal flexion, however I recommend doing both. Each position has a role to play in achieving spinal stabilization.

The term *bracing* is often used to describe the action of the muscles in stabilizing the pelvis and spine. This is different to the *scooping* or *hollowing* action of the abdominals often preferred in the abdominal and spinal articulation blocks. Some argue that bracing is more effective in stabilizing and protecting the spine than hollowing. I believe that all forms of muscle control contribute to the vast movement vocabulary that allows us to enjoy life to its fullest and perform our daily activities and athletic endeavors effectively and efficiently.

Note that front support, leg pull front, and push-up share the same characteristic of the pelvis being lifted off the mat with the limbs acting as support structures with the other exercises. However, they differ from the other exercises in that the trunk is facing down versus up. In this position, the abdominals need to work to prevent gravity drawing the lower back into an arch. Biasing the pelvis toward a slight posterior tilt helps maintain abdominal engagement and achieve pelvic-lumbar stabilization.

Shoulder Bridge Prep

This exercise combines pelvic–lumbar stabilization with hip disassociation. It places the body in a challenging bridge position, starting from the up phase of the Mat Work: Pelvic Curl and continuing with the lifting of one leg. The hip extensors of the supporting leg are fundamental to maintaining this challenging bridge position. The pelvic stability in this exercise relies greatly on the hamstrings and the abdominal muscles, which together hold the pelvis stable with a bias toward a posterior tilt: the abdominals pulling the pubic symphysis upward and the hamstrings pulling the ischial tuberosity downward.

Feel an energy line running through the body: diagonally outward and upward through the knees and diagonally downward from the knees through the trunk and shoulders. Use this sense of oppositional forces to keep the body aligned and to balance the work of the flexors and extensors of the trunk, which are co-contracting.

Imagery

Visualize a suspension bridge on which a mechanical arm goes up and down without affecting the stability and strength of the bridge. Also visualize a straight line that runs from the shoulders through the hips to the knees. This energy line provides the foundation for the exercise.

☐ Keep a consistent 90-degree angle in the knee of the moving leg.

☐ Initiate the movement from the hip joint.

☐ Maintain hip extension in the supporting leg together with a stable pelvis.

Muscle Focus
- Abdominal muscles
- Hamstrings

Objectives
- To strengthen the hip extensors
- To develop pelvic–lumbar stabilization
- To develop hip disassociation
- To improve back extensor control

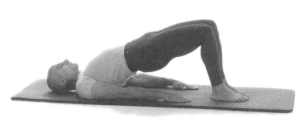

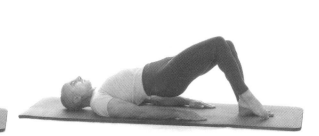

Lie supine with the spine in a neutral position. Bend the knees and place the feet hip-width apart. Keep the scapulae in a neutral position, the arms straight by the sides, the fingers reaching toward the feet.

Exhale. Draw in the abdominal muscles and tilt the pelvis in a posterior direction. Lift the spine off the mat, one vertebra at a time, while extending the hips. Create a straight line from the shoulders to the knees.

Inhale. Hold this position, distributing the weight evenly on the feet and keeping the legs parallel. Elongate the hip flexors while engaging the shoulder extensors to support the structure and to accentuate the mid- and upper-back work.

Exhale. Lift one leg from the hip joint, maintaining a 90-degree angle in the knee. Keep the pelvis stable and level throughout, with minimal shifting of weight to the supporting leg.

Inhale. Lower the lifted leg and touch the mat lightly with the foot.

Exhale. Lift the leg. Keep the hip extensors of the supporting leg working, and avoid lowering or tilting the pelvis. After several repetitions, place the foot on the mat and switch legs, again with minimal shifting of weight, and repeat the exercise with the other leg.

Inhale. Complete the exercise by placing both feet on the mat and exhaling while rolling down, vertebra by vertebra, from the top of the spine through the lumbar region to the sacrum.

Shoulder Bridge

Muscle Focus
- Abdominal muscles
- Hamstrings
- Hip flexors

Objectives
- To strengthen the hip extensors
- To develop pelvic–lumbar stabilization
- To develop hip flexor control and flexibility
- To improve hamstring flexibility

This challenging exercise builds on the Mat Work: Shoulder Bridge Prep and the Mat Work: Pelvic Curl. The key to the exercise is maintaining a stable pelvis that is not affected by the leg swinging up and down. You should feel the front of the moving leg elongating on the way down (stretching the hip flexors) and the back of the leg elongating on the way up (stretching the hamstrings). The stretching of the hamstrings is enhanced by the dorsiflexion of the foot.

Orient the pelvis toward a posterior tilt when in the bridge position. This helps to prevent the pelvis from tilting anteriorly, which could cause hyperlordosis and pressure on the lumbar spine, particularly when the leg is lowered. The tendency to anteriorly tilt the pelvis is exacerbated when the hip flexors are tight.

Imagery

Visualize a ride at an amusement park featuring a carriage on the end of a girder that swings like a pendulum. The leg is the girder that swings in an arc shape, and the foot is the carriage.

☐ Maintain consistent height of the pelvis from the mat.

☐ Avoid tipping the pelvis to one side.

☐ Keep the pelvis neutral or in a slight posterior tilt.

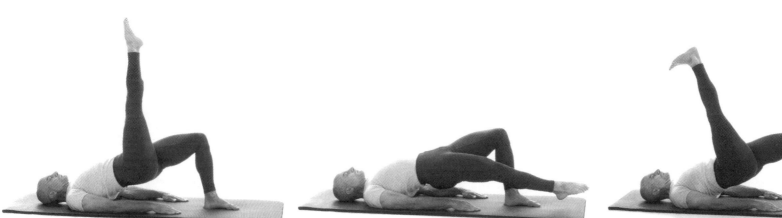

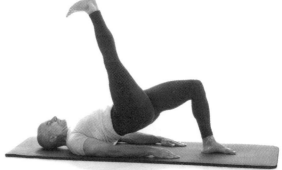

Inhale. Lie supine with the knees bent and the feet firmly placed on the ground. Perform a pelvic curl, pausing in the top position. Lift one foot off the ground, bending the knee toward the chest, and then straighten the leg directly toward the ceiling.

Exhale. Lower the straight leg toward the floor with the foot plantarflexed.

Inhale. Kick the straight leg upward, dorsiflexing the foot. After 5-10 repetitions, pause with the leg reaching toward the ceiling and plantarflex the foot. Bend the knee and place the foot on the floor to return to the start position (up phase of the pelvic curl). Switch legs and repeat the sequence with the other leg. Complete the exercise by placing both feet on the mat and rolling down to the mat as in the pelvic curl.

Scissors

The scissors is a challenging exercise, in large part because of the arched position of the lower back. This position feels precarious and demands a high level of pelvic–lumbar stabilization. The same position is used for Step Barrel: Scissors, except that here the arms take the place of the barrel making it more challenging. However picturing the spine being supported by a rounded barrel is helpful. The pelvis should be stable and anchored as the legs perform a scissors action, alternating as they pass through the centerline (the starting point) perpendicular to the floor.

Note that the elbows should be directly under the pelvis (not splaying); without their support, the pelvis would sink and the whole structure would begin to collapse. Keeping an equal degree of split in each leg creates the desired wide V-position and an equal stretch of the hip flexors and hamstrings.

Imagery

Imagine the legs opening wide like a handheld fan, then closing and opening to the other side. I use this image frequently, as it seems to help create the desired movement and dynamic.

- ☐ Maintain an arc shape of the spine.
- ☐ Keep the elbows parallel to each other (or as close to parallel as possible).
- ☐ Cradle the pelvis in the hands.

Muscle Focus

- Hip extensors
- Hip flexors
- Abdominal muscles

Objectives

- To develop hip flexor and hip extensor control
- To improve hip flexor and hip extensor flexibility
- To develop shoulder and pelvic–lumbar stabilization

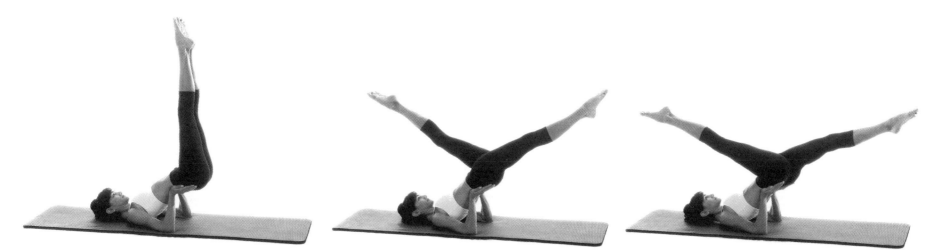

Inhale. Lie in a supine position and draw the knees toward the chest. Create a ball shape with the body and roll over onto the shoulder girdle. Place the hands under the pelvis, as if holding a bowl, and create an arc shape with the trunk. Now straighten the legs up toward the ceiling.

Exhale. Open the legs (one forward, one backward; equidistant from the centerline) into a wide V-position. Pulse the legs twice in the open scissors position, exhaling on each pulse.

Inhale. Switch legs, passing through the start position, and repeat the pulses in the open V-position on the opposite side, again exhaling on each pulse.

Bicycle

Muscle Focus

- Hip extensors
- Hip flexors
- Abdominal muscles

Objectives

- To develop hip flexor and hip extensor control
- To improve hip flexor and hip extensor flexibility
- To develop shoulder and pelvic–lumbar stabilization

The bicycle is an extension of the Mat Work: Scissors, therefore proficiency in doing the scissors is required. Although both legs perform a large cycling action (one bending and the other straightening simultaneously), at one point in each cycle they are in the straight-legged scissors position, which can be a reference point. Try to touch the floor with the back leg as the knee bends—a position that demands a high degree of spinal extension and flexible hip flexors. Avoid compromising pelvic–lumbar stabilization, and possibly creating excessive pressure on the lower back, in order to achieve more range. Emphasis should be placed on the abdominal muscles to protect the lower back and achieve the support needed for this exercise. Flexibility, awareness, and strength developed from previous exercises will assist you in executing this challenging exercise.

Imagery

The large, fluid, circular motion of the legs conjures up an image of cycling a penny-farthing bicycle (an old-fashioned bike with one large wheel in front and a small one in back).

- ☐ Maintain an arc shape of the spine.

- ☐ Perform elongated movements with maximum fluidity.

- ☐ Keep the legs parallel, avoiding external rotation of the hip, particularly when bending the knee of the leg that is in hip extension.

- ☐ Keep the elbows parallel to each other (or as close to it as possible).

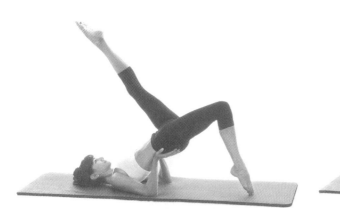

Inhale. Lie in a supine position and draw the knees toward the chest. Create a ball shape with the body and roll over onto the shoulder girdle. Place the hands under the pelvis, as if holding a bowl, and create an arc shape with the trunk. Now straighten the legs up toward the ceiling. Open the legs (one forward, one backward; equidistant from the centerline) into a wide V-position.

Exhale. Extend the back leg (furthest from the face) toward the floor. Bend the knee and touch the floor with the toes (or as close to the floor as possible).

Inhale. Flex the hip and bring the bent leg toward the chest. At the same time, take the straight leg over to replace the previous back leg.

Begin straightening the bent leg in front of the face as the straight one starts bending to touch the floor with the toes. Continue this large cycling action. After several repetitions, reverse the direction of the cycling (no need to touch the floor with the toes in the reverse direction).

Back Support

This exercise emphasizes the co-contraction of the trunk flexors and extensors in creating a stable trunk. It directly strengthens the back, shoulders, and hip extensors, and it indirectly addresses the need for flexibility and control of the opposing flexors, particularly the shoulder and hip.

The initial movement, once the setup position has been achieved, is hip extension supported by shoulder and back extension. During the hip extension, the hamstrings must engage before the gluteal muscles. Deviating from this sequence of muscle recruitment (by recruiting the gluteals first) may lead to incorrect positioning of the pelvis (tucking) and lack of hamstring activation.

Finally, although "vertebra-by-vertebra" articulation of the spine is often used in Pilates, in this case you must strive to keep the spine in a stable, neutral position and hinge from the hip and shoulder joints, lifting the trunk as one solid unit.

Imagery

Think of the hips as the hinge of a door (on its side), opening (as the pelvis lifts) and closing (as the pelvis lowers). Alternatively, visualize two poles (or energy lines): one running from the head through the trunk to the hip joint, and the other running from the ankles through the knee to the hip joint. As the pelvis lifts, the two poles connect and become one. As the pelvis lowers, the joined pole, that spans head-through-ankles, splits in two.

☐ Avoid flaring the ribs.

☐ Lift the pelvis from the hip joint in a hinging action, keeping the back and legs straight.

☐ Allow the head to follow the line of the spine.

Muscle Focus
- Shoulder extensors
- Hip extensors
- Back extensors

Objectives
- To develop trunk stabilization
- To strengthen the shoulder and hip extensors
- To improve back extensor control

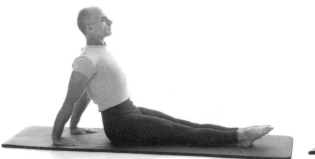

Inhale. Sit with the arms extended about a foot behind the pelvis with fingers facing the pelvis. Straighten the legs out in front and softly plantarflex the feet. Engage the back extensors and scapular stabilizers.

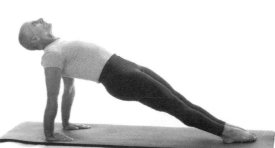

Exhale. Lift the pelvis off the floor, hinging at the hip and shoulder joints, until the body is in a straight line.

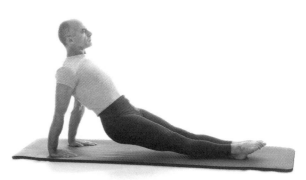

Inhale. Lower the body without quite touching the mat, hinging at the hip and shoulder joints. Repeat 5 times. After the final repetition return to the start position.

Leg Pull Back

Muscle Focus

- Hip, back, and shoulder extensors
- Hip flexors

Objectives

- To strengthen the hip and shoulder extensors
- To develop trunk stabilization
- To improve hip flexor control

The Mat Work: Back Support is a necessary prerequisite to learning and mastering this exercise. As with the leg pull front, the key to the exercise is maintaining stillness in the body, except for the one leg that lifts and lowers.

Flexibility is a major factor in the success of this exercise. Without it, your ability to perform the exercise will be limited. The flexibility of the shoulders is already challenged by the back support position. As the leg lifts forward and up, hip flexor strength and hamstring flexibility play a vital role.

Imagery

Use the concept of the poles or energy lines discussed in Mat Work: Back Support. Keep the head-through-ankles pole stable and straight, and visualize the lifting leg as yet another pole attached to the side of the pelvis. The leg swings up and down without affecting the large, stable central pole.

☐ Isolate the movement of the leg as you lift it and lower it.

☐ Keep the hip extensors of the supporting leg and the back extensors engaged.

☐ Align the head with the spine.

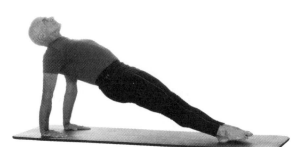

Inhale. Sit with the arms extended about a foot behind the pelvis with fingers facing the pelvis. Straighten the legs out in front and softly plantarflex the feet. Engage the back extensors and scapular stabilizers. Lift the pelvis off the floor, hinging at the hip and shoulder joints, until the body is in a straight line.

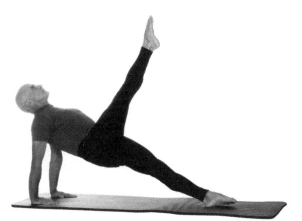

Exhale. Flex the hip, lifting one leg up toward the ceiling.

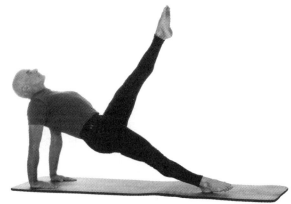

Inhale. Lower the leg, lightly touching the mat. Repeat several times before changing to the other leg. Return to the start position.

Front Support

Also known as the plank or push-up position, the front support exercise utilizes two critical areas of stabilization: the pelvic–lumbar region and the shoulder girdle. Strengthening these two areas and establishing good muscle activation provides efficient stabilization for subsequent and more challenging exercises in a similar position on all the apparatus. When good alignment and solid stabilization are not present, the trunk and the shoulder region "collapse," resulting in inefficient and sometimes harmful positions. This may take some relearning, since many people are accustomed to doing a great many push-ups—incorrectly.

Imagery

Imagine the body as a strong, solid bridge or ramp that will not budge under immense weight.

☐ Keep the body in a straight line from head to toe.

☐ Maintain pelvic–lumbar and scapular stabilization throughout the exercise.

VARIATION

To further challenge yourself in this position, exhale and bend one leg in toward the chest, kneeling lightly if necessary. Inhale, and straighten the leg back to the front support position. Exhale, and bend the other leg. Inhale, and return to the front support position. Repeat 5 times on each leg.

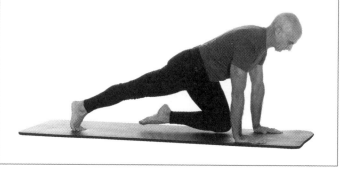

☐ Keep the hands directly under the shoulders.

Muscle Focus

- Abdominal muscles
- Scapular stabilizers

Objectives

- To develop trunk and shoulder stabilization
- To strengthen the upper body

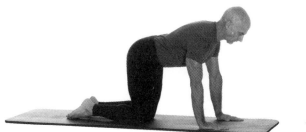

Inhale. Kneel in a quadruped position, with the knees hip-width apart and the hands shoulder-width apart. Establish a neutral position of the spine, with the weight evenly distributed between the upper and lower body.

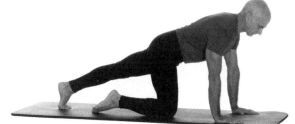

Exhale. Reach one leg back with minimal weight shift. Further stabilize the shoulder region.

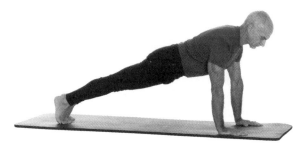

Inhale. Extend the other leg back into the front support position, with the arms and legs firm and straight. Hold this position for 30-60 seconds while further engaging the internal support system, maintaining stability throughout the body.

Muscle Focus

- Elbow extensors
- Abdominal muscles

Objectives

- To strengthen the elbow extensors and shoulder girdle
- To develop trunk stabilization
- To practice spinal articulation

Push-Up

Unlike a typical push-up, the Pilates push-up is a movement sequence that involves the entire body, shifting from the front support position, through a roll up, to standing upright and back again. Within this sequence are the actual push-ups, which, with the elbows kept close to the sides of the body, emphasize the elbow extensors. Of primary importance is keeping the scapulae stable as the elbows bend and the body is lowered and then lifted back up. The level of scapular stabilization determines the depth of the elbow flexion—as soon as the scapulae start to elevate or adduct, lift the body back up and regroup.

Few people are initially able to keep the scapulae stable in a neutral position. Many a "muscle man" has crumbled trying to do push-ups while keeping the scapulae still. During a presentation at a large forum in China in 2003, I asked for a volunteer to do no more than 10 push-ups correctly. (I defined correctly as holding the trunk and scapulae absolutely stable and moving only the arms.) A hulk of a man with muscles bulging everywhere came up. I must admit I thought that I'd met my match and my experiment would fail. As he proceeded with the utmost confidence, I stopped him each time his scapulae began to move. He did not get very far, and when I feared that the pool of sweat that had built up under him was about to drown us both, he collapsed and, with a slight smile, conceded that he needed to learn how to do push-ups again (after doing 500 a day for 20 years!).

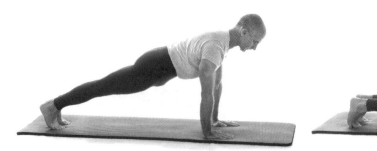

Exhale. Kneel in a quadruped position, with the knees hip-width apart and the hands shoulder-width apart. Establish a neutral position of the spine, with the weight evenly distributed between the upper and lower body. Reach one leg back with minimal weight shift then extend the other leg back into the front support position, with the arms and legs firm and straight.

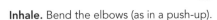

Inhale. Bend the elbows (as in a push-up).

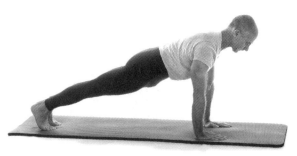

Exhale. Extend the elbows. Repeat the push-up twice.

We gave each other a hug, and no words were necessary to express the understanding, camaraderie, and respect we felt for each other—and the work.

Once you have mastered moving from the front support position to standing and back again, I advise that you gradually decrease the number of arm walks until you can do the movement with no "arm walking"—just one swoop up and then a dive back to the front support position. This demands pushing off from the arms and simultaneously lifting the pelvis high into the air, transferring the weight to the feet, and then rolling up through the spine. Reverse this sequence to return to the front support position.

Imagery

Imagine the body as a strong, solid bridge that will not budge under immense weight. When the pelvis is lifted, visualize the body as a pyramid, with the tailbone as the tip and the feet and hands as the base. When lifting into the roll up, the sense should be of a band around the midsection of the body with an external force like crane pulling you up from the back and then lowering you again following the upright standing position. The dynamic should be brisk.

☐ Engage the abdominal muscles throughout the exercise.

☐ Keep the elbows close to the sides of the body.

☐ Do not allow the scapulae to adduct or elevate.

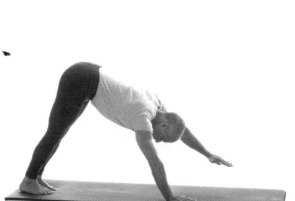
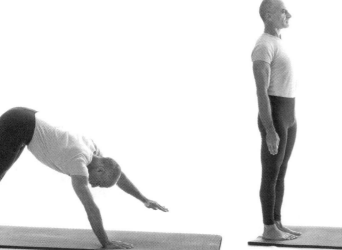
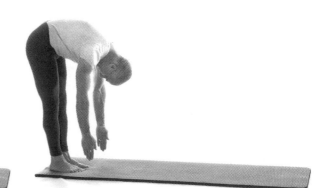
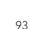

After the second repetition lift the pelvis upward and walk the hands toward the feet, transferring the weight to the feet.

Roll up to a standing position.
Inhale. Establish good upright alignment.

Exhale. Roll down and walk the hands forward to the front support position. Repeat the sequence 3 to 5 times.

Muscle Focus

- Hip extensors
- Abdominal muscles
- Scapular stabilizers

Objectives

- To strengthen the shoulder girdle
- To develop hip extensor control
- To develop trunk stabilization

Leg Pull Front

Mastering the Mat Work: Front Support before learning this exercise is imperative, because it is the foundation on which the leg pull front exercise is built.

The key to the exercise is maintaining stillness in the body, except for the leg that lifts and lowers. Using only one leg for support while moving the other makes this difficult position less stable and therefore more challenging. Note that when the leg lifts to the back (extends) the pelvis remains stable, which means that the leg may extend no more than a few degrees (depending on hip flexor flexibility) before the pelvis starts tilting anteriorly. Dancers may be tempted to do a full arabesque, tilting the pelvis anteriorly, but I urge you to keep the pelvis neutral and maximize height without tilting the pelvis. This translates into pure hip extension. Then, when the pelvis is allowed to tilt both anteriorly and rotate to maximize turnout and height, the leg will be higher and stronger than ever before.

Imagery

Create a drawbridge as described in the Mat Work: Front Support. One part of the bridge remains stable as another section lifts to allow tall ships to pass under it. The fixed section of the bridge does not move when the other section lifts.

- ☐ Maintain the plank position of the body throughout the exercise.

- ☐ Keep the pelvis neutral with a bias toward a slight posterior tilt.

- ☐ Maintain scapular stabilization.

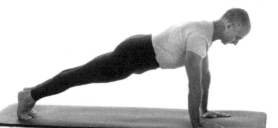 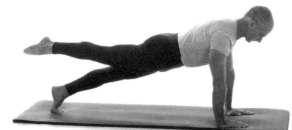 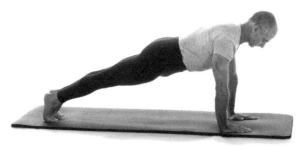

Inhale. Kneel in a quadruped position, with the knees hip-width apart and the hands shoulder-width apart. Establish a neutral position of the spine, with the weight evenly distributed between the upper and lower body. Reach one leg back with minimal weight shift, and then extend the other leg back into the front support position, with the arms and legs firm and straight. Lift one leg slightly off the ground, plantarflexing the foot.

Exhale. Extend the hip, lifting the leg higher.

Inhale. Lower the leg so the toes touch the ground lightly, maintaining plantarflexion. On the final repetition, dorsiflex the foot and place it on the ground, returning to the front support position. Repeat on the other side.

Lateral Flexion and Rotation

The focus of the exercises in this block are movements that involve lateral flexion and rotation of the spine. These movements place greater emphasis on the oblique abdominals versus the rectus abdominis. The oblique abdominals, located more toward the sides of the trunk versus the front, and in particular the internal oblique muscles, work with the transversus abdominis to stabilize the spine and protect the back from injury. Many athletic and recreational endeavors, such as swimming, kayaking, golf, throwing sports, and tennis, involve extensive use of the very powerful obliques. Greater strength and coordination in the oblique muscles can enhance athletic performance.

The oblique abdominals are key lateral flexors of the spine, however, the quadratus lumborum and spinal extensors can also produce lateral flexion. Excessive contraction of the obliques combined with inadequate use of the spinal extensors causes the trunk to round forward (spinal flexion) as it flexes laterally. Conversely, excessive contraction of the spinal extensors causes the back to arch (spinal extension) as it flexes laterally. Therefore, finely coordinated contraction of the anterior and posterior muscles of the spine is required to achieve the desired position for lateral flexion. Exercising in this side position provides valuable practice for maintaining neutral alignment of the pelvis and spine during everyday activities, and learning to brace the muscles of the core allows you to support and protect the spine during those activities.

Certain exercises in this chapter use rotation of the spine in some form: some from a sitting position as in the spine twist and the saw, others from a supine position as in the corkscrew, and even from a side plank position as in the twist. All the exercises emphasize the oblique abdominals, yet each is unique in its pattern of coordinated recruitment of the spinal flexors, lateral flexors, rotators, and extensors. I have divided this block into two sub-sections for further clarity. The first encompasses the exercises that focus on lateral flexion. The second is exercises that highlight rotation.

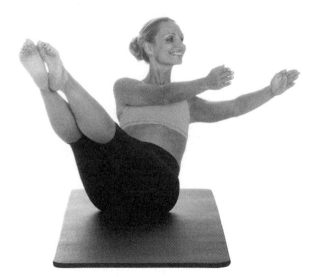

Muscle Focus

- Oblique abdominals

Objectives

- To strengthen the lateral flexors
- To stabilize the pelvic–lumbar region
- To develop hip adductor control

Side Leg Lift

Every good, well-balanced exercise program should include lateral flexion of the trunk. The side leg lift is a fundamental exercise that is relatively simple to execute and teach yet profound in its effect. Significant imbalances in strength and range of motion between the two sides of the trunk are common, and this imbalance should be addressed by working each side independently. This exercise also develops pelvic–lumbar stabilization.

The ideal alignment of the body in this exercise is a straight line, with the spine in a neutral position, the trunk flexors and extensors co-contracted and the lateral flexors on both sides engaged. As the lateral flexors on the topside contract concentrically and shorten, the lateral flexors on the underside contract eccentrically and elongate. However, the lower back extensors tend to overpower and dominate the abdominals. To avoid this, shift the legs slightly forward of the centerline. Do not allow the legs to move too far forward however, as this results in flexion of the trunk.

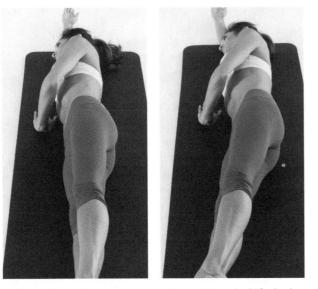

If the ideal plumb alignment cannot be achieved, shift the legs slightly forward of the centerline, creating a banana shape.

Imagery

Imagine a long energy line reaching from the top of the head through the trunk, legs, and feet. The body creates an elongated bow shape as the legs lift. Another helpful image is that of a fish on its side with its tails swooping upward.

☐ Keep the oblique abdominals on both sides recruited.

☐ Keep the adductors engaged, moving the legs and pelvis as one unit.

☐ Maintain a sense of lengthening the lower leg, keeping it alongside the top leg.

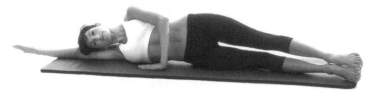

Inhale. Lie on one side with the bottom arm straight in line with the body and the head resting on it. The pelvis is "stacked" perpendicular to the mat and the legs are pressing together. The top arm is either bent, with the palm down on the mat in front of the body, or straight and palm resting on the top thigh (more challenging).

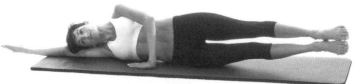

Exhale. Lift both legs by flexing the trunk laterally (tilting the pelvis), keeping the legs together and the body aligned.

Inhale. Lower the legs without allowing the feet to touch the mat. Following the final repetition lower the legs to the start position and repeat on the other side.

Side Kick

This exercise reinforces the concept of trunk and pelvic stabilization with hip disassociation. In a side-lying position, you rely on a much smaller and narrower base of support than you do in exercises in which you are supine or prone. Consequently, the level of difficulty is increased and the lateral stabilizers of the body are more fully activated. By focusing on scapular and trunk stabilization, you minimize the pressure on the elbow and maximize stability. As the leg swings back and forth, spinal flexors and extensors are in a state of balanced co-contraction, holding the trunk and pelvis stable. When the leg swings forward, the extensors work to prevent spinal flexion; when it swings back, the abdominal muscles work to prevent spinal hyperextension. These subtle internal adjustments are hardly visible to the eye, but their impact on the pelvis and spine is significant.

This exercise is an excellent example of how the body adapts to changes in the center of gravity. As the leg swings back and forth, the pelvis adapts by shifting slightly in the opposite direction to the leg. This small back and forth motion of the pelvis assists greatly in maintaining a balanced, stable position, both in this exercise and in everyday movements. However this should be differentiated from an anterior or posterior tilt of the pelvis, which is not desirable.

Imagery

Imagine the swinging motion of a pendulum. Now place the pendulum on its side without affecting its movement. The motion of the leg should feel like a pendulum, swinging freely and effortlessly.

☐ Minimize rocking the trunk backward and forward.

☐ Maximize the range of motion of the leg.

☐ Maintain shoulder stability, particularly of the lower shoulder, and keep the underside of the rib cage lifted.

☐ Avoid thrusting the ribs forward as the leg swings back.

Muscle Focus

- Abdominal muscles
- Back extensors
- Hamstrings
- Hip flexors

Objectives

- To develop pelvic–lumbar stabilization
- To increase hip flexor control and flexibility
- To increase hip extensor control and flexibility
- To develop hip disassociation

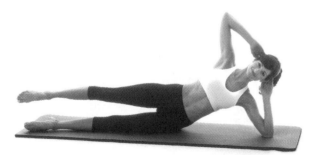

Inhale. Lie on one side, leaning on the elbow of the lower arm with the hands behind the head. Engage the underside oblique abdominal muscles and shoulder stabilizers to support the trunk. Stabilize the bottom leg on the floor and hold the top leg at hip height, engaging the hip abductors.

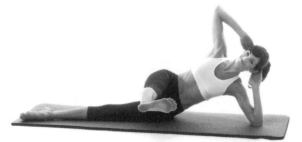

Exhale. Swing the top leg as far forward as possible, dorsiflexing the foot and pulsing twice when reaching the maximum range. Avoid tucking (posteriorly tilting) the pelvis; keep it in a neutral position.

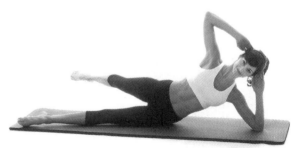

Inhale. Swing the leg back as far as possible, plantarflexing the foot and elongating the leg, pulsing twice when reaching the maximum range. Maintain a neutral position of the pelvis (avoid hyperextending the back and anteriorly tilting the pelvis). Repeat the forward-and-back leg swing several times, finishing in the backward swing position.

Side Bend

Muscle Focus
- Oblique abdominal muscles
- Scapular stabilizers

Objectives
- To develop oblique abdominal strength and control
- To improve trunk flexibility
- To develop shoulder strength and stabilization

As you enter the realm of advanced level work, the base of support becomes smaller and in many cases less stable. The side bend relies primarily on trunk and shoulder strength and stabilization. In this exercise, the pivot point around which much of the movement occurs is a single shoulder joint, which, by its nature, is very mobile and potentially unstable. Therefore, you must focus particular attention on correct mechanics of the shoulder. As the body arcs at the top position, the pelvis should lift as high as possible toward the ceiling while the free arm swoops over the body, accentuating the arc shape. The head must follow the line of the spine, focusing the gaze toward the hand on the floor. Resist the tendency to lift the head and look upward; doing so can result in neck tension.

The musculature should not relax between repetitions—you should keep a sense of continuous movement. Ideally, even in the bottom phase (the "resting" position), there should be room enough for a piece of paper to pass between the pelvis and the mat. Tremendous support must come from the underside, the lateral aspect of the trunk. The oblique abdominal muscles are the engine that drives this exercise.

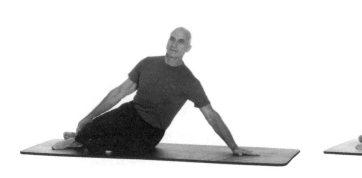

Exhale. Sit sideways with your weight on one side of the pelvis. Bend the legs and place the top foot in front of the bottom one. Rest the upper body weight on the supporting arm while maintaining strong shoulder stabilization and recruiting the abdominal obliques. The other arm rests on the side of the body.

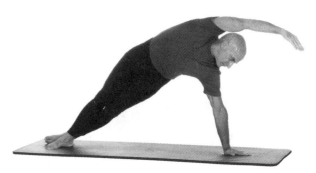

Inhale. Lift the pelvis away from the floor while straightening the legs, and raising the upper arm to shoulder height, fingers directed toward the ceiling. Reach a point where the body is in a straight diagonal line, the arms are straight and aligned with each other creating a T position with the line of the body.

Exhale. Draw in the lateral muscles of the underside of the trunk and lift the pelvis higher toward the ceiling, creating an arc shape with the body as the upper arm reaches overhead.

Imagery

A wonderful image to aid in lifting and arcing the body is that of a dolphin leaping out of the water. This movement of course is on the side, but the action and grace of the movement is similar. Also imagine that the movement is being performed between two panes of glass. This accentuates the two-dimensional quality of the exercise.

- ☐ Initiate the movement from the oblique abdominal muscles.
- ☐ Maintain abdominal engagement throughout the exercise.
- ☐ Keep the scapular stabilizers engaged throughout.

VARIATION

Perform this same movement pattern, but rather than using a straight arm for support with the weight on the wrist, place the forearm on the mat. In this version the legs will remain straight throughout.

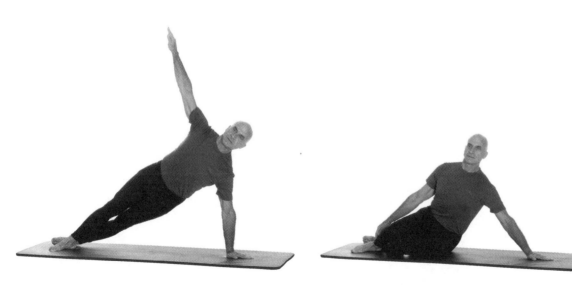

Inhale. Return to the previous position with the body in a straight diagonal line and the arms aligned.

Exhale. Lower the body to the start position (without touching the floor if possible).

Side Kick—Kneeling

Muscle Focus
- Hip abductors, flexors, and extensors
- Abdominal muscles
- Shoulder stabilizers

Objectives
- To develop trunk stabilization
- To develop hip flexor and hip extensor control
- To improve hip flexor and hip extensor flexibility
- To strengthen the hip abductors

This exercise is an extension of the Mat Work: Side Kick, made more difficult by decreasing the base of support to one hand and the lower leg. The primary focus remains on pelvic–lumbar stabilization and hip flexion and extension. Keep the swinging leg as high as possible during the transition from front to back; this increases the hip abductor work exponentially. The head should be aligned with the spine throughout, which decreases the chance of neck tension. A good way to test balance is by lifting the supporting hand slightly off the mat and balancing on only the lower leg: The body should be able to balance momentarily, with a sense of lightness.

Employing effective shoulder and trunk stabilization helps moderate the weight bearing on the wrist. Sometimes pressing the fingertips into the mat and engaging the wrist flexors slightly decreases the extension of the wrist and alleviates some of the pressure on the wrist.

Imagery

Use the pendulum imagery described in the Mat Work: Side Kick, of a pendulum lying on its side swinging, adding the

VARIATION

To decrease or eliminate wrist extension, make a fist with the supporting hand before placing it on the mat. This alternate support hand position decreases or eliminates excessive wrist extension.

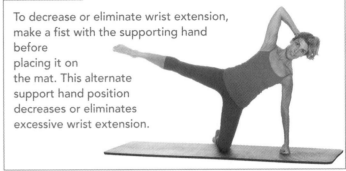

feeling of being suspended like a bridge. The body does in fact create a bridge, which should be lifted high off the ground, and the leg swings freely back and forth.

- ☐ Maintain a neutral pelvis.
- ☐ Do not sink into the supporting shoulder or the underside of the rib cage.
- ☐ Try to keep the leg above hip height (as high as possible).

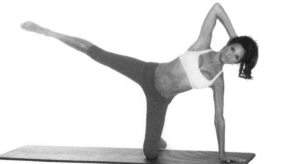

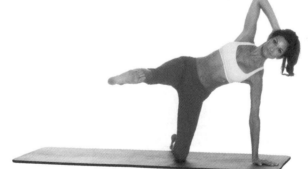

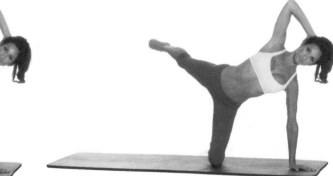

Inhale. Kneeling, shift the weight to one knee with the lower leg reaching directly back. Place the supporting hand (on the same side of the body as the weighted knee) on the floor directly under the shoulder, and lift the other leg out to the side at hip height or higher if possible. Place the free hand behind the head.

Exhale. Swing the top leg as far forward as possible, dorsiflexing the foot and avoiding a posterior tilt of the pelvis (tuck). Perform two pulses together with the breath when the leg is at maximum forward reach.

Inhale. Swing the leg back as far as possible and plantarflex the foot; avoid hyperextending the lumbar spine and anteriorly tilting the pelvis. Elongate the leg backward, doing two pulses at maximum reach before swinging it forward again. End the exercise with the leg reaching back.

Spine Twist—Sitting

This exercise emphasizes organized rotation of the spine around the longitudinal axis. Proper engagement of the oblique abdominal muscles allows correct rotation of the spine. Incorrect rotation in daily activities that demand sound rotation, such as cleaning and gardening or recreational activities such as golf, volleyball, and tennis, can lead to backache or more severe injuries. People tend to use the shoulders and arms excessively to compensate for lack of mobility in the trunk, rather than using the powerful muscles of the trunk and focusing on spinal rotation. Tremendous improvement in performance can be gained when rotation of the trunk is maximized and the powerhouse is employed, rather than relying primarily on the arms and shoulders.

Imagery

Imagine two poles or energy lines: one is longitudinal, running up and down the back, and the other is in the transverse plane reaching across the shoulders from the fingertips of one hand to the fingertips of the other. The transverse pole rotates around the longitudinal one, while both poles remain in their respective planes of motion.

☐ Keep the pelvis and legs still throughout the exercise.

☐ Initiate the movement from the waist, not from the shoulders, keeping the arms aligned in a straight line with the shoulders.

☐ Move the head and trunk as one unit.

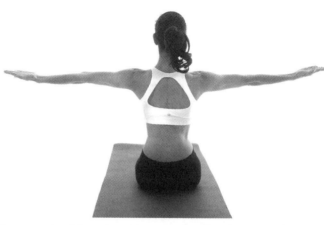

The arms should reach out in opposite directions, creating a straight line across the shoulders.

Muscle Focus
- Oblique abdominals
- Back extensors

Objectives
- To strengthen the oblique abdominal muscles and back extensors
- To improve trunk mobility and stability

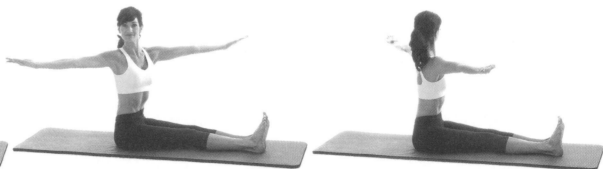

Inhale. Sit upright with the legs straight and together and the feet dorsiflexed. Hold the arms in a T position with the palms facing upward (shoulders in external rotation).

Exhale. Rotate the trunk to one side and do two pulses when you reach maximum range.

Inhale. Pass through the center and repeat the movement to the other side. Complete the exercise by returning to the start position.

Saw

Muscle Focus
- Hamstrings
- Adductors
- Back extensors

Objectives
- To improve flexibility of the hamstrings and adductors
- To develop control of the back extensors
- To develop control of the oblique abdominals

The saw involves an intricate interplay of extending and rotating the trunk and stretching the hamstrings and adductors. Maintain an extended back, rather than a rounded back, as the trunk and arm reach forward over the leg during the stretch phase. This maximizes the hamstring stretch and offers the added benefit of strengthening the back extensors. This exercise is at times taught with flexion of the trunk, in an endeavor to engage the abdominals more and stretch the back. In my opinion this position is ineffective at doing either. It will not challenge the abdominals enough to achieve any significant strength gain and will not be a profound stretch for the back muscles. The only part of the back that might stretch is the mid- and upper back, a region that few people need to flex—quite the contrary, many people today suffer from round shoulders and kyphotic-type posture.

When reaching forward over the leg, keep the spine aligned over the leg and the head aligned with the spine, looking down toward the leg. Some instructors recommend rotating the trunk in this position and looking toward the back arm. However, people typically have enough difficulty achieving straight alignment of the trunk; adding rotation to this difficult position often results in severe compensations and bad alignment.

Note that the saw requires that the trunk move with the pelvis from the hips, as one unit, when stretching over the leg, rather than through segmental articulation of the spine. In addition, remain true to the longitudinal axis when rotating the spine in the initial phase, and return to this exact position, on the longitudinal axis, in the final stage of the exercise before returning to face center. In the sitting upright positions, whether facing front or rotated, keep the spine elongated over the stable base of the pelvis.

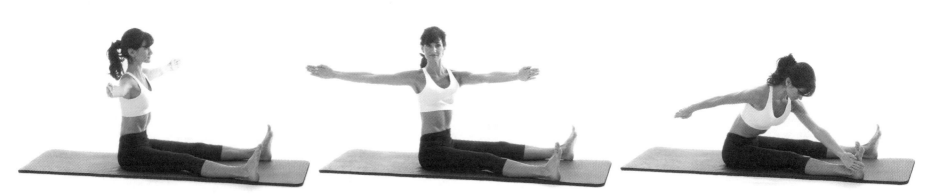

Exhale. Sit upright, with the legs straight and open slightly beyond shoulder-width and the feet dorsiflexed. Hold the arms in a T position, reaching them as far out to the sides as possible, palms facing forward.

Inhale. Rotate the trunk around the longitudinal axis. Keep the pelvis anchored, and move the arms and head with the trunk.

Exhale. Reach forward over the leg with the trunk. The front hand extends past the small toe, and the back hand reaches back with the palm facing the body. Feel the oppositional pull of the arms.

Imagery

Visualize a pole strapped to the back, which you rotate around when in the upright position before folding over the leg. When folding the trunk over the leg for the stretch, maintain the feeling of the pole strapped to the back to accentuate spinal extension and straight alignment.

☐ Keep the back extensors engaged when reaching forward.

☐ Keep the feet dorsiflexed with the toes reaching toward the ceiling.

☐ Anchor the pelvis and distribute your weight evenly on the sit bones throughout the exercise.

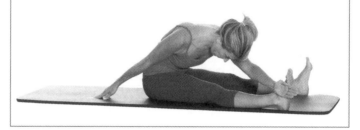

VARIATION

In order to assist with the stretch phase, when the trunk is over the leg, place the back hand on the ground and press forward with the back arm. This offers support for the trunk and increases the stretch.

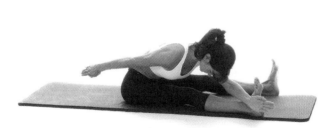

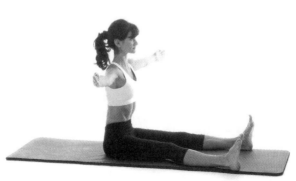

Inhale. Extend the spine further to accentuate the hamstring stretch as the body begins lifting up. Continue lifting to the longitudinal axis while facing the side.

Exhale. Rotate back to the center start position. Repeat the movement to the other side.

Muscle Focus

- Abdominal muscles

Objectives

- To strengthen the abdominal muscles
- To develop pelvic–lumbar stabilization

Corkscrew

This exercise builds on the principles of the Mat Work: Supine Spine Twist but incorporates a longer lever (the legs), intensifying the hip flexor work and the abdominal work, particularly that of the oblique abdominals. The pendulum motion and circling of the legs demand intricate control of the spine and coordination of the abdominal muscles and hip flexors, which act alternately as movers and stabilizers at various points in the exercise. Note that the pelvis rocks from side to side with the movement of the legs, with one side of the pelvis briefly lifting off the mat as the legs move to the opposite side. However, the pelvis anchors soon afterward, as the legs pass through the center of the arc to the other side. The lower back should imprint into the mat as the legs pass through the center and should leave the mat only momentarily, as the legs go out to the sides before returning to the center.

Imagery

Visualize drawing a big circle on the ceiling as the legs arc around in one direction and then in the reverse.

☐ Keep the legs and feet together and aligned throughout the exercise.

VARIATION

The pendulum is a corkscrew variation in which the legs move from side to side, rather than in circles. It is less demanding on the hip flexors and abdominals, but there is tremendous focus on the oblique abdominals.

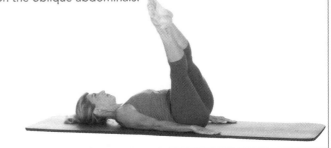

☐ Keep the shoulder girdle, neck, and head still and relaxed.

☐ Focus the movement in the waist region.

☐ Bend the knees to reduce strain on the hip flexors and lower back (if necessary).

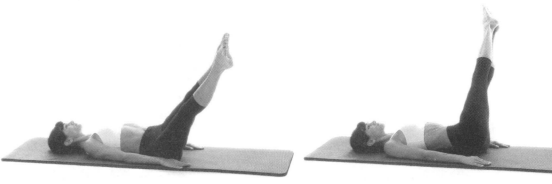

Exhale. Lie supine, with the arms in a T position or at the sides of the body, which tends to be a more challenging position as it offers less stability, and the legs at a 90-degree angle to the floor. Imprint the lower back into the mat.

Inhale. Shift the pelvis and both legs to one side, keeping the shoulders stable and relaxed. The top leg must reach out further to stay aligned with the lower leg.

Exhale. Circle the legs downward in an arc through the center and around to the opposite side. As the legs pass through the center, imprint the lower back into the mat.

Once the legs reach the opposite side of the arc, bring them back to the start position. Alternate the direction. Use the starting point (12 o'clock) as the reference position that you always return to and pause in.

Hip Circle Prep

Certain elements of the Mat Work: Corkscrew apply to this exercise; however, the sitting V-position of the body requires a higher level of stabilization, strength, and control. The shoulder girdle must remain stable, and abdominal support must be maintained in order to avoid excessive stress on the lumbar spine as the legs reach out, circle down and around to the other side, and return to center.

The trunk rotation and the power it demands can enhance athletic performance, as well achieving a deeper understanding of the power encapsulated in the powerhouse.

Imagery

The image of drawing a cone shape from the pelvis out through the feet, with the feet tracing the large part of the cone, describes the movement clearly. The bigger the cone, the more support and stabilization you need.

☐ Avoid hyperextending the lumbar spine as the legs circle.

☐ Keep the shoulder girdle stable, and the mid- and upper-back extensors engaged.

Muscle Focus
• Abdominal muscles

Objectives
• To strengthen the abdominal muscles with an emphasis on the oblique abdominals.
• To promote pelvic–lumbar and shoulder stabilization
• To develop trunk rotation

VARIATION

In the advanced version of this exercise, the arms move with the upper body as one unit in one direction, while the legs and pelvis move as one unit in the opposite direction. The arms reach forward together with the legs, then move to one side and circle up and around to the other side; the legs reach to the opposite side, and then circle down and around to meet the arms back in the center. The arms describe one cone and the legs another: one clockwise and the other counterclockwise. Reverse directions after 3-5 repetitions.

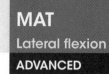

☐ Move the pelvis from side to side as the legs draw a large circle.

☐ Keep the legs together as they move with the pelvis as one unit.

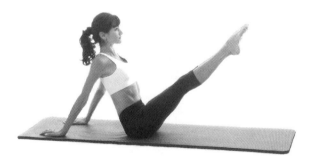

Exhale. Sit in a V-position with the arms extended behind you and the hands resting on the floor. Face the fingers away from the body. The arms should support the body only lightly, like training wheels on a bicycle. Bend the knees toward the chest and straighten the legs at approximately a 60-degree angle to the floor, keeping them together.

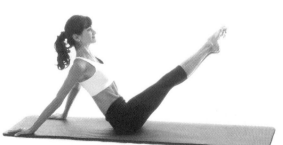

Inhale. Shift the pelvis and the legs as a unit to one side.

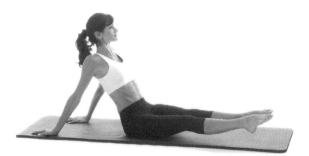

Exhale. The legs circle down and around to the opposite side as the pelvis moves through the center to the opposite side. Return to the start position. Repeat the movement several times to achieve a sense of flow, then change the direction of the circle.

Muscle Focus

- Oblique abdominal muscles

Objectives

- To strengthen the abdominal muscles, with an emphasis on the obliques
- To develop pelvic stabilization and trunk rotation

Criss-Cross

The action of the lower body in this exercise is identical to that of the Mat Work: Single-Leg Stretch: a pumping motion, keeping the feet at the same level and creating a sense of internal resistance for the hip flexors as you draw the knee of the straight leg toward the chest.

The rotation of the trunk is key because it emphasizes the work of the oblique abdominal muscles. There is a tendency to laterally flex the trunk and flare the ribs on the side of the bent leg during the rotation, resulting in a swivel-type motion as opposed to a true rotation. You can prevent this by contracting the internal obliques on the bent-knee side, drawing the lower ribs towards the pelvic crest. In addition, as fatigue sets in due to the intensity of the exercise and the load on the abdominal muscles, the height of the trunk in forward flexion sometimes progressively decreases and the lower back starts to lift off the mat into hyperlordosis.

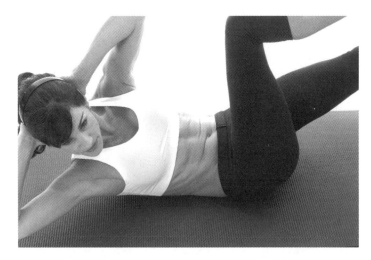

This close-up illustrates the rotation of the trunk and the stability of the pelvis, resulting in strong abdominal oblique activation.

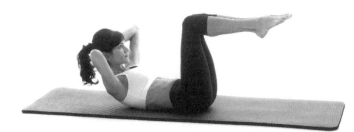

Inhale. Lie supine and draw the knees to the chest. Lift the trunk into forward flexion with the scapulae off the mat, the thighs at approximately 100-degrees of hip flexion, and the shins parallel to the floor. Interlace the fingers behind the head and hold the elbows wide.

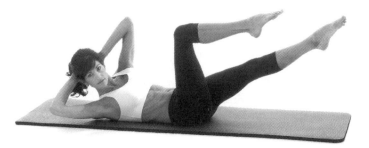

Exhale. Straighten one leg, rotating the trunk toward the bent knee.

If this occurs, immediately pause and reestablish the proper position, lifting into forward flexion, before continuing. It is preferable to stop rather than to compromise good form. Practicing incorrect form, even with the best of intentions, is counterproductive and can lead to negative habitual movement patterns and possible physical ailments. If the fatigue is excessive, cease working the abdominals and move onto the next block.

One other common mistake is flapping the elbows back and forth in an attempt to reach for the knee, with minimal or no rotation of the trunk. The upper body, including the head and arms, must move as one unit. Keeping the elbows opposite the ears is typically a good, comfortable position.

Imagery

The piston imagery describing the precise leg movements in the Mat Work: Single-Leg Stretch applies here. The feeling in the waist should be like a rotating disc with the lower section (the pelvis) held absolutely stable and the top section (the trunk) rotating on an axis. Or imagine a chicken turning on a skewer that runs longitudinally through its body.

☐ Keep the elbows wide and stable.

☐ Imagine rotating from the waist, avoiding lateral flexion.

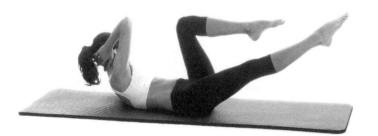

Inhale. Simultaneously change legs as the trunk passes through the center.

Exhale. Complete the straightening of the second leg and rotate the trunk to the other side.

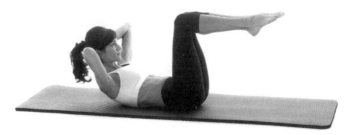

Inhale. Return to the start position.

Muscle Focus

- Oblique abdominal muscles

Objectives

- To develop oblique abdominal strength and control
- To improve trunk flexibility
- To develop shoulder strength and stabilization

Twist

This exercise adds the element of rotation to the Mat Work: Side Bend, making the movement three-dimensional. The rotation involves not only the trunk, but also, very significantly, the shoulder. A single shoulder supports the weight of the body in a suspended position and accommodates its rotation, with most of the movement occurring in the glenohumeral joint. This is a tall order for this small, relatively unstable, muscle-dependent joint.

I like to teach the Mat Work: Side Bend before teaching the twist. Once both have been learned I often combine them, doing three repetitions of one and then three of the other. As stated in chapter 3, the level of an exercise is determined by the complexity of its coordination, stabilization, and movement. The twist has it all!

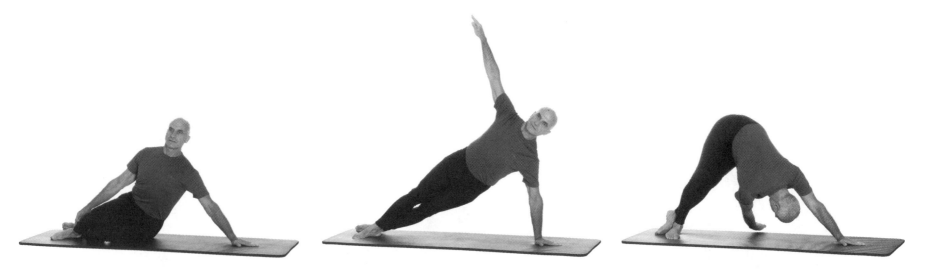

Exhale. Sit sideways with your weight on one side of the pelvis. Bend the legs and place the top foot in front of the bottom one. Rest the upper body weight on the supporting arm while maintaining strong shoulder stabilization and recruiting the abdominal obliques. The other arm rests on the side of the body.

Inhale. Lift the pelvis away from the floor while straightening the legs, and raise the upper arm to shoulder height, fingers pointing toward the ceiling. The body is in a straight diagonal line and the arms are straight and aligned with each other.

Exhale. Lift the pelvis as high as possible and rotate the trunk as the free arm reaches under the body.

Imagery

I use several images in this exercise. The visual I give for the top position of the twist is a pyramid—the trunk creates one side of the pyramid and the legs, as one unit, the other side. When the arm reaches under the body, the movement is like threading a needle, and the energy should be spiraling. The return to the diagonal position should create a well-defined line. In this T position, feel the strong energy line running through the body and a second line running through the arms from the floor up to the sky. Line is everything in this wonderful and challenging exercise.

- ☐ Minimize the use of the legs and maximize the activation of the lateral flexors and rotators of the trunk.

- ☐ Keep the scapula stable, rotating around the gleno-humeral joint.

- ☐ Maintain correct alignment of the head with the spine.

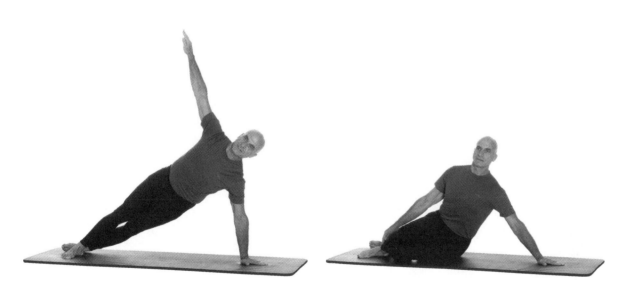

Inhale. Return to the previous position with the body in a straight diagonal line and the arms aligned.

Exhale. Lower the body to the start position, keeping the pelvis slightly off the mat (if possible) or placing it lightly on the mat.

Back Extension

The importance of this block cannot be overemphasized. The following exercises focus on improving all aspects of function of the back extensors: strength, muscular endurance, and controlled activation. The spinal extensors are used to produce or maintain spinal extension, while the abdominals function as stabilizers to distribute the work through the entire back and reduce the potentially harmful forces on the lower back. Integrating spinal extension into your Pilates program is vital for maintaining muscle balance, particularly because so many Pilates exercises emphasize spinal flexion. In addition, many everyday activities of modern day living and many recreational activities draw the spine forward into flexion, further underscoring the need for strength and endurance of the spinal extensors. Conditioning these muscles properly may also reduce the risk of osteoporosis and lower back injury.

However, it is important to note that spinal extension is a common mechanism for producing injury to the back, particularly the lower back. Optimal technique and a careful and well-planned progression to the more demanding exercises must be implemented to reap the benefits and reduce the risks of these exercises. The advanced exercises presented in this block should be attempted only after you have achieved proficiency with the more fundamental exercises, assuming you experience no back discomfort and do not have a condition that contraindicates extension of the spine.

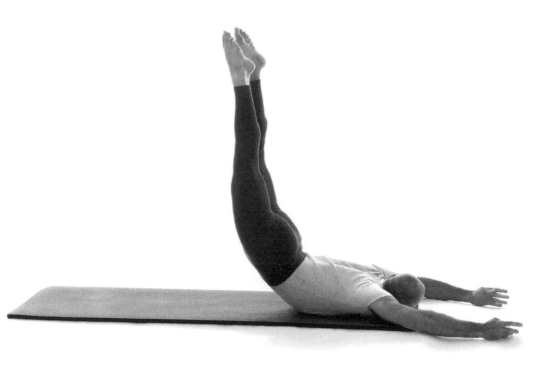

Back Extension

This exercise provides a good foundation for subsequent mat work back extension exercises, such as Swimming, Double-Leg Kick, Rocking, and Swan Dive. Proper abdominal recruitment plays a crucial role in supporting the back and achieving correct alignment during this exercise. Distributing the movement through the entire vertebral column and mobilizing each intravertebral joint helps to prevent the shearing forces on the spine that commonly occur when extension is isolated to the lower back. Abdominal recruitment assists in achieving this distribution of forces and in protecting the lower back.

Just as the abdominals help stabilize the lumbar spine, so the scapular stabilizers help stabilize the thoracic spine. These muscles, particularly the lower trapezius, not only serve as scapular stabilizers but also as mid-back extensors. Take advantage of the muscular interplay at work in back extension exercises and practice establishing good alignment and movement mechanics of the back and shoulders. Allow the pelvis to serve as an anchor for the movement.

Imagery

Use the image of an airplane hovering just above the ground to help achieve an elongated position, as opposed to an excessively arched position, and a feeling of flight.

☐ Maintain abdominal support throughout the exercise.

☐ Keep the head aligned with the spine.

☐ Utilize the scapular stabilizers, press the arms against the sides of the body, and reach the fingers toward the feet.

Muscle Focus

- Back extensors

Objectives

- To strengthen the back extensors
- To develop abdominal and scapular control

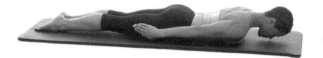

Exhale. Lie prone with the forehead on the floor. Keep the arms by the sides, pressing the palms against the legs. Keep the legs together and the feet gently plantarflexed.

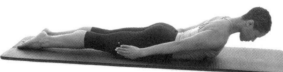

Inhale. Lift the upper trunk, head, and chest slightly off the mat. Keep the legs, including the gluteal muscles, relaxed and together. Press the pubic symphysis gently into the mat while engaging the abdominal muscles.

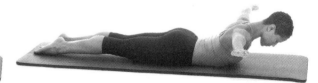

Inhale. Reach the arms out to the sides into a T position, then exhale and return the arms to the sides of the body, keeping the trunk stable throughout.

Exhale. Lower the upper body (not all the way to the mat), keeping the back extensors and abdominals activated. After the final repetition, lower the body to the start position.

Cat Stretch

Muscle Focus
- Abdominal muscles
- Back extensors

Objectives
- To develop abdominal control
- To increase flexibility of the lower back
- To improve shoulder stabilization and control
- To strengthen the mid- and upper-back extensors

This exceptional exercise achieves two important goals: spinal flexion (focusing on the abdominals) and spinal extension (focusing on the back extensors). It has the added benefit of stretching the muscles of the lower back during the flexion phase and improving pelvic–lumbar stabilization during extension. The cat stretch can prove particularly valuable for low-load abdominal and back work, like that required during pregnancy, rehabilitation, and for the older population.

This exercise is often performed with excessive rounding of the upper back during the flexion phase and hyperlordosis during the extension phase. The version offered in this book counters those tendencies by focusing the flexion in the lower back, and the extension in the mid and upper back. The pelvis is held in a neutral position during the extension, as opposed to hyperextension.

Imagery

Spinal flexion invokes an image of a ball of energy, or a whirl-pool that stirs up in the abdominal region, creating a firm, round shape. Spinal extension evokes a feeling of elevating the sternum to create the distinctive look of a sphinx, proud and determined. Also, as the name implies, the image of a cat awakening and taking a lengthy stretch is essential to the dynamic of this exercise. Visualize the cat's spine rounding and arching, displaying its phenomenal mobility and elasticity.

- ☐ Keep the hips above the knees and the shoulders above the hands throughout the exercise.

- ☐ The movement occurs in the trunk, between the hip joints and shoulder joints.

- ☐ Maximize flexion of the lower back during the first phase and extension in the mid- and upper back during the second phase.

- ☐ During the first phase, avoid rounding the upper back excessively, dropping the head too far between the arms, or tucking the pelvis aggressively.

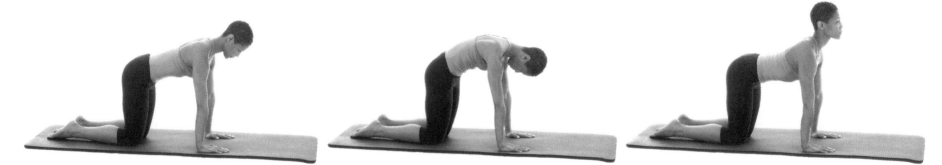

Inhale. Kneel in a quadruped position, with the knees hip-width apart and the hands shoulder-width apart. Establish a neutral position of the spine, with the weight evenly distributed between the upper and lower body. Sense the elongation of the spine from the tailbone to the top of the head, while drawing awareness to the internal support system.

Exhale. Engage the abdominal muscles and draw the spine into flexion while accentuating the curve in the lower back region, allowing the head and pelvis to respond and follow the natural line of the spine.

Inhale. Return to the neutral elongated spinal position. Do not release the abdominal or back muscles during this phase; they continue co-contracting to create a stable trunk.

Exhale. Extend the back, accentuating the arch in the mid- and upper spine, while maintaining stability of the pelvic–lumbar region. Externally rotating the shoulders slightly helps to facilitate the upper back extension.

Inhale. Follow the extension by returning to the start position (neutral spine).

Single-Leg Kick

The setup in this exercise is important, because the positioning of the body can place excessive pressure on the lower back if good abdominal support is not present. The back extensor work should focus on supporting the mid- and upper back. The arms, of course, also add support, and good scapular stabilization is imperative. Position the lower arms either in a triangular shape with the fingers interlaced or parallel to each other. In either case, place the elbows directly under the shoulders and stabilize the scapulae.

Imagery

The body position for the single-leg kick should be like a sphinx. The leg movement should be disassociated from the rest of the body's stable position, with the lower legs bending and straightening like the opening and closing of a handheld fan (when viewed from the side).

VARIATION

In case of discomfort or excessive pressure in the lower back, I recommend performing this exercise in a prone position with the hands together and the forehead resting on the hands.

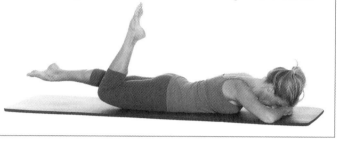

☐ Maintain scapular stabilization throughout the movement.

☐ Keep the pubic symphysis tilting up toward the sternum.

☐ Keep the lower legs lifted off the mat throughout.

Muscle Focus
- Back extensors
- Hamstrings

Objectives
- To develop hip extensor control
- To strengthen the mid- and upper-back extensors
- To improve trunk stabilization

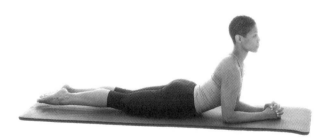

Inhale. Lie prone and, while engaging the abdominal muscles, lift the chest and extend the back. Place the elbows under the shoulders, positioning the forearms in a triangular shape with the fingers interlaced. Keep the legs straight and lift them slightly off the mat.

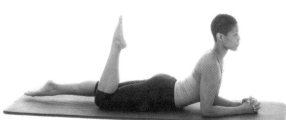

Exhale. Bend one leg and pulse it twice (exhaling on each pulse) then straighten it while simultaneously bending the other leg.

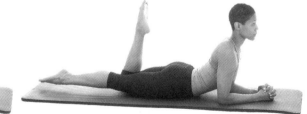

Pulse the other leg twice (continuing to exhale on each pulse). Repeat the same pattern of alternately bending and pulsing the legs, this time inhaling on each pulse, without changing the body position.

Muscle Focus

- Back extensors

Objectives

- To strengthen the back extensors
- To develop hamstring control
- To stretch the muscles of the chest

Double-Leg Kick

This is an exceptional back extension exercise with several important benefits in addition to strengthening the back extensors. First, the arms add support to the back extension, monitoring the load on the back. Second, holding the arms together provides an excellent chest and shoulder stretch. This exercise also provides good hamstring work and prepares you for Mat Work: Rocking. An elongated body position emphasizes the activation of the mid- and upper back as opposed to a high arched position, which would focus the work in the lower back.

Imagery

This is one of several exercises in which I like to visualize an archer's bow. The body is the bow and the arms form the twine. This powerful image also reinforces the elongation desired in this exercise.

☐ Keep the legs lifted slightly off the mat throughout.

☐ Relax the elbows to the floor during the down phase, placing the hands high up on the back.

VARIATION

Those with tight chest muscles and tight shoulders may lack the mobility to interlace the hands behind the back. Holding a small towel will enable them to execute the exercise and reap the benefits without placing excessive strain on the shoulders.

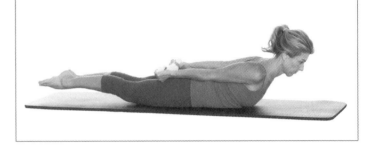

☐ Keep the head aligned with the spine when lifting into back extension.

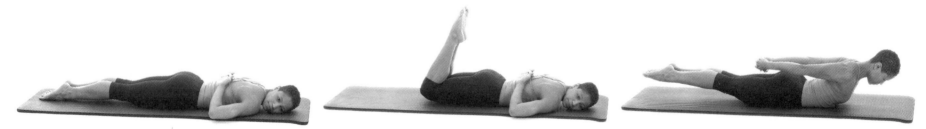

Inhale. Lie prone with the fingers interlaced behind the back. Allow the elbows to fall to the floor, and turn the head to one side, resting it on the cheek. Keeping the legs straight and together, lift them slightly off the mat.

Exhale. Bend both legs together and pulse them three times (exhaling a puff of air on each pulse), keeping the thighs lifted.

Inhale. Extend the back, lifting the chest off the mat. Simultaneously straighten the arms and the legs, and bring the head to the center.

Lower the body to the start position, resting the head on the opposite cheek.

Swimming

I love this exercise! It is so valuable in terms of developing strength and cross-pattern coordination of the back extensors and hip extensors. When the right side of the back is working, the left hip extensors are activated, and vice versa. This pattern is used frequently in everyday movements and recreational activities, most commonly in the normal gait cycle (walking). As we stride forward with the right leg, the left leg goes backward while the trunk rotates slightly to the right, resulting in the exact pattern of the swimming exercise—the back extensors of the right side working with the left hip extensors.

The breathing pattern for this exercise is similar to the Hundred, 5 counts to inhale and 5 counts to exhale, moving the limbs throughout.

Imagery

Imagine doing little flutter kicks with the arms and legs, as if both were doing the leg movement of the crawl swimming stroke in opposite directions. The trunk, from head to tailbone, is like a plank, with the arms and legs hinging around

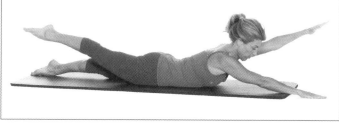

VARIATION

Beginners can make this exercise easier by allowing the arm and leg that are not being lifted to remain on the mat. This provides some support and recuperation time for the limbs.

small, independent axes and having no effect on the stability of the plank.

☐ Maintain trunk and pelvic stability throughout the movement.

☐ Avoid elevating the shoulders.

☐ Keep the movements of the arms and legs small.

Muscle Focus

- Back extensors

Objectives

- To strengthen the back extensors
- To develop trunk stabilization
- To build coordination and cross-patterning
- To improve shoulder flexor and hip extensor control

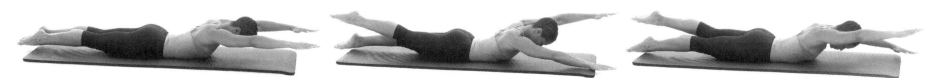

Exhale. Lie prone with the arms reaching forward and the legs together. Lift the chest, arms, and legs slightly off the mat.

Inhale. Lift the left arm and right leg concurrently. Return to the starting position and then lift the right arm and left leg. Start slowly and then speed up the movement, alternating arms and legs, until the movement is continuous. Perform this movement cycle while inhaling for five counts.

Exhale. Repeat the arm and leg movement cycle while exhaling for five counts. Continue this pattern for 10 breath cycles (inhalations and exhalations).

Complete the exercise by suspending the body in back and hip extension for a moment before lowering legs and upper body to the mat.

Muscle Focus

- Back extensors
- Hip extensors

Objectives

- To strengthen the back and hip extensors
- To improve hip flexor flexibility
- To stretch the muscles of the chest

Rocking

Rocking relies on the stable shape of the body and an inner energy to "get the ball rolling." It is difficult to articulate verbally how this happens; once you establish the shape, you shift the center of gravity slightly forward and away you go! Once in motion, it is about maintaining a solid position and utilizing momentum. I cannot overemphasize the importance of the hip extension. Reach the feet to the ceiling at the same time as you extend the back. I recommend actually engaging the knee extensors as if straightening the legs; however, with the hands holding onto the ankles, it forces the legs higher toward the ceiling and lifts the trunk higher into an arc shape. To start the rocking, use the hip extensors to lift the legs even higher and the body will tip forward. Once it has tipped forward, use the back extensors to lift back up. Alternate between lifting the legs higher and the trunk higher to keep the momentum going. Like the Mat Work: Swan Dive, this exercise relies more on stability and intricate muscle coordination than on pure flexibility.

Imagery

The body is the shape of an archer's bow: the body is the bow; the arms the twine. This is similar to the image in the Mat Work: Double-Leg Kick, however in this case the bow

VARIATION

A good preparation for this exercise is to lift into the rocking position and then lower down to the floor. Repeat this action several times without the rocking to develop flexibility, strength, and coordination.

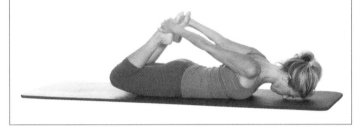

is taut in preparation for shooting the arrow. The position is much more arched. Another good image is that of a boat rocking forward and backward as it sails through the waves.

- ☐ Keep the head still and aligned with the spine.
- ☐ Maintain scapular stabilization with the arms straight.
- ☐ Keep the legs adducting, only opening as much as is needed to avoid pressure on the pelvis and the lower back.

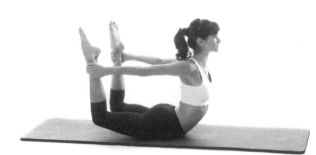

Inhale. Lie prone. Bend the knees and reach back with the arms, taking hold of the legs just above the ankles. Lift the trunk and legs into an arch.

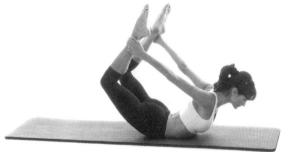

Exhale. Rock forward.

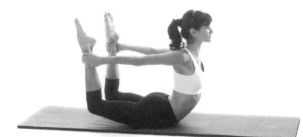

Inhale. Rock backward.

Swan Dive

The swan dive is a beautiful exercise to watch and a very difficult one to execute well. It embodies many of the movement principles of Pilates, particularly flow. This exercise is all about harnessing energy and keeping it moving. Although it appears to rely primarily on flexibility of the spine in extension, this is only part of the story. Flexibility is certainly important, but the essence of doing it well is stabilizing the trunk and activating the correct muscles in the correct sequence with immaculate timing.

You must hold the trunk in a firm position, created by the back extensors and hip extensors and supported by the abdominals. The abdominals assist in providing a firm surface and in distributing the extension through the entire back, working each vertebral joint, rather than concentrating the forces in the lumbar region.

I have seen many a young dancer, with a spine like rubber, struggle to do this exercise well. I am not blessed with a spine like rubber, particularly now as my body gallops toward 60 years of age. Yet I can still manage to achieve more height and flow in this exercise than many young and far more flexible movers. Success comes from years of practice in harnessing the enormous energy that becomes available when the body is unleashed into the forward dive. Hold the body stable, keep all the necessary muscles activated, and maximize the range of every vertebral joint in the spine, as well as the hip joints and even the shoulder joints.

Imagery

Visualize a big, well-inflated tire rolling back and forth. If it is not fully inflated, it will make jarring movements, getting stuck at certain points. So it is with the body: It will stop and start, even with the back extensors and hip extensors engaged, if the trunk is not held firmly in an arc shape. Many joints and muscles work harmoniously together to create this beautiful shape.

☐ Engage the abdominal muscles throughout the exercise.

☐ Maximize momentum and fluidity of movement.

☐ Maintain the arc shape of the body.

Muscle Focus

- Back extensors
- Hip extensors

Objectives

- To strengthen the back and hip extensors
- To develop trunk stabilization
- To harness energy

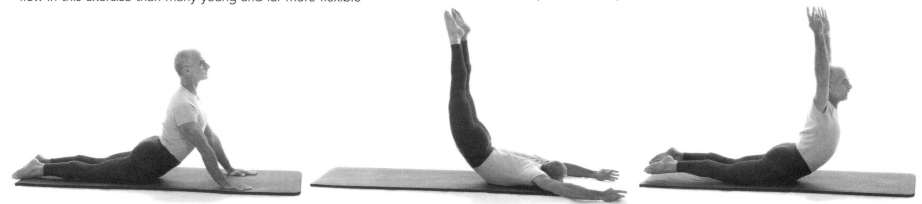

Inhale. Lie prone with the hands under the shoulders and the elbows on the mat. Contract the abdominals and extend the back. Keeping the elbows by the sides, straighten the arms and lift high into the arc position.

Exhale. Release the arms, dropping the body forward toward the mat. Reach the arms beyond the head, in line with the ears, and extend the legs up toward the ceiling.

It is helpful on the first drop forward to place the hands on the forehead with the arms bent and to straighten them as you rock back in the next step. From this point on, they remain straight overhead.

Inhale. Rock backward in an arc shape with the trunk upright, reaching the arms toward the ceiling and lowering the legs to the mat. Maintain the momentum and continue rocking, increasing the height of the legs and arms on each repetition.

On the final repetition, place the arms down and return to the supported arc position. Bend the arms and lower the body to the prone position.

Muscle Focus

- Lower back extensors

Objectives

- To relax the back and shoulders
- To rest the body
- To stretch the muscles of the back, particularly those of the lower back

Rest Position

This position is usually offered after back extension work. The rest position serves as a necessary pause, as well as a good transition into the exercises that follow in the mat work sequence. In a kneeling position, drape the upper body over the thighs. Allow the pelvis to sink toward the heels, releasing the neck, shoulders, and lower back muscles. This position is similar to the child's pose in yoga.

Imagery

Imagine the back spreading or melting over the legs. The back, pelvis, and shoulders are draped over the thighs and with each breath the back expands laterally and the relaxation deepens.

- ☐ Breathe naturally and deeply.
- ☐ Allow the pelvis to sink toward the heels.
- ☐ Allow the eyes to close if it feels more comfortable.

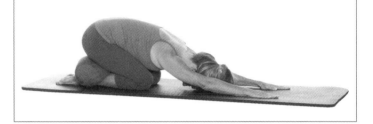

VARIATION

If you have a pre-existing knee condition, place a cushion between the pelvis and the legs so that the flexion of the knees is not as extreme. If you have back problems or other discomforts, you can drape yourself, prone, over a large ball. This will offer support to the trunk and reduce the stress on the knees, hips, and back.

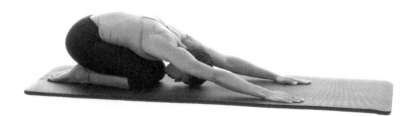

Kneel with the chest on the thighs and the pelvis resting on the heels. Place your forehead on the ground with the arms reaching forward or at the sides of the body, whichever feels more comfortable. Comfort is key.

5

Universal Reformer

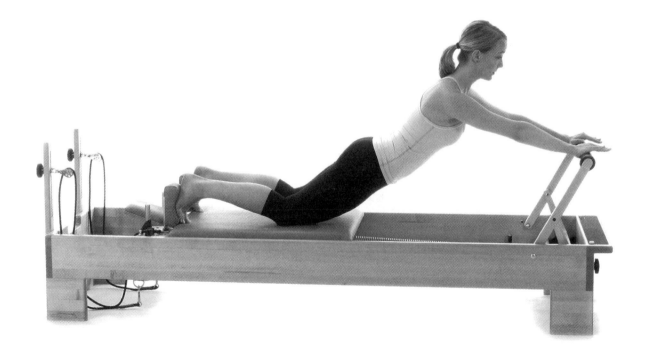

The universal reformer, commonly known simply as the reformer, is undoubtedly the most recognizable and popular piece of equipment in the Pilates menagerie. The scope of this piece of equipment is infinite, limited only by our own creativity and knowledge of the human body. It is the creation of a genius, a man way ahead of his time. The movements performed on the reformer range from fundamental to extremely advanced; they are performed in every conceivable position and for every possible purpose. This versatility exemplifies the method itself.

Each piece of Pilates apparatus has specific advantages and unique features. Just as a good carpenter chooses the correct screwdriver according to the head of the screw, so it is with the choice of Pilates apparatus—the device should be well suited to the task at hand. For instance, the reformer is probably the most user-friendly apparatus on which to perform the foot work; it places the body in a comfortable, non-weight-bearing supine position, facilitating balanced muscle recruitment. Performing the foot work on the reformer is less demanding than doing the same exercises on the cadillac or wunda chair, and the stabilization of the pelvis and trunk, although emphasized on all the apparatus, is most easily achieved on the reformer. The reformer also provides the teacher with a good vantage point to observe and correct alignment and muscle action.

The upper-body exercises that can be done on the reformer are unsurpassed in their diversity and comprehensiveness. The stretches performed on the reformer for the hip flexor, hamstring, and adductor muscles cannot be duplicated as effectively on the other apparatus. The reformer readily accommodates full ranges of motion, with a wide array of body position and resistance options.

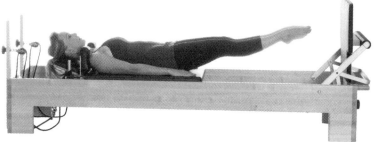

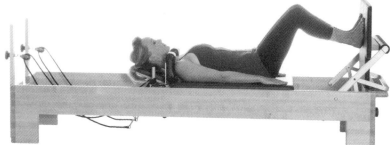

Jumping exercises, which are unique to the reformer, involve literally jumping, as you would on a trampoline, on the jumpboard (also called the foot platform), while lying supine. The jumboard offers exercises for athletes, dancers, and fitness enthusiasts who prefer to use the jumpboard to practice jumping and increase challenge. However, it can also be used by those who have difficulty placing their feet on the foot bar.

Foot Work

Foot work is a fundamental part of the Pilates workout. It can be done on the reformer, cadillac, and wunda chair. In order to be consistent, I teach the same comprehensive foot work routine on each apparatus. In the block system, the foot work typically follows the warm-up, because I see the foot work as an extension of the warm-up, providing a transition into the main body of the session. Although I label it foot work, it clearly involves the entire leg. In fact, it involves the entire body.

Focus initially on the positioning of the pelvis and the spine, because this forms the foundation of the work. I recommend maintaining a neutral pelvis and neutral spine position throughout the foot work. However, this *ideal* cannot always be achieved. In specific cases—for example, if hyperlordosis is present and the lower back muscles are hypertopic—it may be best to deviate from a neutral pelvis and spine in order to achieve correct muscle activation, void of excessive tension.

The position of the pelvis and trunk is essentially the same throughout the foot work. The aspect that changes is the positioning of the feet and legs. The musculature of the lower body is challenged in subtly different ways while the core remains constant. The focus of the muscle activation in this block is the hip extensors and knee extensors, with particular bias toward the hamstrings. Because of the overpowering quality of the larger and typically stronger quadriceps muscle group, it's important to ensure that the hamstrings engage. I prefer that the gluteals, which are also hip extensors, be relaxed during these exercises. This allows smooth, unrestricted hip movement and increases the probability of maintaining a neutral pelvic position.

Be sure to focus on both the concentric and eccentric contraction as the legs straighten and bend. The eccentric contraction, as the legs bend, is often overlooked. This dual focus is among the factors that make Pilates such an excellent regimen for functional training, as both concentric and eccentric contractions are employed continually throughout our daily activities.

When doing the foot work, I encourage straightening the legs completely. There is a tendency to stop short of fully straightening the legs out of fear of "locking" the knees. Failing to fully straighten the legs can lead to both muscular and neuromuscular problems. Not only are the muscles not strengthened in the last few degrees of their range, but the sensation of completely straightening the legs fades from memory, and *almost* straight begins to feel like *completely* straight. The knee joint was built to reach *full* extension and it should be used to its maximum potential.

In the exercise descriptions in this book, I sometimes speak of straightening the legs, or conversely of drawing the legs in, from the abdominals. Anatomically, this is clearly not accurate—there is no muscular connection between the abdominals and the legs. Yet, conceptually, the movement of the legs, when straightening and when bending, emanates from the powerhouse. Visualizing pushing the legs out or drawing the legs in from deep in the pelvic bowl—essentially recruiting the muscles of the internal support system (ISS)—encourages a stable foundation and smooth, flowing movement. I like to visualize the ISS as a steam engine, and the legs as cranks that are driven by that engine This image helps create the desired movement pattern as well as a sensation of warming up.

The foot work offers the teacher and the student a great deal of information regarding strength, flexibility, stabilization, alignment, asymmetries, and movement habits. In many ways the foot work resembles the gait cycle and as such gives insight into the way a person walks and runs. It is a fascinating area of study and should be observed from various angles.

Muscle Focus

- Hamstrings
- Quadriceps

Objectives

- To strengthen the hip extensors and knee extensors
- To warm up using the larger muscle groups
- To develop pelvic–lumbar stabilization

RESISTANCE

Light — Medium — Heavy

Parallel Heels

The heel position has two major benefits. The first is that it allows you to align and use the legs while initially taking the complex mechanism of the foot partially out of the equation. Although the foot is the foundation, it remains still; the movement occurs primarily in the ankle, knee, and hip joints. The second benefit of bearing weight on the heel is that you can more readily connect with the hamstrings when straightening the leg.

In the various heel positions, the foot should remain still, as if there were a floor beneath it. The pivot point is the ankle joint; in contrast, if the foot were in full dorsiflexion, the ankle would be stable and the foot would rock back and forth on the heel.

Imagery

Visualize a rubber band connecting the heels to the sit bones. As the legs straighten, the band stretches, creating a strong pull between the heels and the sit bones. Once the legs are straight, imagine the band overpowering your musculature and pulling the heels backward, despite your attempts to keep the legs straight. This process of creating internal resistance magnifies the eccentric contraction.

☐ Maintain a neutral spine and pelvis.

☐ Initiate the movement with the hamstrings.

☐ Keep the feet partially dorsiflexed and still, as if standing on the floor.

☐ Use the ankles as the pivot point of the movement.

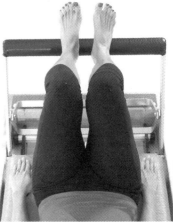

The parallel heels position allows full use of the ankle, knee, and hip joints.

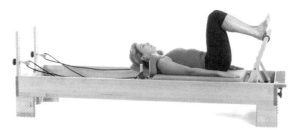

Inhale. Lie supine in a neutral spine position, with the heels on the foot bar, feet 2 to 4 inches (5 to 10 centimeters) apart, and the legs parallel. Relax the arms by the sides of the body, with shoulders positioned firmly against the shoulder rests. Place the head on the headrest (adjusted to provide optimal spinal alignment, free of tension).

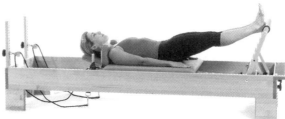

Exhale. Straighten the legs completely, extending the hips and knees while maintaining stability in the pelvis and trunk.

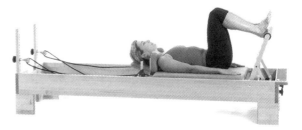

Inhale. Bend the knees and flex the hips, returning toward the stopper without hitting it or halting the movement. Maintain a consistent angle between the feet and the foot bar throughout.

Parallel Toes

During foot work exercises in the toe positions on the reformer, cadillac, and wunda chair, the foot should remain active, maintaining a consistent degree of plantarflexion—determined by the maximum plantarflexion that can be achieved when the knees are fully extended. As the knees bend, maintain this same angle of the foot to the foot bar, keeping the heels still and pivoting at the ankle joint (not the metatarsal–phalange joint). There is a tendency, particularly among dancers, to maintain maximum plantarflexion throughout the movement. This results in a rocking back and forth on the balls of the feet, eliminating the ankle as the pivot point.

Pressure should be evenly distributed throughout the front of the foot when pushing off the ball of the foot and the toes. The toes wrap gently around the foot bar.

The toe positions are more challenging than the heel positions. Not only are they more complex, with more joints involved, but they also feature greater resistance because of the added height of the foot. There is a tendency to drop the heel as the leg straightens, releasing the resistance, and then to lift the heel as the leg bends, placing the foot in full plantarflexion. This typically occurs when there is a lack of strength and the resistance is too high. Lower the resistance and focus on keeping the heel still. Working with less resis-

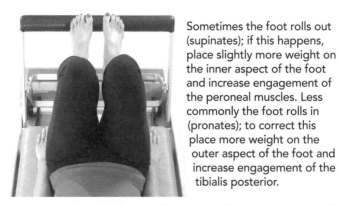

Sometimes the foot rolls out (supinates); if this happens, place slightly more weight on the inner aspect of the foot and increase engagement of the peroneal muscles. Less commonly the foot rolls in (pronates); to correct this place more weight on the outer aspect of the foot and increase engagement of the tibialis posterior.

tance in order to maintain the correct foot position is preferable to loading on the weight and compromising the form.

Imagery

Visualizing a rubber band connecting the heels to the sit bones works for all the foot work positions. When pushing off the toes you should feel a lifted sensation, as if you are pushing off a springboard.

☐ Initiate the movement from the hamstrings.

☐ Keep the heels still and the angle of the feet consistent throughout the movement.

Muscle Focus
- Hamstrings
- Quadriceps

Objectives
- To strengthen the hip extensors, knee extensors, and feet
- To warm up using the larger muscle groups
- To align the foot, leg, and related joints
- To develop pelvic–lumbar stabilization

RESISTANCE

Light   Medium   Heavy

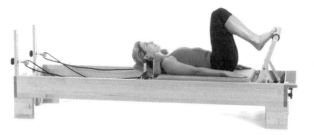

Inhale. Lie supine in a neutral spine position, with the toes softly wrapped around the foot bar, feet 2 to 4 inches (5 to 10 centimeters) apart, and the legs parallel. Relax the arms by the sides of the body, with shoulders positioned firmly against the shoulder rests. Place the head on the headrest (adjusted to provide optimal spinal alignment, free of tension).

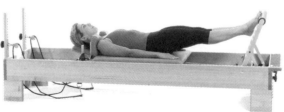

Exhale. Straighten the legs completely, extending the hips and knees while keeping the pelvis and trunk stable.

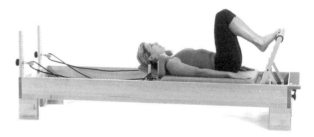

Inhale. Bend the knees and flex the hips, returning toward the stopper without hitting it or halting the movement. Maintain a consistent angle between the feet and the foot bar throughout.

Muscle Focus

- Hamstrings
- Quadriceps

Objectives

- To strengthen the hip extensors and knee extensors
- To warm up using the larger muscle groups
- To develop ankle control
- To bring awareness to the hip adductors

RESISTANCE

Light — Medium — Heavy

V-Position Toes

The extent of external rotation of the hips between the two hip joints in this exercise is not great, approximately 30 degrees, although this will vary somewhat with the individual. Dancers who are accustomed to working with much greater hip external rotation (turnout) should not compare this position to a first position in ballet—it is not. It is a classic Pilates position that can be more accurately compared to a military stance. (Dancers can add exercises that are specifically adapted to incorporate turnout, but it is not the norm.)

The exact position can be achieved when transitioning from the parallel toes position by simply bringing the heels together without adjusting the distance between the feet. Note that the V position is typically done on the toes only, making the transition to it from the parallel toes position seamless.

Imagery

Imagine straightening the legs and squeezing them together at the same time, as if you were holding a big ball or balloon between the legs.

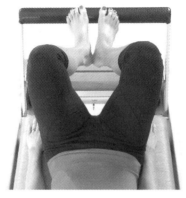

The V position offers comfortable, rather than maximal, hip external rotation.

☐ Initiate the movement from the hamstrings.

☐ Keep the heels still while squeezing them together.

☐ Straighten the legs completely, focusing on the co-contraction of the quadriceps and the hamstrings.

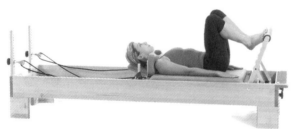

Inhale. Lie supine in a neutral spine position, with the toes on the foot bar 2 to 4 inches apart and the heels together, creating a V position with the feet. Relax the arms by the sides of the body, and touch the shoulders to the shoulder rests. Place the head on the headrest (adjusted to provide optimal spinal alignment, free of tension).

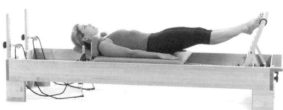

Exhale. Straighten the legs completely, extending the hips and knees while maintaining stability in the remainder of the body.

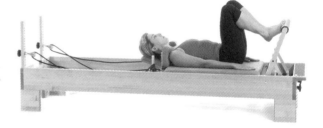

Inhale. Bend the knees and flex the hips, returning toward the stopper without hitting it or halting the movement. Maintain the same degree of hip rotation and a consistent angle between the feet and the foot bar throughout.

Open V-Position Heels

The wide V positions, of both the heels and toes, are not from the classic Pilates repertoire but offer valuable benefits. They take the hip joint into a wider, more challenging range of motion than most people are used to, in terms of both hip abduction and external rotation. I encourage you to explore this range as a means of achieving and maintaining optimal function of the hip joint. These open V positions also allow dancers (and other athletes who use similar movements) to correct their technique and develop strength in this range.

Imagery

As with the V-position toes, imagine straightening the legs and simultaneously squeezing them together, emphasizing the involvement of the hip adductors as the legs straighten and bend. When the knees bend, visualize them reaching out to the sides of the body along a diagonal energy line.

☐ Focus on engaging the hip adductors.

☐ Keep the feet partially dorsiflexed and still, as if standing on a floor.

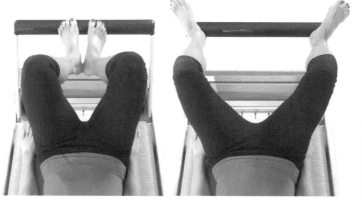

I suggest finding the position by keeping the shape of the V-position toes (consistent hip external rotation), then opening the legs wider and placing the feet toward the outside of the foot bar.

☐ Maintain correct tracking of the leg, aligning the hip, knee, and foot.

Muscle Focus

- Hamstrings
- Quadriceps
- Hip adductors

Objectives

- To strengthen the hip extensors and knee extensors
- To control the hip adductors
- To increase the range of motion of the hip joint
- To warm up using the larger muscle groups

RESISTANCE

Light　　Medium　　Heavy

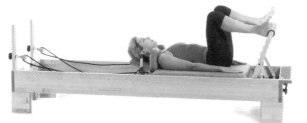

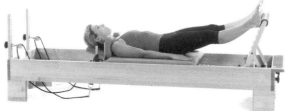

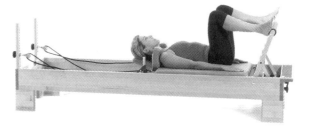

Inhale. Lie supine in a neutral spine, with the heels on the ends of the foot bar and the hips externally rotated, creating an open V position with the legs. Relax the arms by the sides of the body, with the shoulders positioned firmly against the shoulder rests. Place the head on the headrest (adjusted to provide optimal spinal alignment, free of tension).

Exhale. Straighten the legs completely, extending the hips and knees while maintaining stability in the pelvis and trunk.

Inhale. Return toward the stopper without hitting it or halting the movement. Maintain the same degree of hip external rotation and a consistent angle between the feet and the foot bar throughout.

Muscle Focus

- Hamstrings
- Quadriceps
- Hip adductors

Objectives

- To strengthen the hip extensors and knee extensors
- To develop hip adductor and foot control
- To increase the range of motion of the hip joint
- To warm up using the larger muscle groups

RESISTANCE

Light   Medium   Heavy

Open V-Position Toes

This wide V position on the toes is possibly the most complex position in the foot work block, because it requires tremendous control of the hip and knee joints and the feet. In addition, it offers the most stretch in the hip joint and a unique angle of challenge for the hamstrings and quadriceps. Although dancers will find this position particularly familiar and beneficial, many people can benefit from this "opening" of the hip joint.

Imagery

Employ the rubber band, springboard, and straightening-while-squeezing concepts used in the previous foot positions. In addition, the image of an open-leg squat may help you release tension in the hip joint and create a sensation of the pelvis opening and relaxing.

☐ Straighten the legs completely.

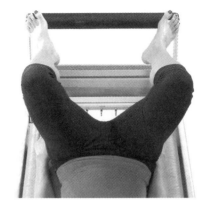

The vastus medialis oblique muscle (VMO) can be distinctly felt and strengthened (often a goal in corrective work of the knee) during this exercise.

☐ Keep the heels still throughout the movement.

☐ Maintain correct tracking of the leg; aligning the hip, knee, and foot.

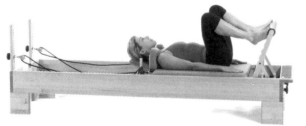

Inhale. Lie supine in a neutral spine, with the toes on the ends of the foot bar and the hips externally rotated, creating an open V position with the legs. Relax the arms by the sides of the body, with the shoulders positioned firmly against the shoulder rests. Place the head on the headrest (adjusted to provide optimal spinal alignment, free of tension).

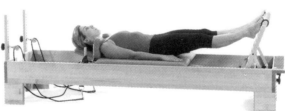

Exhale. Straighten the legs completely, extending the hips and knees while maintaining stability in the pelvis and trunk.

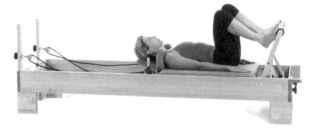

Inhale. Return toward the stopper without hitting it or halting the movement, keeping the heels still. Maintain the same degree of hip external rotation and a consistent angle between the feet and the foot bar throughout.

Calf Raise

This is an exceptional exercise for developing range of motion and strength of the foot, including the many muscles and joints that contribute to its movement. It also allows you to focus on correcting alignment of the foot, which is so important in walking, running, other everyday movements, and many athletic pursuits. Imagine the importance of exact and efficient foot alignment for a marathon runner, who repeats the same movement pattern thousands of times in one event, not to mention countless repetitions during training.

Pay particular attention to the eccentric contraction as you lower the heel. Do not succumb to the pull of the springs by dropping the heel; instead, resist the pull and actively dorsiflex the feet at the end range. Avoid the tendency to roll onto the outside or inside of the foot as you reach maximum plantarflexion. Limiting the range of the ankle joint and maintaining correct alignment, with weight proportionately distributed through the toes, is preferable to going higher and deviating from the centerline.

Imagery

The image of pushing the foot bar away from the body helps to achieve the desired amount of plantarflexion. The more stable the body is, particularly the pelvis, the more powerful each thrust will be. Think of 50 percent of the weight being concentrated around the big toe and the remaining 50 percent distributed through the remaining toes proportionately, according to size of the toe. This is an approximation but provides a good image.

- ☐ Use the full range of motion of the ankle.
- ☐ Maintain correct tracking of the hip, knee and foot.
- ☐ Align the foot correctly, focusing on the subtalar joint.
- ☐ Actively dorsiflex the foot when lowering.

Muscle Focus
- Foot plantarflexors

Objectives
- To strengthen the foot plantarflexors
- To develop foot control and correct alignment
- To warm up the muscles of the lower leg

RESISTANCE

Light   Medium   Heavy

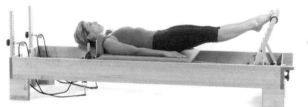

Inhale. Lie supine in a neutral spine position, with the toes softly wrapped around the foot bar 2 to 4 inches (5 to 10 centimeters) apart and the legs parallel. Relax the arms by the sides of the body, with the shoulders positioned firmly against the shoulder rests. Place the head on the headrest (adjusted to provide optimal spinal alignment, free of tension). Straighten the legs completely.

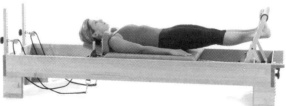

Exhale. Dorsiflex the feet, pressing the heels under the foot bar.

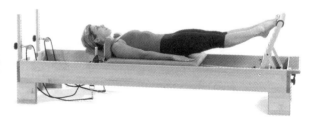

Inhale. Plantarflex the feet.

Muscle Focus

- Foot plantarflexors

Objectives

- To strengthen the foot plantarflexors
- To develop foot control and range of motion
- To develop pelvic–lumbar stabilization
- To warm up the muscles of the lower leg

RESISTANCE

Light   Medium   Heavy

Prance

Like the Reformer: Calf Raise, this exercise begins with the legs straight and the feet in maximum plantarflexion. One foot dorsiflexes while the other plantarflexes, both return to the start position, then the feet switch roles. Before the feet switch, it is important to go through the start position, with legs completely straight and both feet in maximal plantarflexion, to achieve a sense of height and elongation through each cycle. The stability of the pelvis and the profound work of the feet give this exercise the desired sense of flow, elevation, and lightness. The breath pattern also helps greatly in creating the desired flow.

Imagery

This movement is often used in dance training, and the image of a horse prancing is commonly given. Aim to achieve the grace, flow, and proud, upright feeling of a beautiful dancer or horse, barely touching the ground. Another image is of the foot bar as a trampoline, adding lift and buoyancy to the movement and emphasizing the upward thrust.

- ☐ Maintain a stable pelvis throughout the movement.

- ☐ Work both feet equally in their respective full ranges of motion; as one lifts into plantarflexion, the other presses down into dorsiflexion.

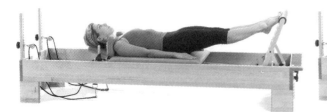

Inhale. Lie supine in a neutral spine position, with the toes softly wrapped around the foot bar 2 to 4 inches (5 to 10 centimeters) apart and the legs parallel. Relax the arms by the sides of the body, with the shoulders positioned firmly against the shoulder rests. Place the head on the headrest (adjusted to provide optimal spinal alignment, free of tension). Straighten the legs completely.

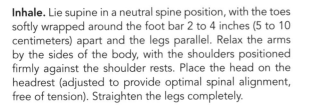

Exhale. Dorsiflex one foot and plantarflex the other. Switch the feet after transitioning through the start position.

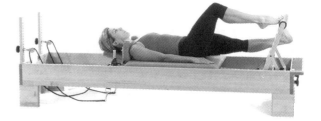

Inhale. Repeat the cycle twice. Continue for 10 complete cycles.

Prehensile

The prehensile position is one of the classic Pilates positions. Even so, I regard it as a unique and specialized position, and I don't necessarily offer it to students early in their training. Because of the unusual position of the foot and a relatively complex movement pattern, it is difficult to execute well. When used appropriately, it is certainly a very valuable position. It provides an effective stretch for the faciae and intrinsic muscles of the foot. When doing the prehensile as part of the foot work, I recommend it follow Prance.

Imagery

The most effective image is a bird wrapping its claws around a branch and holding it firmly.

☐ Keep reaching the heels under the foot bar throughout the movement to maximize the calf stretch.

☐ Wrap the forefoot around the foot bar, stretching the top of the foot.

☐ Keep the toes spread out rather than clenched.

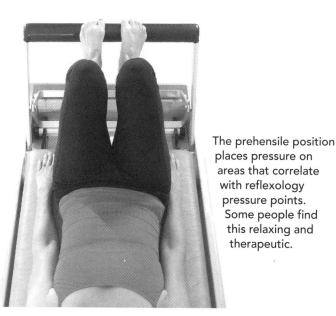

The prehensile position places pressure on areas that correlate with reflexology pressure points. Some people find this relaxing and therapeutic.

Muscle Focus
- Hamstrings
- Quadriceps

Objectives
- To strengthen the hip extensors and knee extensors
- To stretch the calf muscles
- To stretch the intrinsic muscles of the foot

RESISTANCE

Light   Medium   Heavy

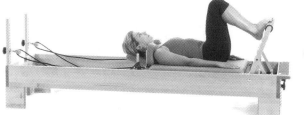

Inhale. Lie supine in a neutral spine position, with the forefeet wrapped around the foot bar 2 to 4 inches (5 to 10 centimeters) apart and the legs parallel. Relax the arms by the sides of the body, with the shoulders positioned firmly against the shoulder rests. Place the head on the headrest (adjusted to provide optimal spinal alignment, free of tension).

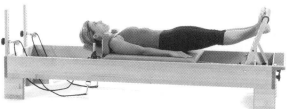

Exhale. Straighten the legs, while pushing the heels under the foot bar.

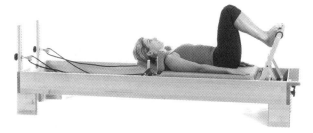

Inhale. Bend the knees, returning toward the stopper without hitting it or halting the movement. Continue pushing the heels under the foot bar.

Muscle Focus

- Hamstrings
- Quadriceps

Objectives

- To strengthen the hip extensors and knee extensors
- To develop pelvic–lumbar stabilization
- To warm up using the larger muscle groups

RESISTANCE

Light   Medium   Heavy

Single-Leg Heel

Working a single leg is invaluable for several reasons. First, it allows each leg to work independently, without relying on the other. Often one leg is dominant and will take over the work, continuing to get stronger while the less dominant side becomes weaker. This is particularly common following an injury or surgery. Working unilaterally (typically starting with the weaker side) will strengthen the weaker leg in an endeavor to create balance. It will also magnify compensations and misalignments, making it easier to detect them. Finally, exercising a single leg increases the challenge of keeping the pelvis stable. The single-leg series should be included in your program, if at all possible. I recommend preparing by placing both feet on the foot bar, then once good alignment has been achieved, you can lift one foot off without readjusting the other foot, the pelvis, and trunk.

Imagery

Imagine that both legs are on the bar and that you are pushing off both legs. In this way everything remains the same as in the double-leg positions. Visualizing the invisible leg helps keep the structure stable and balanced.

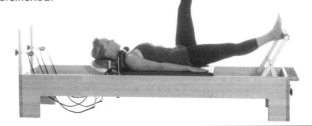

VARIATION

Many single-leg footwork variations are very beneficial. A good option for single-leg heel is to straighten the supporting leg toward the ceiling, as close to perpendicular as possible, as you straighten the working leg. The legs straighten and bend simultaneously. Keep both feet dorsiflexed.

- ☐ Keep the working foot dorsiflexed as if standing on the floor.
- ☐ Keep the supporting leg stable in a tabletop position.
- ☐ Maintain correct alignment and stability of the pelvis.

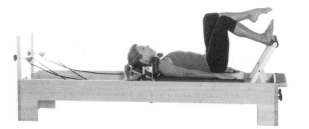

Inhale. Lie supine in a neutral spine position, with the heels on the foot bar 2 to 4 inches (5 to 10 centimeters) apart and the legs parallel. Relax the arms by the sides of the body, with the shoulders positioned firmly against the shoulder rests. Place the head on the headrest (adjusted to provide optimal spinal alignment, free of tension). Lift one leg and hold it in a tabletop position.

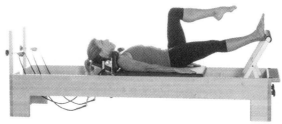

Exhale. Straighten the leg that is on the foot bar completely, extending the hip and knee while maintaining stability in the remainder of the body.

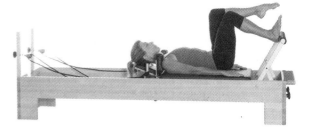

Inhale. Bend the leg, returning toward the stopper without hitting it or halting the movement.

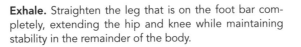

Single-Leg Toes

In this exercise, the feet and legs begin in a parallel position, with the toes wrapped around the bar, which is the most challenging position in the foot work in terms of load. Remember, working with a lighter load and correct alignment is always preferable to compromising good form for the sake of load. However, once you have achieved good form and control, increasing the load to challenge the foot musculature and improve strength can prove valuable.

Imagery

The desired sense of elongation of the movement is easier to feel in the toes position than in the heel position (see also single-leg heel).

☐ Keep the heel of the working foot still throughout.

☐ Straighten the working leg completely with each repetition.

☐ Keep the supporting leg stable in a tabletop position.

☐ Maintain correct alignment of the foot and stability of the pelvis.

Muscle Focus

- Hamstrings
- Quadriceps

Objectives

- To strengthen the hip extensors and knee extensors
- To strengthen the plantarflexors
- To warm up using the larger muscle groups

VARIATION

A good option for single-leg toes is to straighten the supporting leg just above the foot bar. As the working leg straightens, lift the other leg up so that it is perpendicular to the floor. In this position, dorsiflex both feet, plantarflex both feet, then bend the working leg and lower the supporting leg. Return to the start position.

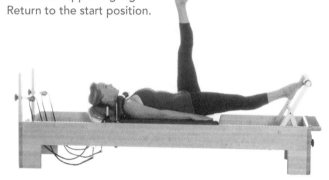

RESISTANCE

Light   Medium   Heavy

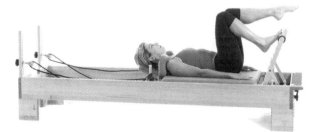 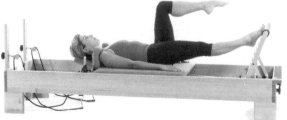 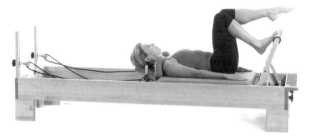

Inhale. Lie supine in a neutral spine position, with the toes softly wrapped around the foot bar 2 to 4 inches (5 to 10 centimeters) apart and the legs parallel. Relax the arms by the sides of the body, with the shoulders positioned firmly against the shoulder rests. Place the head on the headrest (adjusted to provide optimal spinal alignment, free of tension). Lift one leg and hold it in a tabletop position.

Exhale. Straighten the leg that is on the foot bar completely, extending the hips and knees while maintaining stability in the remainder of the body.

Inhale. Bend the leg, returning toward the stopper without hitting it or halting the movement. Maintain a consistent angle of the foot to the foot bar as the knee bends.

Abdominal Work

It is difficult to overemphasize the abdominal work in Pilates. The abdominal muscles are part of the powerhouse and they play a prominent role in a healthy functioning ISS. Even so, the abdominals are only part of the whole and not the entire picture. Because of the strong focus on abdominal work, people sometimes view abdominal exercises as the be-all and end-all of a strong core and of Pilates. They are not! A healthy balance of the musculature of the body, in particular the muscles of the ISS, is the goal, and therefore it is important to create some guidelines from the outset.

There are four layers of abdominal muscle: the rectus abdominis, the external oblique, the internal oblique, and the deepest layer, the transversus abdominis (TA). The TA is a fundamental ingredient in the powerhouse concept, which is part of every movement in Pilates.

The TA should be engaged throughout the Pilates session, as it plays a fundamental role in the stabilization and protection of the spine. Engaging the TA is a prerequisite to achieving the desired effect from abdominal work and the correct quality of movement.

It is interesting to compare, for instance, the typical abdominal crunch to the Mat Work: Chest Lift. They are seemingly so similar, yet the quality and arguably the outcome of each are entirely different, in large part because of the emphasis on TA engagement in the chest lift. The emphasis on the TA should not in any way devalue the importance of the other abdominal muscles, which, when working together as an integrated complex, serve as both an immaculate brace for the trunk and a powerful motivator for any trunk movement. Working the abdominals all together, precisely and with clear intention, is challenging to say the least. I have witnessed many tough and seasoned athletes who were

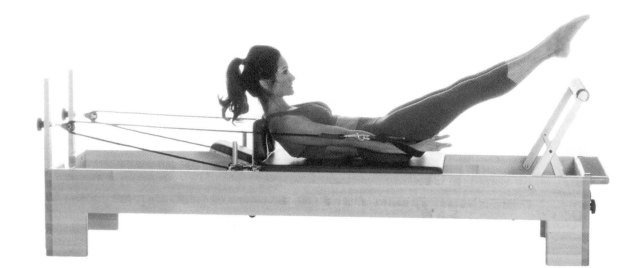

accustomed to performing hundreds of repetitions of abdominal crunches crumble after attempting 10 well-executed chest lifts.

When compiling the abdominal section of the Pilates session, take care to make it balanced. Use both isometric and isotonic (dynamic) exercises because each type of exercise develops the muscles differently and is important for optimal function. In addition, integrate sequences that are biased toward developing strength and those that are biased toward muscle endurance. Remember that the abdominals are recruited and trained not only during forward flexion, but during all ranges of motion, including spinal extension.

An image commonly used in Pilates to achieve the correct recruitment of the abdominal muscles is that of "hollowing" the midsection, specifically the abdominal cavity, of the body. It is this drawing in of the navel to the spine that encourages the recruitment of the TA. I like to visualize a hollow, deep, carved-out wooden bowl. The bowl is solid and stable, able to hold large amounts of energy and life force within it. Some teachers prefer to promote the concept of bracing the midsection as opposed to hollowing, similar to the effect of a corset. This is certainly valid. The common goal is a stable, supportive trunk forming the foundation of the movement, so use whichever image you prefer.

Finally, although we speak a great deal about the importance of spine stabilization and of the vital role the abdominals play in this process, it is important to keep in mind that stabilization is dynamic and ever-changing. The work of the abdominals, although powerful, is not rigid but pliable. Dynamic stabilization also facilitates natural breathing as it provides support for the spine.

Muscle Focus

- Abdominal muscles

Objectives

- To strengthen the abdominal muscles and shoulder extensors
- To develop pelvic–lumbar stabilization

RESISTANCE

Light   Medium   Heavy

Hundred Prep

The hundred preparation, or prep, is simple and very effective. You can immediately feel the abdominal muscles working and sense the synergy between the trunk flexors and the shoulder extensors. This exercise is a challenge for people of every fitness level, and it has many variations to meet different goals. It serves as an excellent preparation for the more advanced Reformer: Hundred and Reformer: Coordination, as it includes elements of both. Hundred prep is an isotonic exercise, which complements the many isometric abdominal exercises.

Imagery

The movement of the upper body and the arms during this exercise can be likened to a seesaw, alternately lifting and lowering as one unit. Achieving this integrated feeling that the abdominal muscles and the arms are working synergistically early in the abdominal work is important, because it is a recurring theme throughout the abdominal series and Pilates in general.

☐ Maintain a stable position of the pelvis throughout.

☐ Avoid hyperlordosis and bulging of the abdominal region.

☐ Keep the head aligned with the spine.

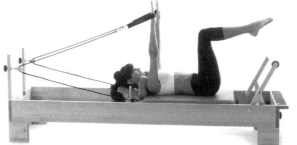

Inhale. Lie supine on the reformer with the legs in a table-top position (hips and knees at a 90-degree angle). Place the hands in the straps with the arms perpendicular to the body, maintaining slight tension in the straps. At this point the spine should be in a neutral position.

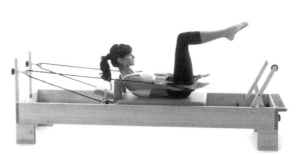

Exhale. Lift the head and chest, while pressing the arms down to the sides of the body and keeping the legs in the tabletop position. Coordinate the movement by first contracting the abdominals (which should remain engaged throughout), and then lifting the upper body while lowering the arms.

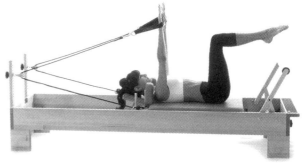

Inhale. Lower the upper body and lift the arms. Return to the starting position, maintaining muscle engagement and slight tension in the straps as you do so.

Hundred

This exercise is a signature exercise of the classic Pilates repertoire. Like the Reformer: Hundred Prep, it emphasizes integration of the abdominals and shoulder extensors. The slight up-and-down beating motion of the arms adds movement to the isometric activity of the abdominals and stimulates circulation and deep breathing.

This challenging exercise demands a high level of awareness, control, abdominal strength, and understanding of the concept of the ISS. The hundred and several other similar abdominal exercises involve isometric contraction of the abdominal muscles in the same position. Therefore supplementing them with isotonic exercises is important in creating a balanced abdominal conditioning program.

Imagery

Visualize the pumping action of the arms as a generator creating energy that gushes through the body, with the epicenter in the abdominal region. The hollow bowl image mentioned previously also helps to fortify the position of the trunk.

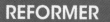
Muscle Focus
- Abdominal muscles

Objectives
- To strengthen the abdominal muscles
- To develop pelvic–lumbar stabilization

RESISTANCE

Light　　Medium　　Heavy

VARIATION

To make the hundred easier on the abdominals and alleviate potential strain on the lower back, keep the legs in a tabletop position.

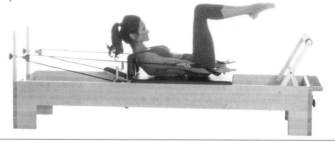

☐ Imprint the lower back into the mat throughout.

☐ Keep the head aligned with the spine and the eyes focused forward.

☐ Keep the carriage as still as possible as the arms pump up and down with small, calm movements.

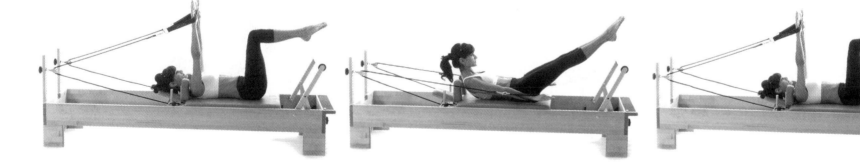

Inhale. Lie supine on the reformer with the legs in a tabletop position. Place the hands in the straps with the arms perpendicular to the body, maintaining slight tension in the straps. At this point the spine should be in a neutral position.

Exhale. Lift the head and chest while pressing the arms down to the sides of the body and straightening the legs. The position of the legs and angle of the hip joints will be dictated by your abdominal strength and control. The classic position, as Joseph Pilates performed the hundred, is with the feet opposite the eyes. However, if you are unable to maintain this difficult position it is quite legitimate to lift the straightened legs higher.

Inhale. Pause, deepening the abdominal contraction.

Exhale. Pump the arms up and down in a small rhythmic motion for five counts.

Inhale. Continue pumping the arms up and down for five counts. Repeat for 10 breath cycles, a total of 100 counts (hence the name *hundred*). Focus on the stabilization of the trunk and pelvis, maintaining forward flexion throughout. Return to the starting position.

Muscle Focus

- Abdominal muscles

Objectives

- To strengthen the abdominal muscles
- To increase pelvic–lumbar stabilization
- To improve coordination

RESISTANCE

Light   Medium   Heavy

Coordination

The name of this exercise hints at its complexity, particularly the coordination of breath with the movement, which is especially challenging. Although coordinating four distinct breaths with four movements might seem to make more intuitive sense and be simpler, I prefer to use two breaths for the four movements. Doing so creates better flow and continuity and encourages deeper breathing, with more active use of the respiratory muscles. It also makes it more challenging, which I personally enjoy.

During the movement, the body can either remain in trunk flexion (isometric contraction) or the trunk and head can be lowered after each repetition (isotonic contraction). Each version has its benefits, however, the head should never go halfway up and down (an area I call *the danger zone*) because this position will inevitably create excessive tension in the neck. Note the coordinated movement pattern of the shoulder extensors working in concert with the trunk flexors. This powerful partnership forms the foundation of this exercise.

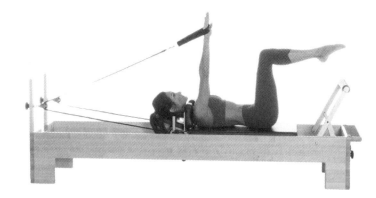

Inhale. Lie supine on the reformer with the legs in a tabletop position. Place the hands in the straps with the arms perpendicular to the body, maintaining slight tension in the straps. At this point the spine should be in a neutral position.

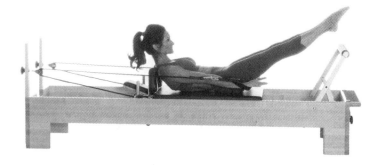

Exhale. Lift the head and chest while pressing the arms down to the sides of the body, straightening the legs, and keeping the feet at eye level.

The sequencing of the movements and muscle recruitment is of utmost importance.

Imagery

This exercise requires a rub-your-stomach-while-patting-your-head type of action. Picture a closed-loop mechanical toy that repeatedly goes through an identical sequence of movements. However, making your actions too mechanical will sacrifice the dynamic of the exercise and flow of the move-ment. The motion should be smooth, with the opening and closing of the legs a little sharper in dynamic than the lifting and lowering of the body as the legs straighten and bend.

☐ Keep the feet opposite the eyes when the legs are straight. Imprint the lower back into the mat when lifted in trunk flexion.

☐ Draw the knees in toward the chest before lifting the arms and then lowering the trunk and head.

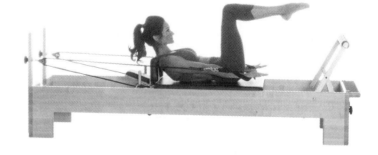

Continue to exhale, opening and closing the legs (no wider than the foot bar) in a brisk motion.

Inhale. Bend the legs into the tabletop position, then lift the arms and lower the trunk and head. Return to the start position.

Muscle Focus

- Abdominals

Objectives

- To strengthen the abdominals
- To develop hip flexor control

RESISTANCE

Light	Medium	Heavy

Round Back—Short Box

The round back exercise introduces the short box series, in which the Pilates box is placed on the reformer sideways to the carriage. The Flat Back and Climb-a-Tree, are also from this same series and lay the foundation for the Tilt, Twist, and Round-About, which involve lateral flexion and rotation. Although the entire series focuses on the muscles of the trunk, particularly the abdominal muscles, each exercise uses the abdominals in a slightly different way, and certain exercises fit comfortably into more than one block. "Borrowing" exercises from the short box series to fulfill a block other than the abdominal work block is quite legitimate. For instance, because of the actions involved, the Tilt, Twist, and Round-About exercises can be allocated as part of the lateral flexion and rotation block (where they appear in this book), as well as the abdominal work block.

The round back comprises two distinct positions: the initial upright position and the round-back C-curve position. To create the C curve, engage the abdominals focusing the flexion of the spine in the lumbar region. Allow the thoracic spine and the pelvis to respond to the action in the lower back while keeping the shoulders above the hips. The back extensors contract eccentrically, working in concert with

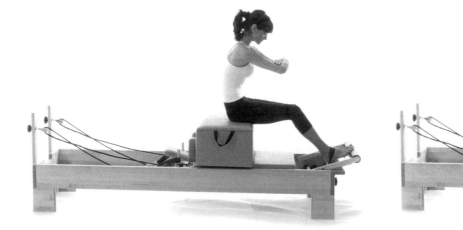

Inhale. Place the foot bar in the down position. Sit upright on the box close to the front. Place the feet under the foot strap with the toes on the foot bar (this will not work on all reformers), and cross the arms in front of the body. The legs are bent and stable and the feet are well secured so that all the movement occurs in the pelvis and trunk. All the springs are attached during the entire series to prevent the carriage from moving.

Exhale. Round the trunk, simultaneously lifting the arms away from the chest.

Still exhaling, lower the body backward with the trunk in the rounded position until the lower back rests on the box (or as close to it as possible).

Inhale. Pause in this position.

the abdominals to create the elongated C curve. Once you have established the shape (and only then), take the trunk back, pivoting at the hip joint, ideally to the point where the lower back rests on the box. Then lift the trunk again, returning to the position in which the shoulders are above the hips. At this point, extend the trunk into the original upright position. Imprinting these two positions of the trunk, upright and round back, in the muscle memory is important, because they form the basis of many of the abdominal exercises in Pilates.

Imagery

In the sitting position, the placement of the shoulders is above the hips. As the trunk is rounded, you should feel that the spine is being stretched from the back like a rubber band, creating the C curve. The spine continues being pulled back until the lumbar spine rests on the box, and then rises again so the shoulders are above the hips. Only at this point is the rubber band released, and the trunk returns to the upright position. Visualizing the opening of the vertebrae in the round position will make the spine feel longer and will help prevent it from collapsing. You should feel even more lifted and taller in the round back position than in the upright position. When tipping back, in the round back position, the action resembles pouring tea from a teapot.

☐ Establish the round back position prior to tipping back.

☐ Maintain the stable, round position of the trunk as it tips back and then lifts up again.

☐ Straighten into an upright position to conclude the exercise only after the shoulders are above the hips.

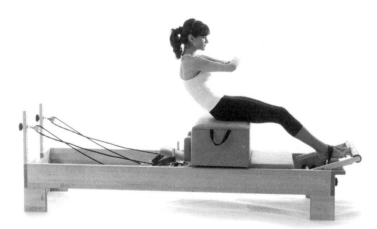

Exhale. Raise the body, maintaining the C curve of the trunk, until the shoulders are above the hips.

Inhale. Extend the trunk, sitting upright. Return to the start position.

Muscle Focus

- Abdominals
- Back extensors

Objectives

- To strengthen the abdominal muscles
- To develop control of the back extensors
- To develop control of the hip flexors
- To develop trunk stabilization

RESISTANCE

Light — Medium — Heavy

Flat Back—Short Box

The flat back exercise has similarities to the Reformer: Round Back exercise in terms of the action of the abdominals and the hip joint being the pivot point of the movement. Both exercises work the abdominal muscles, maintain a stable trunk as the body is lowered and lifted and feature movement in the same plane of motion, the sagittal plane. However, in the flat back exercise the abdominals contract isometrically together with the back extensors to hold the trunk in a neutral spine position (not a literal "flat back") as it is lowered and lifted. In the round back exercise, the abdominals do the bulk of the work to maintain the C-curve position as the body is lowered and lifted, and are supported by the back extensors only in so far as creating the C-curve shape. The hip flexors play an important role in both exercises, contracting eccentrically as the body is lowered and concentrically as it returns to the upright position, but they bear a greater load in the flat back exercise due to the longer lever arm.

The back and forth movement of the trunk is relatively contained and should not exceed 45 degrees when lunging back. Beyond this angle, there is a high risk of hyperextending the back; to avoid this, the pelvis and the trunk must move as one unit, hinging at the hip joint. If the pelvis stops and the upper body continues to tilt back, the result is hyperlordosis and excessive pressure on the lower back.

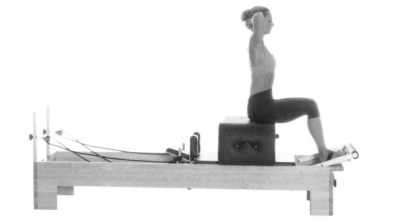

Exhale. Place the foot bar in the down position. Sit upright on the box close to the front. Place the feet under the foot strap with the toes on the foot bar (this will not work on all reformers) and the hands behind the head. The legs are bent and stable. Every effort should be made to keep the lower body uninvolved in the exercise.

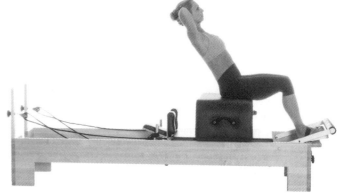

Inhale. Lunge back, moving the trunk and pelvis as one unit.

Imagery

The image of a closed door lying on its side, opening slightly on its hinge and then closing again, helps achieve the correct movement and form.

☐ Co-contract the abdominals and back extensors.

☐ Move the pelvis and trunk as one unit, hinging at the hip joint.

☐ Keep the head aligned with the spine.

Alternatively, the flat back—short box can be performed with the arms overhead holding a pole. This lengthens the lever arm greatly and, as a result, increases the challenge exponentially.

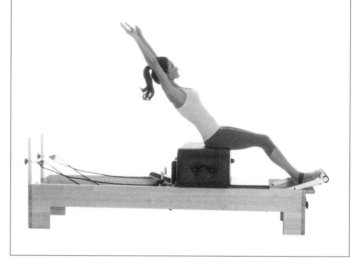

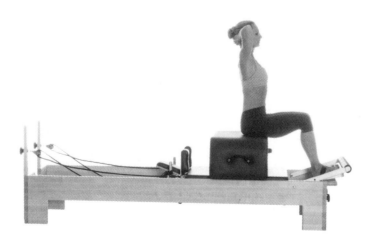

Exhale. Lift the trunk, returning to the start position.

Muscle Focus

- Abdominal muscles

Objectives

- To strengthen the abdominal muscles
- To develop control of the back extensors
- To stretch the hamstrings and chest

RESISTANCE

Light   Medium   Heavy

Climb-a-Tree—Long Box

Although this exercise in its classic form is performed on the short box (box sideways to the carriage) and is regarded as a part of the short box series of exercises, I recommend learning it (and prefer practicing it) on the long box (box longways on the carriage). The long box offers far more support for the lower back and facilitates a better stretch for the thoracic region. This makes it accessible to far more people. Whereas when performing it on the short box the hinge point is centered on the lumbar spine, potentially creating a shearing force on the vertebrae of the lower back. I recommend mastering this exercise on the long box before attempting it on the short box.

I encourage you to maximize the stretch of the hamstrings in the sitting position when the leg is straight by keeping the back extensors engaged and the trunk as upright as possible. It is important to maintain abdominal contraction throughout the exercise, particularly during the arm-circling phase, due to the potential for excessive pressure on the lower back at this point. Achieve deep flexion of the trunk as you climb down and then up the "tree" (leg), highlighting abdominal

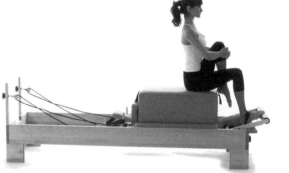

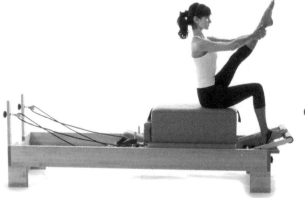

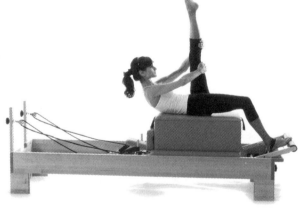

Inhale. Sit upright on the box close to the front. Place one foot under the foot strap with the toes on the foot bar (this will not work on all reformers). Bend the other leg, hold the knee, and draw the thigh to the chest.

Exhale. Pull the thigh to the chest and do three pulses, elongating the back and sitting more upright with each pulse.

Inhale. Hold the ankle and straighten the leg, while keeping the back as straight as possible.

Exhale. Walk the hands down the leg, lowering the trunk to the box in flexion. The upright leg moves to a position perpendicular to the box and holds still (like a tree trunk).

activation. It is important for the leg to be perpendicular to the box. When it is not high enough there is excessive load on the hip flexors and a tendency to hyperextend the lower back. This typically occurs when the hamstrings are tight. When the leg is taken beyond perpendicular, there is a tendency to hang on the leg. This scenario occurs when the hamstrings are very flexible.

Imagery

Imagine climbing down and then up a tree, keeping the body close to the trunk of the tree as possible by maximizing spinal flexion. The tree (leg) must be firm and stable in an upright position, reaching toward the ceiling.

- ☐ Begin the movement by sitting upright with the back extensors engaged.

- ☐ Emphasize trunk flexion when "climbing" down and up the leg.

- ☐ Keep the abdominals engaged, particularly during the arm-circle phase to avoid thrusting the ribs forward.

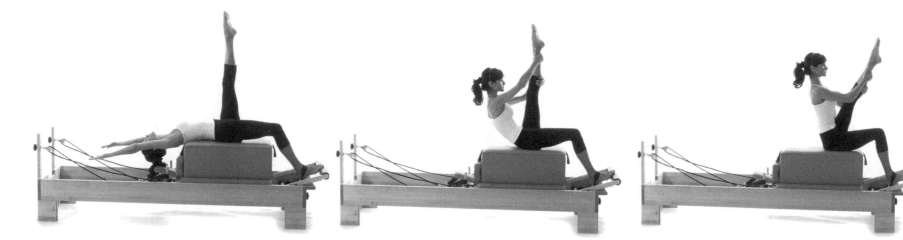

Inhale. Arch the mid- and upper back over the box while reaching the arms overhead and circling them around to the sides of the box.

Exhale. Return to trunk flexion and place the hands on the back of the leg. Climb up the leg, maintaining flexion of the trunk.

Inhale. Extend the spine while keeping the leg straight. Continue inhaling, bend the leg, and return to the start position.

Muscle Focus

- Abdominal muscles

Objectives

- To strengthen the abdominal muscles
- To develop pelvic–lumbar stabilization
- To develop shoulder control

RESISTANCE

Light   Medium   Heavy

Backstroke—Long Box

The backstroke is a complex, high-level exercise that demands coordination and strength. The potential for undue neck strain is great in this exercise, because of the perched position on the box, with the shoulder girdle hanging over the edge, and the resistance from the straps. This results in an enormous demand on the abdominals. Keeping a stable trunk and neck, as the arms and legs move independently is the key to the success of this exercise. In many instances, introducing this exercise on the mat or box without the straps is advantageous, adding resistance only when good coordination, muscle recruitment, and strength have been achieved. The eyes must focus forward throughout the exercise and not follow the arms as they straighten up toward the ceiling and then circle around.

Imagery

Imagine the trunk being a rowing boat, sturdy and stable. Think of the legs and arms as oars moving independently of the trunk in a circular motion. The pause following the circling of the arms and legs, with the arms pressing against the legs, places the body in a streamlined position. This is the point you should feel as if you are a boat gliding through the water after a powerful stroke of the oars.

- ☐ Keep the eyes focused directly forward throughout the exercise.

- ☐ Maintain maximum trunk flexion with the head aligned with the spine.

- ☐ Synchronize the movement of the arms and legs.

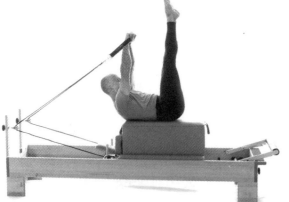

Exhale. Lie supine on the long box, facing the footbar, with the base of the scapulae placed at the back edge of the box. Lift the trunk into maximal spinal flexion and the legs into a tabletop position. Hold the straps with the hands in a fist position, palms facing up and elbows pointing outward. The hands are held opposite the forehead and above the sternum. Eyes are focused forward.

Inhale. Straighten the arms and legs directly up toward the ceiling (perpendicular to the box).

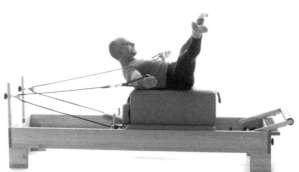

Externally rotate (turn out) the legs.

Exhale. Circle the arms and legs out and around.

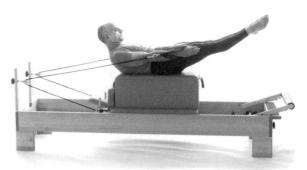

Still exhaling, complete the circle by bringing the legs together and the arms to the sides of the legs.

Pause with the legs straight ahead at eye level and the arms pressing against the outer thighs.

Inhale. Bend the legs and arms, simultaneously rotating the hips back to a parallel position. Return to the start position.

Abdominals With Legs in Straps

An understanding of the concepts of trunk stabilization and hip disassociation are prerequisites to proper execution of this exercise. If you have already learned the Reformer: Scooter and Reformer: Knee Stretch exercises, described later in this chapter (and I highly recommend that you do so), you can apply the previously learned movement patterns to this exercise, which is essentially the knee stretch in a supine position.

Because of the significant load on the hip flexors this exercise can create potentially hazardous stresses on the spine, particularly if the spinal stabilization, provided largely by the abdominals, is insufficient. This makes the exercise very challenging. Developing a good strength ratio between the hip flexors and the abdominals is important. Problems arise when one group (usually the hip flexors) overpowers the other.

A distinction must be made between the rectus femoris, a two-joint hip flexor, and the psoas and iliopsoas, which are single-joint hip flexors. The objective should be to focus on the latter, which is often overshadowed by the former.

To encourage use of the psoas iliopsoas, the feeling should be that the movement is emanating from deep in the pelvic bowl, rather than from the legs. It sometimes helps to imagine the legs being almost weightless and the abdominals pulling the legs in (in reality the abdominals only stabilize).

Imagery

Combine two images: the abdominal muscles creating a hollow bowl, anchored into the carriage, and the legs moving like pistons pumping in and out (with the emphasis on the "in" phase toward the body). The feet remain at eye level, moving along a horizontal plane.

☐ Draw the knees in toward the forehead.

☐ Move the feet along a horizontal plane, avoiding them dropping down or the knees bending excessively.

☐ Maintain pelvic–lumbar stabilization while imprinting the lower back into the carriage.

Muscle Focus

- Abdominal muscles

Objectives

- To strengthen the abdominal muscles
- To strengthen the hip flexors
- To develop pelvic–lumbar stabilization

RESISTANCE

Light	Medium	Heavy

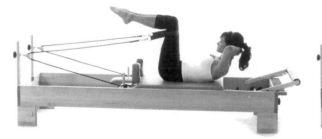

Inhale. Lie supine, with the back of the head close to the foot bar (it may feel more comfortable lowering the foot bar). The pelvis should be in front of the shoulder rests, touching the shoulder rests with the tips of the fingers. The arms are straight. Thread the legs through the straps, placing them just above the knees, and bring the legs into a tabletop position. Hold the trunk in forward flexion and place the hands behind the head.

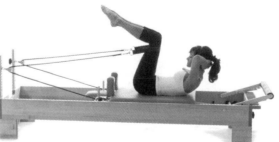

Exhale. Draw the thighs toward the chest.

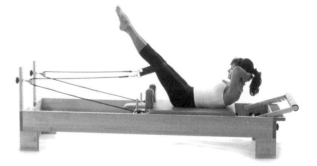

Inhale. Straighten the legs, maintaining pelvic–lumbar stabilization.

Exhale. Perform 5 to 10 repetitions, then return to the start position.

Muscle Focus

- Oblique abdominal muscles

Objectives

- To strengthen the oblique abdominals and hip flexors
- To develop pelvic–lumbar stabilization

RESISTANCE

Light   Medium   Heavy

Oblique Abdominals With Legs in Straps

This exercise is very similar to the Reformer: Abdominals With Legs in Straps but has the added component of trunk rotation. The element of rotation increases the challenge of maintaining pelvic stability—and works the oblique abdominals intensely. The upper body should move as one unit, with the elbows absolutely stable and pointing outward. Although the rotation of the vertebrae occurs largely in the thoracic spine, the sense should be that the upper body moves as a unit while the lower body is stable, with the movement occurring in the area of the waist. Think of the body as a series of discs; the lower disc (the pelvis) is stable while the upper disc (the trunk) rotates around the center, which is the waist. Mastery of the Mat Work: Criss-Cross is a recommended prerequisite for this variation.

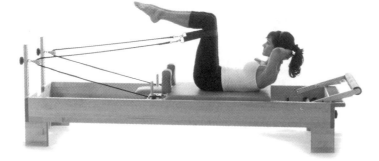

Inhale. Lie supine, with the back of the head close to the foot bar (it may feel more comfortable lowering the foot bar). The pelvis should be in front of the shoulder rests, touching the shoulder rests with the tips of the fingers. The arms are straight. Thread the legs through the straps, placing them just above the knees, and bring the legs into a tabletop position. Hold the trunk in forward flexion and place the hands behind the head.

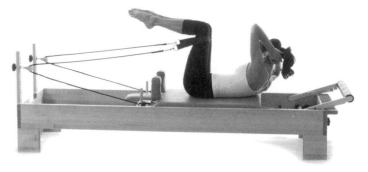

Exhale. Draw the thighs toward the chest and rotate the trunk simultaneously, bringing the upper shoulder toward the knees.

Imagery

As with the Reformer: Abdominals With Legs in Straps, think of the abdominal region as a hollow bowl, and the legs as moving pistons of an engine. Emphasize the inward movement of the legs toward the body.

☐ Rotate the trunk, as opposed to swiveling it (lateral flexion).

☐ Try to keep the lower scapula off the carriage during the rotation.

☐ Keep the elbows wide and stable and the shoulders relaxed.

☐ Maintain pelvic-lumbar stabilization.

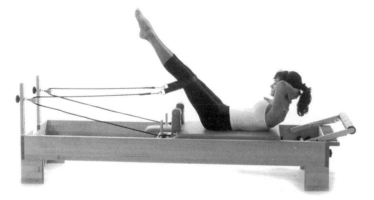

Inhale. Straighten the legs and keep the feet at eye level as the trunk returns to center, preparing to rotate to the opposite side.

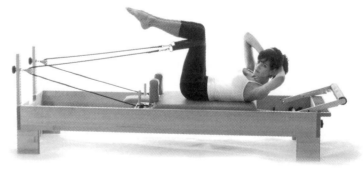

Exhale. Draw the thighs toward the chest and simultaneously rotate the trunk to the other side, bringing the upper shoulder toward the knees. Continue alternating sides, straightening the legs and bringing the upper body to center prior to each rotation. Perform 5 to 10 repetitions, then return to the start position.

Hip Work

The hip joint deserves special consideration and has earned a block unto itself. Its close proximity to, and profound influence on, the pelvis affects the whole body, up and down the kinetic chain. The hips play a key role in the gait cycle and many other daily activities, from climbing stairs to sitting down and rising up from a chair. Many muscle groups act on the hip joint, and they are prone to imbalance. For instance the gluteus medius, so vital in hip support and pelvic alignment, tends to be weak in relation to the other gluteals. The hip flexors often become tight while the hip extensors become relatively weak, due in part to a modern lifestyle that has many of us spending hours a day sitting. Imbalances of the musculature in this region are further compounded by activities with highly repetitive motions, such as cycling and running, as well as dance (particularly classical ballet), in which the hip joint is in external rotation (turn out) much of the time.

A concept that is emphasized in the hip work block is *hip disassociation*—the performance of a smooth, uninterrupted movement of the hip joint while the adjacent pelvis is kept absolutely stable. Mastering the concept of disassociation is important, not only in relation to the hip joint, but also to other parts of the body, such as the shoulder joint.

The hip joint can be viewed as a big spoon in a pot. The action used when stirring a pot is similar to the smooth action desired when mobilizing the hip joint. The balance of the musculature is critical, and a good choice of imagery can assist in mastering the often-intricate process of moving and stabilizing with different muscle groups.

Frog

The frog resembles the V-position in the foot work: Stability and alignment of the trunk and pelvis are maintained, and the basic action of the legs is the same. However, here the focus is on the hip adductors in addition to the knee extensors and hip extensors. As with all the exercises in the hip work block, the frog demands a high degree of pelvic stabilization because the feet are in the straps instead of on the stable foot bar. Note that the resistance is light, orienting the work toward stabilization as opposed to strength and requiring the weaker muscle groups of the hip joint to do more of the work. When the resistance is higher, the larger and stronger quadriceps tend to be dominant and the pelvic-lumbar stabilizers are not required to work quite as hard.

Imagery

The image of a frog jumping works well, although the dynamic of the exercise is relatively slow. Focus on squeezing the legs together as you straighten the knees, as if you were holding a big balloon between the legs. This squeezing encourages activation of the hip adductors and prevents overemphasizing the knee extensors.

- ☐ Stabilize the pelvic–lumbar region throughout the exercise.

- ☐ Avoid bringing the knees too close to the chest, causing the tailbone to lift.

- ☐ Squeeze the heels together continuously.

Muscle Focus
- Hip adductors

Objectives
- To strengthen the hip adductors
- To develop pelvic–lumbar stabilization

RESISTANCE

Light	Medium	Heavy

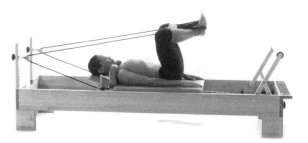 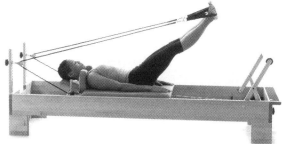 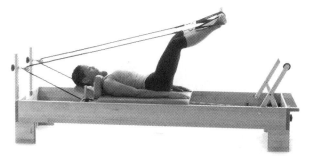

Inhale. Lie supine, with the spine in a neutral position. Place the feet in the straps and bend the knees, with the hips externally rotated. Softly dorsiflex the feet and press the heels together.

Exhale. Straighten the legs on a diagonal line, at an angle of approximately 45-degrees to the carriage.

Inhale. Bend the knees and return to the starting position.

Muscle Focus

- Hip adductors
- Hip extensors

Objectives

- To strengthen the hip adductors and hip extensors
- To develop pelvic–lumbar stabilization

RESISTANCE

Light   Medium   Heavy

Hip Circle Down

The hip circle highlights the concept of hip disassociation and demands a great deal of skill. It also activates the hip adductors prominently, emphasizing control and precision. Softening or even bending the knees slightly can be beneficial, in order to de-emphasize the quadriceps and emphasize the hip adductors. Keeping the pelvis stable and in a neutral position encourages correct muscle activation, with a good balance between the hip adductors and the hamstrings. The hamstrings tend to overpower the adductors at certain points in the exercise, possibly because most people are more familiar with using them and they are generally better conditioned. Be aware of this tendency.

Imagery

Imagine drawing the desired circular shape (two back-to-back semicircles as opposed to two true circles) in space with the feet. The legs squeeze together as they draw a line down the center and then part as they trace the semicircles, meeting again at the top. The size of the circle can be increased as more control is achieved. The movement should be fluid and the lines of the drawing smooth and continuous.

☐ Maximize the hip adductor work.

☐ Engage the hamstrings together with the adductors as the legs are lowered down the center.

☐ Maintain a stable neutral pelvic position.

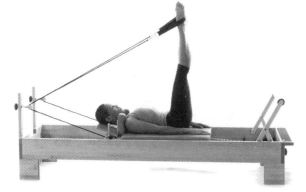

Inhale. Lie supine, with the spine in a neutral position. Place the feet in the straps and straighten the legs toward the ceiling, as close to perpendicular as possible, without tilting the pelvis. Externally rotate the hips and softly plantarflex the feet.

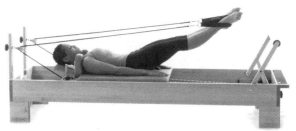

Exhale. Lower the legs straight down the center.

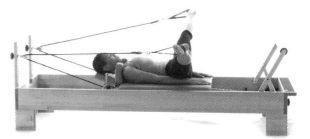

Inhale. Open the legs and circle them around and up to the start position.

Hip Circle Up

It is often easier to feel the adductors working in this version of the hip circle as compared with the circle down version. The load on the adductors is clearly felt as the legs come together to press against the resistance during the concentric phase of the exercise. In the Reformer: Hip Circle Down, the adductors work eccentrically during this phase, resisting the pull of the springs as they open. In both versions, the adductors should work isometrically as the legs press against each other when moving up and down the centerline.

Imagery

Imagine drawing the desired circular shape (two back-to-back semicircles as opposed to two true circles) in space with the feet. An image that I often use when working with the hip is that of a big spoon stirring thick syrup or porridge, the spoon being the femur and head of the femur. This encourages a smooth, fluid motion free of tension. Tension in the hip joint can often restrict the movement of the hip. Note that if the movement of the hip joint is restricted, the pelvis will tend to move around in order to compensate for the limited range of motion in the hip.

☐ Maximize the hip adductor work.

☐ Engage the hamstrings with the hip adductors as the legs are lifted up the center.

☐ Maintain a stable neutral pelvic position.

Muscle Focus
- Hip adductors
- Hip extensors

Objectives
- To strengthen the hip adductors and hip extensors
- To develop pelvic–lumbar stabilization

RESISTANCE

Light　　Medium　　Heavy

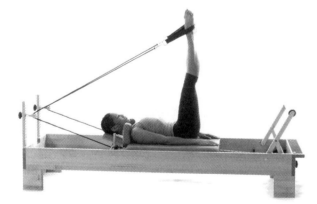

Exhale. Lie supine, with the spine in a neutral position. Place the feet in the straps and straighten the legs toward the ceiling, as close to perpendicular as possible, without tilting the pelvis. Externally rotate the hips (turn out) and softly plantarflex the feet.

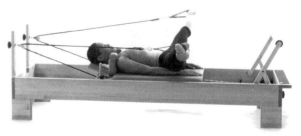

Inhale. Open the legs to the sides.

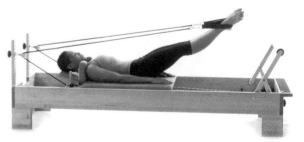

Exhale. Circle the legs down, around, and together to connect with each other, lift the legs up to the start position.

Muscle Focus

- Hip adductors

Objectives

- To strengthen the hip adductors
- To develop hip adductor flexibility
- To develop pelvic–lumbar stabilization

RESISTANCE

Light   Medium   Heavy

Opening

This exercise is a particularly valuable part of the feet-in-straps series because it places the body in an optimal position to explore the hip joint's functional range of motion (ROM)—the maximum ROM that can be achieved while maintaining the integrity of pelvic and spinal alignment. This exercise has the potential to develop control and strength in these extreme ranges, qualities that are particularly important for dancers, figure skaters, and gymnasts. Athletes involved in these endeavors typically have extreme flexibility, but they sometimes lack the muscular strength to support their expansive ranges of motion, which can result in injury.

Imagery

Imagine squeezing the legs against a large balloon.

- ☐ Keep the legs well supported so that they do not drop toward the floor.
- ☐ Maintain a stable neutral pelvic position.
- ☐ Maximize hip adductor ROM and activation.

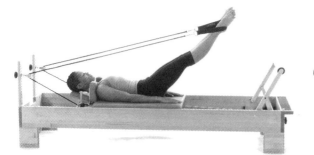

Exhale. Lie supine, with the spine in a neutral position. Place the feet in the straps and straighten the legs on a diagonal line of approximately 45 degrees. Externally rotate the hips and dorsiflex the feet, keeping the knees soft.

Inhale. Open the legs wide.

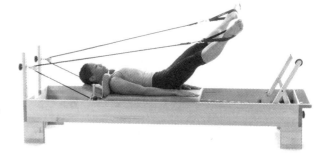

Exhale. Close the legs and return to the start position.

Extended Frog

The extended frog combines the Reformer: Frog with the Reformer: Opening, but it requires more control and coordination than either of those exercises. Maintain tension in the straps as the legs bend from the open-leg position into the frog position in the final phase by keeping the hamstrings engaged and the carriage still. I like to think of the movement as circular rather than linear, originating in the hip joints. The positioning and stability of the pelvis is critical; it provides a foundation for the exercise and accommodates the stretch by serving as an anchor.

Imagery

You should feel as if you were stirring an enormous pot of porridge, performing large circular motions with the feet and legs.

☐ Keep the carriage still as the legs bend in from the open position.

☐ Keep the pelvis in a stable neutral position throughout the exercise.

☐ Maintain hip extensor engagement as the legs bend, to prevent the legs from coming too close to the chest, causing the pelvis to tuck.

Muscle Focus

- Hip adductors

Objectives

- To strengthen the hip adductors
- To develop hip adductor flexibility
- To develop pelvic–lumbar stabilization

RESISTANCE

Light   Medium   Heavy

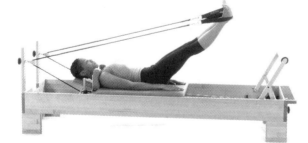

Exhale. Lie supine, with the spine in a neutral position. Place the feet in the straps and straighten the legs on a diagonal line of approximately 45 degrees. Externally rotate the hips and dorsiflex the feet.

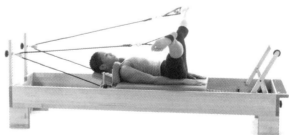

Inhale. Open the legs wide along the line of the pelvis.

Exhale. Bend the knees, bringing the heels together to the frog position, maintaining tension in the straps. When the heels connect, straighten the legs to the start position.

Muscle Focus
- Hip adductors

Objectives
- To strengthen the hip adductors
- To develop hip adductor flexibility
- To develop pelvic–lumbar stabilization

RESISTANCE
Light | Medium | Heavy

Extended Frog—Reverse

The extended frog reverse, although very similar to its sibling the extended frog, feels quite different. The stretch in the adductors is more intense as the legs are straightened out to the sides, and the work of the adductors is more challenging as the legs are brought together. Keeping tension in the straps and the carriage still is important as the legs straighten from the frog position to the open position, with the legs out to the sides. Maintaining hamstring engagement helps keep tension in the straps. Emphasize the circular action that occurs in the hip joints. The position and stability of the pelvis should not be compromised—if it tilts, the full potential of the adductor stretch will be lost.

Imagery

The movement should feel as if you had been stirring an enormous pot of porridge in one direction and have just reversed the direction of the stirring, using large circular motions with the feet and legs.

- ☐ Keep the carriage still as the legs straighten out to the sides.
- ☐ Keep the knees soft as the legs close, focusing the work on the hip adductors.
- ☐ Keep the pelvis in a stable neutral position throughout the exercise.

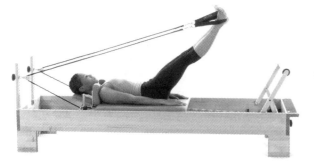

Exhale. Lie supine, with the spine in a neutral position. Place the feet in the straps and straighten the legs on a diagonal line of approximately 45 degrees. Externally rotate the hips and dorsiflex the feet.

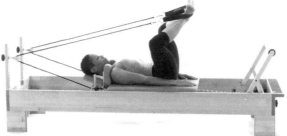

Inhale. Bend the knees to a frog position, keeping the heels together.

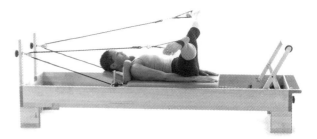

Exhale. Straighten the legs out to the sides into an open position without moving the carriage. Close the legs together, returning to the start position.

Spinal Articulation

The spinal articulation block incorporates the principles, and targets the muscle groups, that are fundamental to Pilates. The spine is the central pillar of the body, not only in terms of bone structure but also in terms of muscular support and neurological well-being. As Joseph Pilates wrote in *Return to Life Through Contrology*, "If your spine is inflexibly stiff at 30, you are old; if it is completely flexible at 60, you are young." Cultivating awareness and control of the intricate intersegmental movements of the spine is a lifelong process. Joseph Pilates specifically addresses the vertebra-by-vertebra movement of the spine in *Return to Life* and claims that this "rolling" and "unrolling" movement "gradually but surely restores the spine to its normal at-birth position with its corresponding increased flexibility."

In order to achieve the desired flowing movement, you must be acutely aware of the small intervertebral muscles and be able to control them. Breath is also an important component in spinal articulation; not only does it provide a rhythm to the movement, but it also encourages the recruitment of key muscles. In addition, spinal articulation can enhance the breathing process by "wringing" the lungs out as you would a sponge, which in turn allows them to fill to their full capacity.

The majority of the spinal articulation exercises move through spinal flexion, and it is typically this range of motion that we associate with the term spinal articulation. However, at times you may reap great benefits by visualizing spinal articulation as the spine extends. This is a difficult concept to grasp and is not recommended in all back extension exercises, but when used at the right time it can serve as an invaluable cue.

The abdominals play a prominent role in spinal articulation, whether it is articulation through spinal flexion or spinal extension, and whether the abdominals are functioning as movers or as stabilizers. Good abdominal control is a required ingredient for successful spinal articulation. Furthermore, the TA has a particularly profound role in facilitating efficient spinal articulation. Thus, spinal articulation should be practiced and mastered at all levels of Pilates work.

The image of a rolling wave describes spinal articulation exceptionally well. It conjures up not only the progressive curling action but also the feeling of the continuous flow of the waves. Being a man who loves the ocean—I swim, surf, and windsurf—any image relating to water inspires me. But even those who do not participate in water sports but have seen the ocean can appreciate the smooth, natural, rhythmic power of a rolling wave!

Muscle Focus

- Abdominal muscles
- Hamstrings

Objectives

- To develop spinal articulation
- To develop hip extensor control

RESISTANCE

| Light | Medium | Heavy |

Bottom Lift

This introductory exercise in the spinal articulation block is essentially a pelvic curl, which is typically the first exercise in the mat work, performed on the reformer. However, the element of instability introduced by the mobile carriage makes the bottom lift far more challenging than the pelvic curl. In addition, the range of motion is greater because the feet are placed much higher, on the foot bar rather than on the floor. Pelvic stabilization and spinal articulation must be mastered on the mat before proceeding to the bottom lift on the reformer. The hamstrings, which are crucial to the lifting and lowering of the pelvis, play an even greater role in this version; they act not only as hip extensors but also as knee flexors in order to keep the carriage in place. The movement of the carriage should be minimal; strive to keep it still and close to the stopper. The lower the spring tension is set, the more difficult it is to keep the carriage still and close to the stopper; also more work will be demanded of the hamstrings. Start with a comfortable spring setting, and as you become progressively proficient at this exercise, lower the tension. Note that the weight is on the balls of the feet, which demands foot stability and exceptional control of the ankle and subtalar joint to maintain good alignment.

Imagery

Use the image of a banana peel being peeled off the fruit, just as the spine is peeled off the reformer, and then the image of the peel being returned to the fruit as the spine is lowered.

☐ Minimize movement of the carriage.

☐ Align the feet, keeping the heels still throughout the exercise.

☐ Keep the legs parallel and the hip adductors engaged.

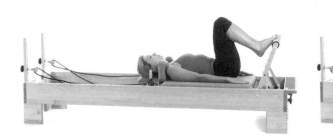

Inhale. Lie supine in a neutral spine position, with the headrest down (flat). Place the balls of the feet on the foot bar, with the legs parallel and the knees bent.

Exhale. Draw in the abdominal muscles and tilt the pelvis in a posterior direction. Articulate the spine upward, one vertebra at a time, extending the hips and lifting onto the shoulder girdle. Align the body along a straight line from the shoulders to the knees, avoiding hyperlordosis.

Inhale. Pause, holding this position.

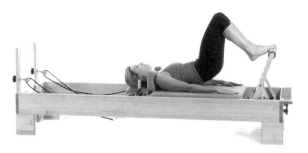

Exhale. Articulate the spine down to return to the start position.

Bottom Lift With Extension

Adding knee extension to the bottom lift accentuates the hip extensor component of the exercise and requires excellent pelvic–lumbar stabilization. Activating the hip extensors and the knee extensors facilitates the straightening of the legs, creating a suspended bridge position. Although the gluteal muscles may be recruited to help support the position, they are not the prime focus. An effort should be made to engage the hamstrings prior to the gluteals during hip extension, as there is a tendency for the gluteals to overshadow the hamstrings.

Avoid straightening the legs completely, as this can place undue strain on the lower back. When returning to the stopper, maintain the strong energy line from shoulders through the trunk to the knees; this helps offset the natural tendency to drop the pelvis and flex at the hip joint.

Imagery

The extended position resembles a suspension bridge—well supported and stable, with no breaks in the line of the body from feet to shoulders.

- ☐ Keep the heels still throughout the movement.

- ☐ Keep the knees soft; do not extend them completely.

- ☐ Lift the pelvis and extend the hips further as you bring the carriage toward the stopper.

Muscle Focus
- Abdominal muscles
- Hamstrings

Objectives
- To develop spinal articulation
- To develop hip extensor control

RESISTANCE

Light   Medium   Heavy

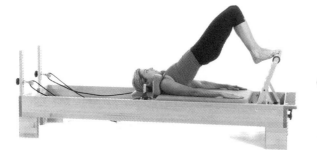

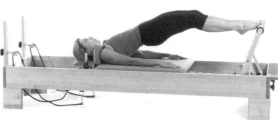

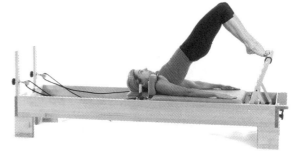

Inhale. Lie supine, with the spine in a neutral position and the headrest down (flat). Place the toes on the foot bar, with the legs parallel and the knees bent.

Exhale. Draw in the abdominal muscles and tilt the pelvis in a posterior direction. Articulate the spine upward, one vertebra at a time, extending the hips and lifting onto the shoulder girdle. Form a straight line from the shoulders to the knees, avoiding hyperlordosis.

Inhale. Pause in this position.

Exhale. Extend the knees (not completely) and the hips, without lowering the pelvis.

Inhale. Bend the knees, keeping the pelvis high and the legs parallel. Repeat this movement 5 to 10 times.

Exhale. Articulate the spine down, returning to the start position.

157

Muscle Focus

- Abdominal muscles
- Hamstrings

Objectives

- To develop spinal articulation
- To strengthen the hip extensors
- To increase upper back and shoulder flexibility

RESISTANCE

Light   Medium   Heavy

Semicircle

The semicircle is a progression of the bottom lift with extension, however the position is more challenging and the ranges of motion are more demanding. Greater control and the recruitment of several additional muscle groups are required. The raised position of the pelvis and the V position of the legs demand increased hip adductor and extensor control to keep the hip flexors stretched and the legs well aligned. (The legs tend to splay due to tight hip flexors and overuse of the gluteal muscles.) Keeping the pelvis lifted and the legs in a moderate V position as the carriage returns toward the stopper ensures an effective stretch of the hip flexors.

This exercise offers an opportunity to take advantage of the range of motion by not stopping in a neutral position of the spine, but continuing into hyperextention. The increased range benefits not only the lower body but the upper body as well. It emphasizes shoulder stability and flexibility, as well as extension of the thoracic spine. This stretch of the thoracic region is particularly beneficial for people who have tight shoulder and chest muscles, and the round-shoulder posture that is so prevalent today.

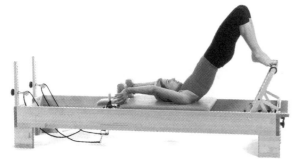

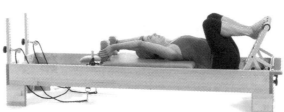

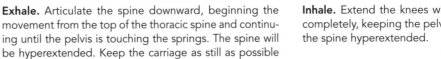

Inhale. Lie on the carriage with the feet in a small V position, toes on the foot bar and heels together. Lift the pelvis and fully extend the hips. Press the hands against the shoulder rests and straighten the arms, lifting onto the shoulder girdle and keeping the pelvis elevated.

Exhale. Articulate the spine downward, beginning the movement from the top of the thoracic spine and continuing until the pelvis is touching the springs. The spine will be hyperextended. Keep the carriage as still as possible during this phase.

Inhale. Extend the knees without straightening the legs completely, keeping the pelvis just above the springs and the spine hyperextended.

Imagery

The movement of the semicircle should feel like a rolling wave with no beginning and no end. The sensation of flow is extremely profound. It is a beautiful exercise to do and watch.

☐ Minimize the movement of the carriage when articulating the spine up and down.

☐ Squeeze the heels together throughout the exercise, maintaining a small V position of the feet.

☐ Keep the arms straight.

<table>
<tr><td>VARIATION</td></tr>
<tr><td>The direction of this sequence can be reversed. From the start position, extend the knees but do not straighten them completely. Roll the spine down, without moving the carriage, placing the pelvis close to the springs. Then bend the knees, bringing the carriage in toward the stopper, and roll up to the start position.</td></tr>
</table>

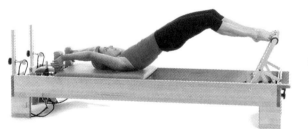

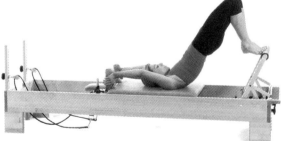

Exhale. Draw in the abdominal muscles, tilt the pelvis in a posterior direction, and articulate the spine upward, one vertebra at a time, lifting onto the shoulder girdle and reaching full hip extension. Keep the carriage as still as possible during this phase.

Inhale. Bend the knees, keeping the hips extended and the pelvis lifted. Return to the start position.

Muscle Focus

- Abdominal muscles

Objectives

- To develop spinal articulation
- To increase flexibility in the lower back and hamstrings

RESISTANCE

Light   Medium   Heavy

Short Spine

This version of the short spine is slightly different from the exercise performed by Joseph Pilates. In the classic version, the roll-up onto the shoulders is performed as the carriage moves toward the stopper. In this version the roll-up is performed with the carriage stationary and positioned firmly against the stopper. Not relying on the springs or straps during the roll-up requires greater abdominal control and a flexible spine. In addition, by taking the carriage all the way to the stopper first, you will achieve a more effective hamstring stretch as you bring the legs over the face. During this phase,

keep the pelvis as stable as possible and the sacrum as close to the carriage as possible. Most people find it impossible to keep the pelvis in a neutral position as the legs go over, but anchoring the sacrum by drawing it toward the carriage helps stabilize the pelvis and ensures a significant hamstring stretch.

When the legs are overhead, bend the knees, keeping tension in the straps and the trunk stable (not collapsing). Keep the feet positioned above the face and the legs in a diamond shape, as the spine rolls down, vertebra by vertebra, onto the carriage. This provides a wonderful stretch for the

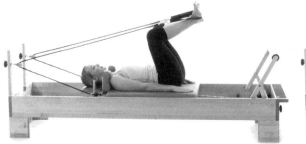

Inhale. Lie supine, with the feet in the straps in the frog position, hips in external rotation, knees bent, heels together, and feet dorsiflexed. Note that the headrest must be down.

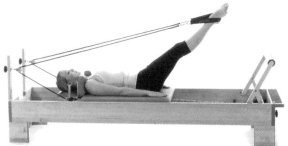

Exhale. Straighten the legs and plantarflex the feet.

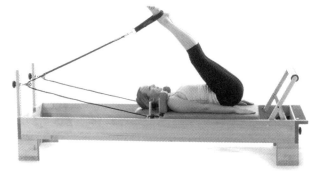

Inhale. Bring the legs overhead, moving the carriage to the stopper.

lower back. Once the pelvis can move no further, dorsiflex the feet and take the legs across the body, extending the hips without bending the knees farther and maintaining the diamond shape. Finally, place the pelvis in a neutral position, returning to the start position.

Note that the extreme flexion of the spine, plus the potential weight placed on the cervical spine, precludes those with back and neck problems—particularly if discs are involved—from performing this exercise.

Imagery

Enjoy the flowing wave-like motion of this exercise. The energy should feel circular and never-ending. The sensation is similar to the Reformer: Semicircle.

☐ Bring the carriage all the way to the stopper before rolling up.

☐ Keep tension in the straps when rolling up onto the shoulders and bending the legs into the diamond shape.

☐ Maintain the diamond shape of the legs during the final phase, emphasizing hip extension and not bending the knees.

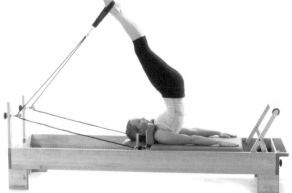

Exhale. Articulate the spine, rolling up onto the shoulders.

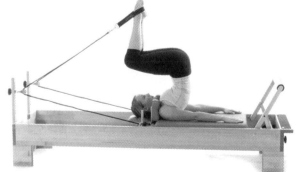

Inhale. Bend the knees, creating a diamond shape with the legs.

Exhale. Articulate the spine downward, keeping the feet above the face.

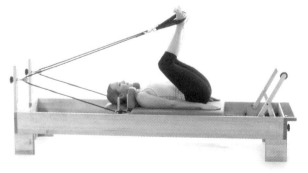

Inhale. Dorsiflex the feet, extend the hips to bring the legs across the body, and place the pelvis on the carriage. Return to the start position.

Muscle Focus
- Abdominal muscles
- Hamstrings

Objectives
- To develop spinal articulation
- To develop hip extensor control

RESISTANCE

Light   Medium   Heavy

Long Spine

This version of the long spine differs from the classic Pilates exercise, in which the carriage is stationary against the stopper during the roll-up onto the shoulders and the straps are lengthened to accommodate this position. In this version, the focus is on balance and stabilization during the roll-up and the roll-down. The carriage is still, but not against the stopper, with the springs in a tensioned state. Performing the exercise this way demands tremendous control of the ISS and the hip extensors, with assistance from the back extensors and shoulder extensors.

Maintaining the straight upright position of the legs, almost perpendicular to the floor, requires great control on the way up and even more on the way down. In the down phase, the eccentric contraction of the hip and back extensors allows smooth articulation of the spine without any movement of the carriage. This is a formidable challenge, particularly when the resistance is light.

I recommend that you start with medium resistance, and lower the resistance to make it more challenging as you gain more proficiency. Because this exercise can potentially

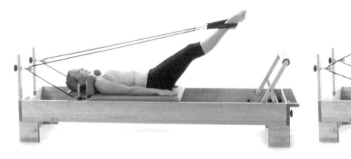

Exhale. Lie supine on the carriage, with the feet in the straps and the legs straight and together, forming a diagonal line at an angle of approximately 45 degrees to the carriage. The headrest must be down.

Inhale. Lift the legs to perpendicular position, keeping the sacrum anchored on the carriage.

Exhale. Roll up onto the shoulder girdle, articulating the spine. Keep the carriage still during this phase.

place weight on the cervical spine as well as on the back, those with back and neck problems—particularly if discs are involved—should not perform this exercise.

Personally this is one of my favorite exercises, but it can only be performed well once you have achieved a high level of proficiency in other less challenging spinal articulation exercises. There is definitely an element of danger in this exercise and it is important to recognize this fact. If you lose control while up on the shoulders, the springs will pull you onto the neck, placing great stress on the cervical spine.

Imagery

Imagine the legs being pulled up a boat's mast like a sail. Once at the top, the body remains as straight as the mast. The body is then lowered, like a sail being lowered down the mast.

- ☐ Keep the carriage still, completely in the balance, while articulating the spine up and down.

- ☐ Use the hamstrings eccentrically during the roll-down phase.

- ☐ Place the pelvis down firmly, anchoring the sacrum on the carriage, before returning to the start position.

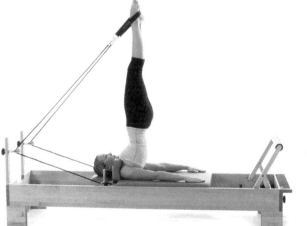

Inhale. Abduct the legs slightly, maintaining the upright position of the body.

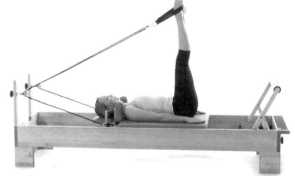

Exhale. Roll down to the carriage, articulating the spine. Keep the carriage still during this phase.

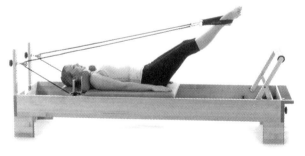

Anchor the sacrum, and then circle the legs down and around to the start position.

Stretching

Few would argue that flexibility is an important aspect of any fitness and conditioning regimen. This block of stretches should always be included in a well-balanced session. It is up to you to decide what part of the body should be emphasized in terms of flexibility. I suggest that a stretch for the hip flexors and hamstrings be included, if at all possible; these two muscle groups tend to be tight with many people and they have a profound effect on the alignment and function of the pelvis. Balance in the pelvic area is crucial. Even if a person is hypermobile, there tends to be an imbalance between the hamstrings and the hip flexors, and the focus may shift from flexibility to control.

Another area that deserves particular attention in terms of flexibility is the shoulder girdle. The shoulders tend to get tight, which severely affects the upper body and the neck, leading to deterioration in function and at times to pain and discomfort. I often add a stretching regimen for this area of the body.

Of course, flexibility of the spine is addressed in the spinal articulation block. Flexibility in general, but particularly that of the spine, deteriorates with age, making this an element of fitness that must be addressed. For optimum function at any level of activity, flexibility and functional range of motion are key.

Stretches need to be held for a relatively extended period of time to achieve relaxation of both the muscle being stretched and the body in general. The optimal duration of a stretch is debatable, but in general I prescribe holding the stretch for three to five breath cycles. Using visual imagery of the muscle elongating like an elastic band can be extremely advantageous. In addition, focusing on long and deep breaths is invaluable in achieving relaxation and a sensation of a deep stretch in the muscle.

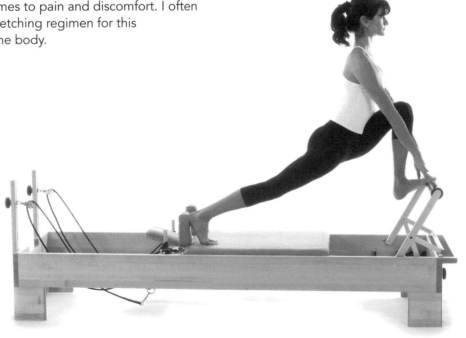

Standing Lunge

This is the first in the series of hip flexor–hamstring stretches. The primary focus of this exercise is flexibility, which is accomplished in two distinct phases: a hip flexor stretch and a hamstring stretch. Coordinated action of these two muscle groups helps create a balance in pelvic alignment and function. During the hip flexor stretch, bias the pelvis toward a posterior tilt by contracting the abdominal muscles (to lift the pubic symphysis) and the hamstrings (to draw down the ischial tuberosity). This position increases the stretch of the hip flexors and alleviates pressure on the lower back.

During the hamstring stretch, maintain a contraction of the back extensors, which draws the pelvis in an anterior direction and creates a deeper stretch of the hamstrings. It also strengthens the muscles of the back, particularly the mid-back, which are so important for healthy posture and yet are often neglected. Note that, throughout this series, the front knee never advances beyond the ankle while in the hip flexor stretch position, and the pelvis travels along a consistent horizontal line (without dropping or lifting) as the front leg straightens and the hamstrings stretch.

Imagery

The basis of every stretch is a stable anchor point. For the hip flexors and the hamstrings, the anchor point is the pelvis. The pelvis is anchored in a position that opposes the direction of the stretch in order to maximize the stretch. The pelvis is oriented in a posterior position for the hip flexor stretch, creating the feeling of a strong force pulling the pelvis up the front of the body and resulting in an arc shape of the trunk. The pelvis is oriented in an anterior position for the hamstring stretch, forming a straight energy line emanating from the back of the pelvis and running up through the spine and out the top of the head, creating a flat back. Thinking of these two shapes—arching in the front for the hip flexors and a flat, straight line in the back for the hamstrings—makes it easier to achieve the correct positions and maximize the stretches.

☐ Tilt the pelvis posteriorly and extend the upper back during the hip flexor stretch.

☐ Travel along a horizontal line with the pelvis when straightening the front leg for the hamstring stretch.

☐ Tilt the pelvis anteriorly, keeping the back flat and the head aligned with the spine, during the hamstring stretch.

Muscle Focus
- Hip flexors
- Hamstrings

Objectives
- To increase hip flexor and hamstring flexibility
- To improve back extensor control
- To develop pelvic-lumbar stability

RESISTANCE

| Light | Medium | Heavy |

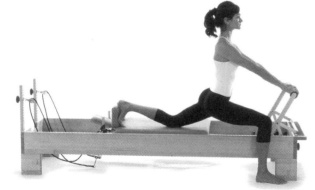

Stand beside the reformer with the hands on the foot bar, feet shoulder-width apart, and arms straight. Place the outside foot on the floor in line with the foot bar and the other leg on the carriage, with the foot against the shoulder rest and the knee on the carriage. Bend the other knee so that it is directly over the ankle, and maintain an upright position of the trunk. Focus on the hip flexor stretch and hold the position for three to five breath cycles.

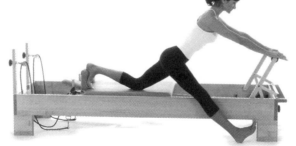

Lift the toes and dorsiflex the foot of the standing leg, pushing the heel into the floor; straighten the knee, keeping the pelvis on the same horizontal line as it travels back, and hinge the trunk forward. Keep the back as flat as possible and the back extensors engaged, focus on the hamstring stretch, and hold the position for three to five breath cycles.

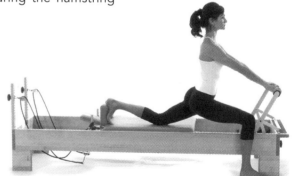

Bend the front knee and lift the trunk, with the pelvis traveling forward along the horizontal line. Return to the start position. Perform the sequence twice on the same side before changing to the other side and performing the sequence twice.

Muscle Focus

- Hip flexors
- Hamstrings

Objectives:

- To increase hip flexor and hamstring flexibility
- To improve back extensor control
- To develop pelvic-lumbar stability

RESISTANCE

Light   Medium   Heavy

Kneeling Lunge

The key principles of the hip flexor–hamstring stretches are consistent throughout the series. To maximize the stretch of the hip flexors, focus on activating the abdominals and tilting the pelvis posteriorly, activating the upper-back extensors, extending the thoracic spine, and creating an arc shape from the back knee through the thigh, pelvis, trunk, and head. To maximize the stretch of the hamstrings, focus on activating the lower-back extensors, tilting the pelvis anteriorly and keeping the pelvis and trunk square. Maintaining the alignment of the spine along a centerline is important. There is a tendency to align the spine over the straightening leg, which results in a lateral curve of the trunk.

In the initial position the front knee is aligned directly above the ankle, which is consistent in all the variations in this series. As the body transitions into the hamstring stretch, the pelvis travels along a consistent horizontal line and does not drop toward the carriage; at the same time, the angle between the kneeling leg and the carriage also remains consistent. This kneeling lunge position necessitates even greater pelvic stability and more flexibility than the standing lunge. A misaligned, unstable pelvis compromises its effectiveness as an anchor and subsequently compromises the stretch itself.

Imagery

The pelvis is the anchor of the stretch, whether stretching the hip flexors or the hamstrings. Align the pelvis to maximize the stretch and feel it pulling on the muscle and elongating it like a rubber band.

- ☐ Tilt the pelvis posteriorly and extend the upper back during the hip flexor stretch.

- ☐ Travel along a horizontal line with the pelvis when straightening the front leg for the hamstring stretch.

- ☐ Keep the back extensors engaged and the head aligned with the spine during the hamstring stretch.

- ☐ Tilt the pelvis anteriorly, keeping the back flat and the head aligned with the spine, during the hamstring stretch.

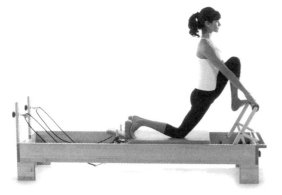 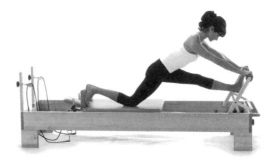 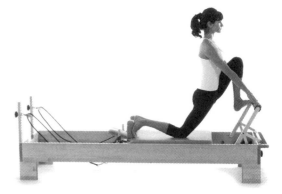

Kneel on the carriage and place one foot on the foot bar, with the knee directly over the ankle. Keep the other knee on the carriage, with the foot against the shoulder rest. Place the hands on the foot bar, shoulder-width apart, and maintain an upright position of the trunk. Focus on the hip flexor stretch of the kneeling leg and hold the position for three to five breath cycles.

Straighten the leg on the foot bar, moving the pelvis along a consistent horizontal line and hinging forward with the trunk to create a "crease" between the back leg and the pelvis at the hip joint. The angle of the back leg to the carriage should remain consistent. While keeping the back extensors engaged, focus on the hamstring stretch and hold the position for three to five breath cycles.

Return to the start position.

Full Lunge

This third stretch of the series is very challenging because it includes an element of balance. The front knee is again aligned above the ankle, but in this version the back leg is completely straight and in mid-air. As the body transitions from the hip flexor stretch into the hamstring stretch, the pelvis travels along a consistent horizontal line. This stretch is particularly difficult to control for hypermobile people, who, despite being very flexible, may lack the strength to support their extraordinary ranges of motion. Such an imbalance can lead to injuries. The full lunge develops strength and flexibility concurrently, resulting in a healthy balance between the two.

Maximize the stretch and protect the lower back during the hip flexor stretch by activating the abdominals and tilting the pelvis posteriorly. Emphasize engagement of the back extensors during the hamstring stretch and tilt the pelvis anteriorly

The added steps described in the variation section further develop control, heightened awareness of the core, functional strength and flexibility of the hamstrings and hip flexors, and, of course, balance.

Imagery

This position is a very powerful one, particularly when the trunk

Muscle Focus
- Hamstrings
- Hip flexors

Objective
- To increase hip flexor and hamstring flexibility
- To develop hip flexor and hamstring control

RESISTANCE

Light — Medium — Heavy

VARIATION

For added challenge, once you have mastered the full lunge, establish a strong start position, remove your hands from the foot bar, take the arms out to the sides, and balance with the trunk upright. Straighten and bend the front leg three to five times before placing the hands back on the foot bar and proceeding with the hamstring stretch full lunge.

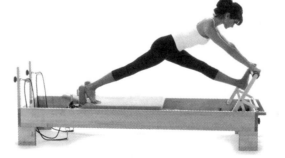

is upright and you are balancing in the lunge position. I like to relate it to the warrior pose in yoga; although the position is slightly different, the sense of strength and power is quite similar. As with all Pilates exercises the powerhouse is important, yet in this position there is a tremendous sense of strength emanating from the legs.

- ☐ Press the heel of the back leg against the shoulder rest.
- ☐ Keep the knee of the back leg straight throughout the exercise.
- ☐ Align the front foot with the hip joint on the same side.

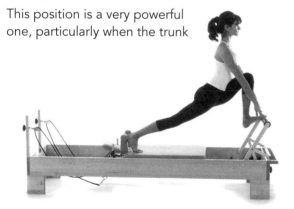

Stand on the carriage, with the hands on the foot bar, shoulder-width apart. Press the heel of one foot against the shoulder rest, with the toes slightly forward, and place the front part of other foot on the foot bar, with the front knee directly over the ankle. Maintain a lifted position of the trunk and keep the back leg straight. Focus on the hip flexor stretch of the back leg and hold the position for three to five breath cycles.

Straighten the front leg, hinging the trunk forward. Maintaining the back extensor engagement, tilt the pelvis anteriorly. Keep the trunk and pelvis square, and the head aligned with the centerline of the body. Focus on the hamstring stretch and hold the position for three to five breath cycles.

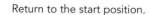

Return to the start position.

Full-Body Integration (FBI)

This block exemplifies the Pilates philosophy possibly better than any other. It is about the body working as an integrated, well-lubricated, and well-calibrated machine. All Pilates exercises are about the body working as an integrated unit, however, the exercises in this block are those that defy categorization by region of the body. The exercises in this block rely on the integration of the whole body for performance.

The many exercises in this block have been further categorized according to level of difficulty and complexity. Full-Body Integration I (Fundamental/Intermediate) includes the fundamental- to intermediate-level exercises. Full-Body Integration II (Advanced/Master) includes the higher-intermediate to advanced and master-level exercises. All exercises in FBI I should be mastered before proceeding to the higher-level exercises of FBI II. Please bear in mind that Pilates is not about learning the higher-level work and then never again doing the more fundamental exercises. Sessions should be a combination of different levels of the work and

include a variety of exercises. All FBI exercises demand a high level of body awareness; the better the understanding of the work, the deeper and more profound the results.

Several of the FBI exercises emphasize the *in* (forward) phase of the movement. In many instances, this will occur as the spring is shortening and the resistance decreasing. Yet the breath pattern dictates that you exhale, which we typically do on the exertion. Therefore, it is the reverse of the norm. I regard the leg going back as a *wind-up* for the leg coming forward, which is the *action*. As you pull the leg forward (hip flexion), you resist the pull of the spring, working the hip and knee extensors eccentrically and creating resistance within the musculature. In some of the exercises, such as the reverse knee stretch, there is an actual increase in the resistance as the legs move toward the trunk, with the hip flexors working concentrically, while, in many other exercises in this group, the resistance diminishes as the legs come forward and it should feel more like you are absorbing the force or the impact (eccentric contraction).

The resistance of the springs must correspond to the objectives of the exercise: whether the emphasis is on strength or stability. Differing tensions will result in very different outcomes. Increasing the tension of the springs emphasizes the leg work or arm work and strengthens the muscles in those limbs, whereas decreasing the tension highlights pelvic and trunk stabilization. I typically recommend starting with an emphasis on stabilization, therefore working with relatively light resistance.

Scooter

The scooter highlights the concept of disassociation, in which one region of the body remains stable, supporting another part of the body that is moving. In this exercise, the trunk, supporting leg, and pelvis remain stable while the opposite leg moves back and forth. The intention is to extend the moving leg to the point of full hip extension, without compromising pelvic stability. Given the positioning of the pelvis in a posterior tilt, this may mean that the knee does not straighten completely, depending on the flexibility of the hip flexors.

In establishing the position of the trunk, the first step is to draw in the abdominals and round the back. The flexion is focused in the lumbar spine, although clearly the entire spine is in flexion. Initiating the flexion from the lumbar region and allowing the pelvis, upper back, and head to respond to this action creates the desired shape and elicits the desired muscle activation.

There is a tendency to recruit the gluteal muscles excessively, as a result of the positioning of the pelvis. The hip joint must move freely in this exercise, and excessive gluteal recruitment often inhibits the movement of the hip joint.

There is also a tendency to round the upper back excessively. This inclination is due in part to the natural shape of the thoracic spine. Excessive rounding during this exercise should be avoided, as it diminishes the focus on the lumbar region and abdominal recruitment and encourages shoulder elevation. Worse, it reinforces the tendency to adopt an undesirable, unhealthy round-shoulder posture during the activities of daily life.

Imagery

The position for the scooter resembles a sprinter pushing back into the starting block before a race. It exemplifies power about to be unleashed. The power surges as the leg comes forward.

☐ Maintain a consistent C curve through the spine, including the head.

☐ Avoid elevating the shoulders.

☐ Focus on hip disassociation and pelvic stability.

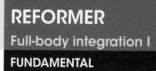
Muscle Focus
- Abdominal muscles
- Hip and knee extensors

Objectives
- To develop pelvic and trunk stabilization
- To strengthen the hip and knee extensors

RESISTANCE

Light   Medium   Heavy

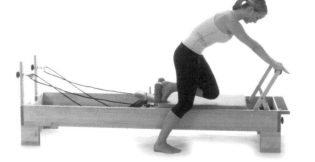

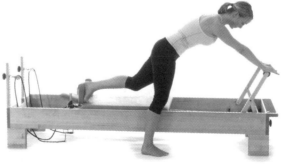

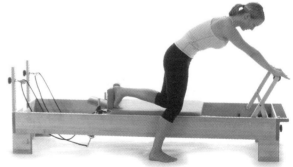

Exhale. Place the hands on the foot bar, shoulder-width apart, with the arms straight. Press one foot against the shoulder rest, with the knee slightly off the carriage. Place the other foot on the ground alongside the reformer. Bend the knee of the standing leg, lining up the heel (vertically) with the heel of the foot against the shoulder rest. Draw in the abdominal muscles and round the trunk.

Inhale. Extend the leg that is on the carriage, moving the carriage away from the stopper. Pause before the point at which the pelvis would start to move in an anterior direction.

Exhale. Draw the leg forward, bringing the carriage toward the stopper. Emphasize the inward motion, maintaining stability of the shoulders, trunk, and pelvis.

Muscle Focus

- Abdominal muscles

Objectives

- To develop pelvic stabilization and trunk stabilization
- To strengthen the hip and knee extensors (medium resistance)

RESISTANCE

Light — Medium — Heavy

Knee Stretch—Round Back

This exercise also utilizes the concept of disassociation, with the trunk in the same position as the Reformer: Scooter, except that now you are kneeling with both knees on the carriage and both legs are moving. The body is no longer supported by having one foot solidly planted on the floor. This makes for a much less stable position, significantly increasing the level of difficulty of the exercise. Maintaining stability of the trunk, including the pelvis, as the legs move backward and forward is crucial. Note that the extension of the legs in this exercise is smaller than in the Reformer: Scooter.

Achieving the desired alignment of the spine involves rounding (flexing) the lumbar spine and allowing the upper back and pelvis to respond, resulting in a gentle curve of the entire spine (including the head). I advise not tucking the pelvis or contracting the gluteals excessively; doing so restricts the movement of the hip joints, which in turn transfers the pivot point of the movement from the hips to the lumbar spine.

Imagery

Imagine the legs swinging back and forth like a pendulum that is placed on a slight diagonal. As the pendulum swings against gravity the movement is slightly slower, and as it returns with gravity assisting the movement becomes more dynamic.

- ☐ Maintain a consistent C curve through the spine, including the head.

- ☐ Emphasize the inward phase of the movement.

- ☐ Draw the carriage forward, as close to the stopper as possible.

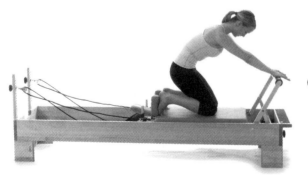

Exhale. Kneel on the carriage and sit on the heels, with the feet against the shoulder rests. Place the hands on the foot bar, shoulder-width apart, with the arms straight. Draw in the abdominal muscles, round the trunk and lift the pelvis slightly off the heels.

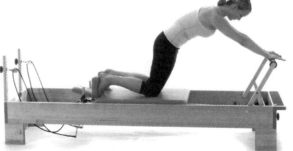

Inhale. Extend the hips, moving the carriage away from the stopper and keeping the arms and trunk stable.

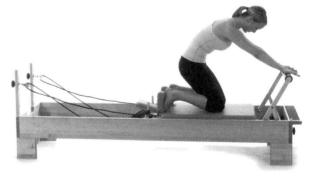

Exhale. Flex the hips, draw the legs forward, and bring the carriage toward the stopper. Emphasize the inward motion, and maintain stability in the shoulders, trunk, and pelvis.

Knee Stretch—Flat Back

In this exercise as in the Reformer: Flat Back—Short Box exercise, *flat back* means a neutral spine position, as opposed to an actual flat back, in which the natural curves of the spine would be eliminated. Co-contraction of the abdominal muscles and the back extensors keeps the spine in a neutral position, as opposed to the flexion of the spine seen in the Reformer: Knee Stretch—Round Back. However, all the other elements are the same, particularly the emphasis on trunk stabilization and hip joint disassociation. A strong sense of an energy line extending from the tailbone, through the trunk to the head helps maintain stability and alignment of the spine.

Imagery

Imagine a donkey kicking its hind legs back while balancing on its front legs and keeping the upper body stationary, then drawing the legs in vigorously preparing to kick again.

☐ Maintain a neutral spine position.

☐ Emphasize the hinging action of the legs from the hip joints.

☐ Keep the wrists neutral and firm, with thumbs and fingers together and straight.

Muscle Focus
- Abdominal muscles
- Back extensors

Objectives
- To develop trunk stabilization
- To strengthen the hip extensors and knee extensors

RESISTANCE

Light | Medium | Heavy

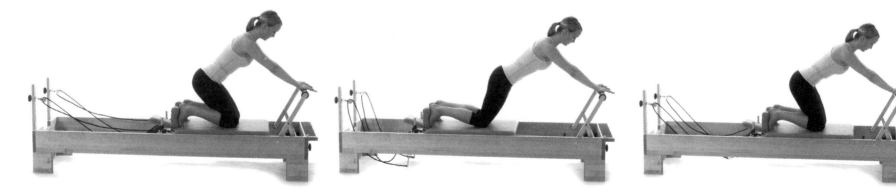

Exhale. Kneel on the carriage, sitting on the heels with the feet against the shoulder rests. Place the hands on the foot bar, shoulder-width apart, with the arms straight. Stabilize the shoulders, maintain a neutral spine and lift the pelvis slightly off the heels.

Inhale. Extend the hips, moving the carriage away from the stopper and keeping the arms and trunk stable.

Exhale. Flex the hips, draw the legs forward and bring the carriage toward the stopper. Emphasize the inward motion, and maintain stability in the shoulders, trunk, and pelvis.

Stomach Massage—Round Back

Muscle Focus
- Abdominal muscles
- Back extensors

Objectives
- To develop trunk stabilization
- To strengthen the knee extensors and foot plantarflexors

RESISTANCE

| Light | Medium | Heavy |

This exercise features vigorous, intense work of the legs (including the feet), while the trunk remains stable. In contrast with the supine position used for the foot work, the sitting position intensifies the demand on the muscles of the trunk, particularly the back extensors, and increases the challenge exponentially. With the trunk in an upright position rather than supine, the exercise is more functional—the muscles are used in a way that more closely simulates common upright movements and enhances postural muscle development. Daily activities such as sitting in a chair, walking, and running are frequently performed without adequate attention to proper muscle activation and support, resulting in misalignment of the trunk and possible muscle imbalance and strain. Proper execution of this exercise develops the stabilizers of the trunk and creates awareness of correct spinal alignment.

Imagery
Push the foot bar away from you as if you were pushing away a heavy box or catapulting a heavy load into the air with your legs.

☐ Press the hands gently against the front of the carriage.

☐ Maintain a moderate C curve of the trunk, with the head following the line of the spine.

☐ Keep the shoulders above the hips throughout the exercise.

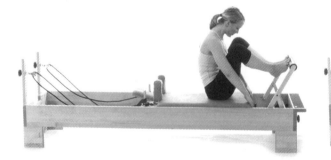

Inhale. Sit on the reformer facing the foot bar. Position yourself on the sit bones in the center of the carriage or closer to the foot bar, if possible. Place the toes on the foot bar, feet in a V position, with the heels together. Press the hands against the front of the carriage and round the trunk, positioning the shoulders directly above the hips.

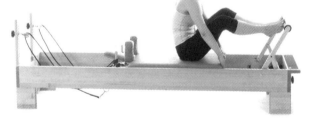

Exhale. Straighten the legs completely, dorsiflex and then plantarflex the feet.

Inhale. Bend the knees, returning to the start position.

Stomach Massage—Flat Back

This version of the stomach massage shares the movement sequence of the Reformer: Stomach Massage—Round Back: pressing the feet against the foot bar, straightening the legs, dorsiflexing and plantarflexing the feet, and keeping the trunk stable. The key difference is that the trunk is in a flat back position, which in this context translates to a neutral spine position, or as close to it as possible The trunk should be fully supported by the musculature, rather than the arms. The arm position simply creates a frame for the body offering support, like flying buttresses of a bridge, and adds a stretch across the front of the chest (also felt in the anterior aspect of the shoulder). Keep the elbows pointing directly back, parallel to each other and slightly bent.

Imagery

The movement can be likened to leaning against a wall and pushing a large load away or lying supine on the floor and catapulting a big bag up into the air with the legs.

☐ Maximize the co-contraction of the back extensors and abdominal muscles.

VARIATION

Perform the movement pattern as described, but rather than placing the hands on the shoulder rests, reach them forward on an upward diagonal line, arms shoulder-width apart. This increases the challenge of the exercise, as the arms no longer offer any support, which places greater demand on the stabilizers of the trunk.

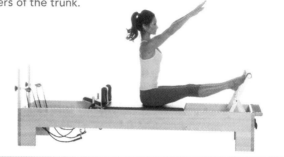

☐ Keep the elbows parallel, slightly bent, and reaching backward.

☐ Keep the trunk stable and upright throughout the movement.

Muscle Focus

- Back extensors
- Abdominal muscles

Objectives

- To develop trunk stabilization
- To strengthen the back extensors, knee extensors, and foot plantarflexors

RESISTANCE

Light   Medium   Heavy

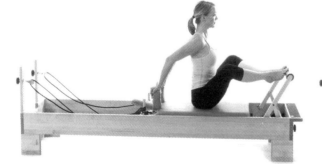

Inhale. Sit on the reformer facing the foot bar. Position yourself on the sit bones in the center of the carriage or closer to the foot bar, if possible. Place the toes on the foot bar, feet in a V position with the heels pressing together. Place the hands on the shoulder rests, with the fingers and elbows facing back and the elbows slightly bent. Keep the trunk upright in a position that is as close to a neutral spine as possible.

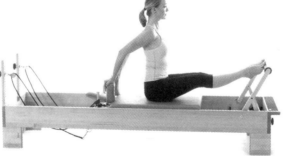

Exhale. Straighten the legs completely, dorsiflex and then plantarflex the feet.

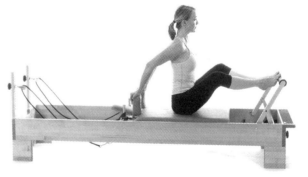

Inhale. Bend the knees, returning to the start position.

Muscle Focus
- Abdominal muscles
- Hip flexors

Objectives
- To develop trunk stabilization
- To strengthen the abdominal muscles and hip flexors

RESISTANCE

Light | Medium | Heavy

Knee Stretch—Reverse

This exercise focuses on three core principles: pelvic–lumbar stabilization, shoulder girdle stabilization, and hip flexor activation. The abdominal support is crucial to prevent excessively loading, and potentially straining, the lower back and to keep the pelvis and trunk stable. The juxtaposed actions—the legs moving forward and back while the upper body and the pelvis remain still—facilitate effective hip disassociation. As with most Pilates exercises, this one can be broken down to the stabilization of one area by way of isometric contractions and the movement of another through the use of both concentric and eccentric contractions.

In this exercise, executing the concentric phase of the hip flexor contraction (in which the legs come forward toward the chest) is easier than doing the eccentric phase (in which the legs move backward and the hip flexors elongate). The latter phase demands strong abdominal support to maintain pelvic–lumbar stabilization while counteracting the pull of the hip flexors as the legs move backward. If the abdominals are not adequately conditioned and the hip flexors do not elongate but rather remain in an isometric contraction, the back will begin to arch as the legs move backward.

Use caution when executing this exercise because the hip flexors are being loaded with resistance, which can potentially stress the lower back. For this reason I prefer to do this exercise in spinal flexion, as opposed to a neutral spine position, giving a mechanical advantage to the abdominals in protecting the spine.

Imagery

The legs move back and forth like pistons of an engine with the driving action on the forward motion and the control on the return. The fuel of the engine is the powerhouse, the core of the body, from which the movement emanates.

- ☐ Maintain spinal flexion throughout the exercise.
- ☐ Avoid elevating the scapulae.
- ☐ Place the arms on a slight diagonal, with the shoulders forward of the hands.

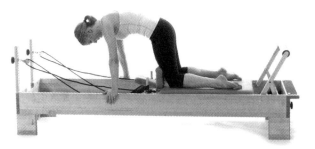

Inhale. Kneel in a quadruped position, placing the knees against the shoulder rests and the hands on the frame of the reformer, with the fingers on the outside of the rail. Position the shoulders slightly forward of the hands. Stabilize the shoulder girdle, and round the trunk.

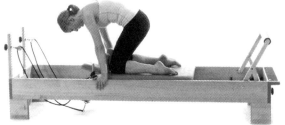

Exhale. Flex the hips, draw the knees toward the chest, and keep the pelvis still, maintaining the C curve of the trunk.

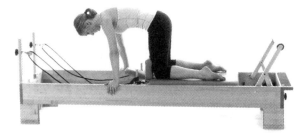

Inhale. Extend the hips without changing the position of the spine or pelvis, returning to the start position.

Down Stretch

Although this exercise appears relatively simple, it demands considerable control and strength. It highlights the concept of stabilization occurring in several key areas at once: the trunk, pelvic-lumbar region, and scapulae. The hips are in an extended position and the abdominal muscles (which draw the pubis symphysis upward) work together with the hamstrings (which draw the sit bones downward) to keep the pelvis stable with a bias toward a posterior tilt. The stable position of the pelvis, together with strong abdominal work, protects the lumbar spine from excessive pressure and amplifies the hip flexor stretch.

The shoulder joint acts as a pivot point for the movement. The shoulder flexors, together with gravity, move the carriage out, and the shoulder extensors, with the assistance of the springs, lift the body from the downward phase to the stopper. Emphasize extension of the thoracic spine as the body rises in the upward phase. Note that the lighter the resistance, the more challenging the exercise becomes.

Imagery

An image I have used in this exercise for many years is the figurehead of an old wooden ship. Imagine it rolling up and down as the ship sails over huge swells in the ocean. Also, I like to visualize a fishing line connected to the sternum. As the line is reeled in from above it helps lift the body, particularly the chest, during the up phase of the movement.

☐ Maintain a slight arc shape of the body.

☐ Keep the back, hip, and shoulder extensors working throughout the exercise.

☐ Press the feet against the shoulder rests, keeping the legs parallel.

Muscle Focus
- Abdominal muscles
- Upper-back extensors

Objectives
- To develop trunk stabilization
- To develop shoulder extensor and upper back extensor control

RESISTANCE

Light   Medium   Heavy

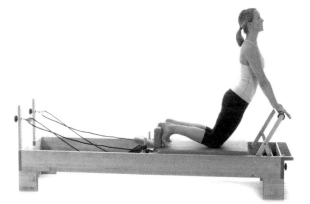

Inhale. Kneel on the carriage facing the foot bar. Place the hands on the foot bar, shoulder-width apart, with arms straight. Place the feet against the shoulder rests, with the legs parallel. Establish a line that runs from the knees through the thighs, hips, trunk, and shoulders and out the tip of the head.

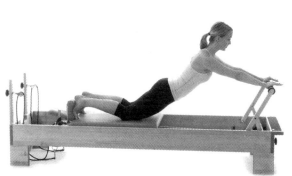

Exhale. Push the carriage back, pivoting from the shoulders and maintaining the arc shape of the body.

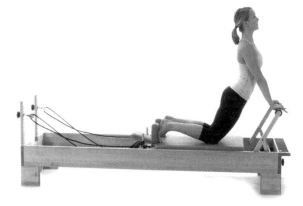

Inhale. Extend the shoulders, pressing down onto the foot bar to bring the body up to the start position. Hold the carriage against the stopper momentarily before repeating.

Muscle Focus

- Abdominal muscles
- Back extensors

Objectives

- To develop trunk and scapular stabilization
- To improve hamstring and shoulder flexibility
- To develop core strength

RESISTANCE

Light   Medium   Heavy

Elephant

The elephant and the Reformer: Up Stretch are almost identical, except that the elephant is performed with the feet flat. This adjustment increases the stretch down the back of the legs, which can be further magnified by lifting the toes. Although this exercise is sometimes performed with a round back, my preference is to keep the back flat, establishing one long line from the hip joints through the trunk, shoulders, arms, and hands. This ensures strong work of the back extensors (in co-contraction with the abdominal muscles), particularly those of the mid- and upper back. Keeping the back flat also accommodates a deep stretch of the shoulders and, by activating the back extensors, pulls the pelvis in an anterior direction, accentuating the hamstring stretch.

The legs should move back and forth fluidly, pivoting from the hip joint and emphasizing the inward phase. The range of motion of the movement and the distance the carriage travels should be relatively small. Two energy lines are present throughout: One runs from the hips through the trunk, shoulders, and arms; the other runs from the hips down the legs and through the heels. Together they form a pyramid, with the tailbone reaching up toward the ceiling as the top point. The carriage forms the solid base of the pyramid.

Imagery

The legs move like a pendulum swinging from the hip joints. The movement should be disassociated from the pelvis and the trunk. The image of using the abdominal muscles to pull in the legs deepens the abdominal work. Physiologically, of course, the abdominals do not pull the legs in; they help stabilize the trunk. The legs are pulled in by the springs and hip flexors (depending on the resistance).

☐ Maintain stability of the arms, shoulders, and trunk.

☐ Align the head with the spine and maintain the pyramid shape throughout the exercise.

☐ Keep the weight on the heels to maximize the stretch down the back of the legs.

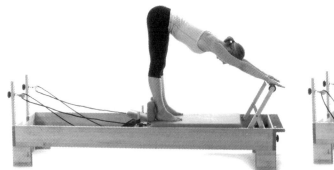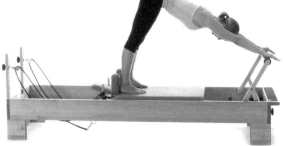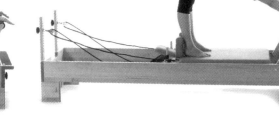

Exhale. Stand on the carriage, with the body in a pyramid shape: pelvis high in the air; hands on the foot bar, shoulder-width apart; and feet flat on the carriage, with the heels against the shoulder rests. (Optional: lift the toes slightly.)

Inhale. Extend the hips, hinging at the hip joint and moving the carriage back.

Exhale. Flex the hips, moving the carriage forward toward the stopper. Return to the start position.

Note that there is no need to actually touch the stopper. Certainly if flexibility and control allows, then you should do so, however, the goal is to bring the carriage as close to the stopper as possible while maintaining perfect alignment.

Up Stretch

This exercise and others like it that are based on the pyramid position are about creating straight lines and pivoting from specific joints. The line of the body extends from the hips, through the trunk, shoulders, arms, and hands. With this line serving as a solid foundation, the legs merely move in and out like a pendulum, creating a second straight line. Trunk stabilization and core strength are the essence of this exercise, with a coordinated contraction of the abdominal muscles (which prevent hyperlordosis as the carriage moves out) and the back extensors (which prevent spinal flexion as the carriage returns toward the stopper). The shoulders should remain firm and stable, establishing a strong connection to the trunk.

As with most of the FBI exercises, using less resistance increases the level of difficulty, particularly challenging the body's core strength and stabilization.

Imagery

As with the Reformer: Elephant, there is a sense of pulling the legs in with the abdominal muscles. I like to visualize a pyramid, with the tailbone as its tip and the feet and hands as the ends of its base. As the legs go back and forth the size of the base changes, but the pyramid shape remains constant, with the tailbone reaching skyward.

☐ Maintain the stability of the arms, shoulders, and trunk.

☐ Align the head with the spine.

☐ Press the heels into the shoulder rests.

Muscle Focus
- Abdominal muscles
- Back extensors

Objectives
- To develop trunk and scapular stabilization
- To improve hamstring and shoulder flexibility
- To develop core strength

RESISTANCE

Light   Medium   Heavy

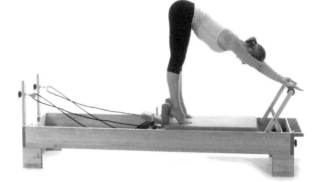

Exhale. Stand on the carriage and place the hands on the foot bar, shoulder-width apart. The pelvis is high in the air, and the heels press into the shoulder rests about halfway up.

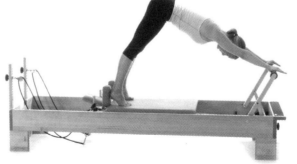

Inhale. Extend the hips, hinging at the hip joint, stabilizing the trunk and shoulders, and moving the carriage back.

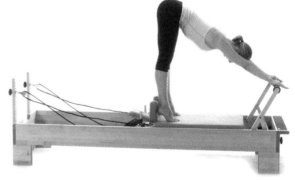

Exhale. Flex the hips, hinging at the hip joint, moving the carriage forward toward the stopper. Return to the start position.

177

Long Stretch

Muscle Focus

- Abdominal muscles
- Scapular stabilizers

Objectives

- To develop trunk and scapular stabilization
- To develop core strength
- To strengthen the shoulder flexors

RESISTANCE

Light   Medium   Heavy

The long stretch begins in the Reformer: Up Stretch position. The pelvis is lowered from this high point to a Mat Work: Front Support position, commonly regarded as a push-up position. This is accomplished by keeping the arms stable and pivoting from the shoulder and hip joints. Then without altering the position of the body and with the arms controlling the movement, the body glides forward over the foot bar, moving the carriage all the way to the stopper (or as close to it as possible) and then returns to the start position.

Unless the reformer has an adjustment for height, tall people may not be able to move the carriage to the stopper without altering the mechanics of the exercise or the position of the body. If the reformer has no adjustment for height, those who are tall should stop the movement at the point where the body position begins to change and compensations become apparent, but continue to strive to reach the maximum range possible. The shoulders should be at least perpendicular to the foot bar, if not slightly beyond, before pushing back to the start position.

The precision, control and core strength achieved in the long stretch can then be incorporated into all forms of the push-up, heightening both its integrity of alignment and intensity.

VARIATION

By repeating the first step of the long stretch—dropping the body from the pyramid position to the push-up position and then back up to the triangular shape of the pyramid—we essentially create a new exercise, which I call Up Stretch 2. Note that you are essentially hinging at the shoulders and hips, keeping the arms remaining absolutely stable. It should feel, moving like a see-saw going up and down.

Imagery

Imagine being catapulted out of a cannon. This powerful image initially seems unstable and perhaps frightening. But once you establish a strong, stable platform with the body, your confidence in using this image—and your enjoyment of performing this challenging movement—will grow. Even if body mechanics and height prevent actually doing so, think of bringing the carriage all the way to the stopper.

☐ Maintain trunk stabilization.

☐ Maintain scapular stabilization, with a focus on scapular depression and abduction.

☐ Align the head with the spine.

☐ Assume a slight posterior tilt of the pelvis to encourage abdominal engagement, to protect the lower back, and to avoid sinking.

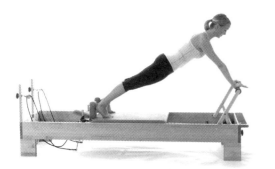

Exhale. Stand on the carriage and place the hands on the foot bar, shoulder-width apart. The pelvis is high in the air, and the heels press into the shoulder rests about halfway up.

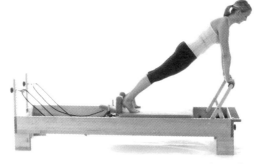

Lower the body to a push-up position, without altering the angle of the arms or shifting the shoulders.

Inhale. Glide the body forward over the foot bar until the carriage reaches the stopper (if possible).

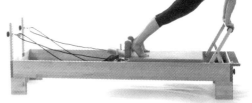

Exhale. Push the carriage back to the start position.

Balance Control Front

This exercise is reminiscent of the classic push-up position and resembles the Reformer: Long Stretch. However, it places the body in a more unstable and somewhat precarious position, which raises the level of difficulty considerably. Co-contraction of the abdominal muscles and the back extensors creates the necessary stabilization of the trunk and pelvis, plus support for the movement, exemplifying the meaning of core strength. In addition, proper form in this exercise requires shoulder stabilization and immaculate control of the shoulder girdle.

I recommend orienting the pelvis toward a posterior tilt, which provides a mechanical advantage to the abdominal muscles and prevents the pelvis from sinking and potentially placing pressure on the lower back. Dropping the pelvis compromises the stability of the entire structure and may result in injury. Likewise, a bias toward depression and abduction of the scapulae reinforces the stability of the shoulder girdle. Allowing this area to collapse may result in strain or injury. I have added plantarflexion of the feet to the positioning of this exercise, which is classically performed with the feet either in a neutral position or dorsiflexed. The plantarflexed position gives the exercise a beautiful line as well as adding an additional dimension of challenge.

Imagery

Visualize the body suspended like a drawbridge. The movement of the arms, like the mobile section of the bridge, occurs independently of the rest of the body. There should be a sensation of floating—the more relaxed you feel, the better. In addition, visualize one strong energy line running through the body from the tips of the toes to the top of the head, and a second line running from the shoulders through the arms, hands, and fingers.

☐ Maintain trunk stabilization.

☐ Maintain scapular stabilization with a bias toward scapular depression and abduction.

☐ Align the head with the spine.

☐ Assume a slight posterior tilt of the pelvis to encourage abdominal engagement, to protect the lower back, and to avoid sinking.

☐ Keep the feet plantarflexed.

Muscle Focus

- Abdominal muscles
- Scapular stabilizers

Objectives

- To develop trunk and scapular stabilization
- To develop core strength
- To strengthen the shoulder flexors

RESISTANCE

Light   Medium   Heavy

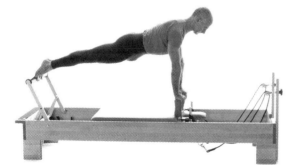

Inhale. Stand on the carriage facing the back of the reformer. Place the hands on the shoulder rests and align the shoulders directly above them. Place one foot on the foot bar in a plantarflexed position. Straighten that leg and lower the body into a plank position, establishing stability and support; then lift the other the leg and place the foot, also plantarflexed, on the foot bar with minimal shifting of weight. Ensure that the body is in one straight line.

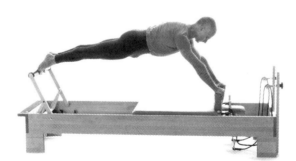

Exhale. Flex the shoulders, pushing the carriage toward the back of the reformer while maintaining a stable, plank-like position of the body. The movement is isolated to the hinge at the shoulder joints.

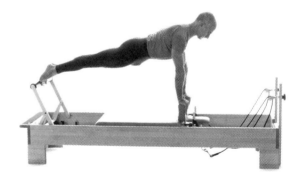

Inhale. Extend the shoulders, controlling the carriage as it returns to the start position.

179

Balance Control Back Prep

Muscle Focus
- Shoulder extensors
- Elbow extensors

Objectives
- To develop trunk and scapular stabilization
- To strengthen the shoulder and elbow extensors

RESISTANCE

Light   Medium   Heavy

This exercise divides the body into two separate and distinct units, in terms of function: the trunk is the upper section and the legs are the lower section. The hinging action occurs at the hip and shoulder joints. The movement is relatively small and the focus is primarily on maintaining an L-shape, formed by the trunk and legs. The L-shape opens slightly as the shoulders extend and the carriage is moved back, but it soon closes as the carriage moves forward toward the stopper.

The back extensors and scapular depressors, fortified by the abdominals, stabilize the scapulae and trunk. The movement is initiated by the shoulder extensors. The hip extensors play an important role in stabilizing the lower body and keeping the body elevated; they should remain engaged throughout the exercise. A common tendency, particularly when the pectorals are tight, is to round the trunk, which eliminates the L-shape and the upright trunk. Avoid rounding, even if it means minimizing the degree of movement.

Imagery

The letter L provides a good image for the initial position. Visualize two spring hinges: one in the shoulder joint and one in the hip joint. These points open slightly and then spring back to position.

VARIATION

By taking the movement further you can do the Balance Control Back, a very challenging and advanced exercise. Initiate the movement as described, with the shoulder, hip, and back extensors. Rather than coming back to the L-shape immediately, continue the movement until the body is in a long straight line, suspended like a bridge. To allow more movement in the shoulders, assume a more open shoulder position by placing the hands on the sides of the shoulder rest.

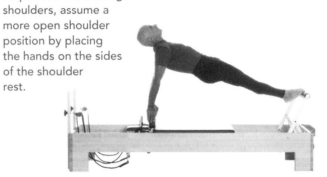

- ☐ Maintain a neutral spine position.
- ☐ Keep the back extensors activated.
- ☐ Maintain scapular stabilization, with a bias toward scapular depression.

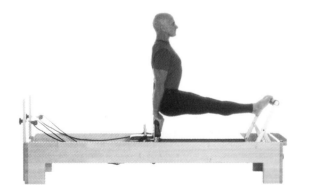

Inhale. Face the foot bar and place the hands on the shoulder rests. Put the feet on the foot bar, with the legs parallel. Establish an L-position with the legs and the trunk.

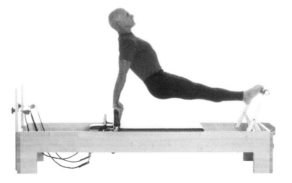

Exhale. Extend the shoulders as you push the carriage back, keeping the back straight.

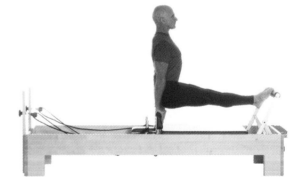

Inhale. Flex the shoulders, controlling the carriage as it returns to the start position.

Arm Work

There are myriad upper body exercises in Pilates, and many are initiated or accomplished through specific movements of the arms. Men often focus their physical training on the upper body and perhaps this general tendency played a role in Joseph Pilates' decision to create numerous options for developing this region. I have arranged the many arm work exercises into series, or groupings, to simplify and enhance the organization of the session. Rather than choose an array of individual exercises, you can choose an entire series. Each offers a well-balanced upper body workout that challenges the body in different ways and offers variety in both execution and effect.

A crucial element in arm work is clearly the shoulder. The shoulder is a wonderfully mobile joint, but at the same time it is potentially very unstable. It relies mostly on the musculature for support, as opposed to bone structure, and thus is often called a *muscle-dependent joint*. Immaculate control of the shoulder mechanism is required to reap the benefits of the arm work. As you enter into the advanced or master level repertoire, and the movements become more difficult, this fact becomes increasingly pertinent. Most of the higher-level work relies heavily on shoulder support.

Correct shoulder mechanics involve a coordinated, linked movement of the humerus and scapula termed the *scapulohumeral rhythm*. Many of the movements of the arm require intricate coordination of the muscles of the scapulae, to prevent undesired movements of the scapulae.

The scapulae provide a stable base on which the arms can move. In addition, coordinated use of the rotator cuff when elevating the arms is essential to prevent undesired upward motion of the head of the humerus into the overlying structures (impingement). Without correct mechanics, it is likely that at some point problems will occur in the shoulder, the neck, or even the back.

I like to advance the notion of one area of the body being stabilized while another area moves freely (disassociation). In the case of the shoulder, the scapulae provide the base of support as the arms move uninterrupted. The scapulae should move in relation to the movement of the arms, but the amount and direction of the movement must be proportional and controlled. The image used in the hip work of a spoon stirring a pot of porridge or syrup can also be used with the shoulder. The movement of the arms should be smooth and uninterrupted, with the scapulae making small, intricate adjustments to accommodate this movement.

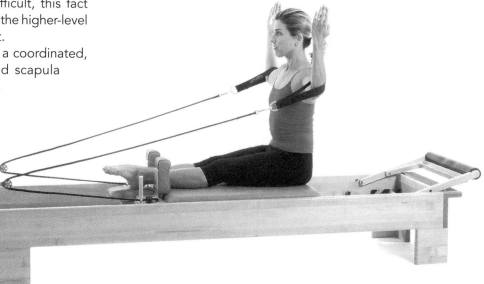

Muscle Focus

- Latissimus dorsi

Objectives

- To strengthen the shoulder extensors
- To develop trunk and scapular stabilization

RESISTANCE

Light   Medium   Heavy

Shoulder Extension—Supine

Performed with the spine in a neutral position, this supine arm work series requires extensive use of the core stabilizers. The emphasis is on developing a rhythmic coordination of the scapular stabilizers—specifically the lower trapezius (which maintains scapular depression) and the serratus anterior (which maintains scapular abduction)—with the muscles that move the arm, specifically the latissimus dorsi. Healthy scapulohumeral rhythm helps prevent excessive elevation and adduction of the scapulae during movement of the arm.

The supine series is particularly valuable because it places the body in a safe, comfortable, non-weight-bearing position, developing arm and shoulder strength together with trunk stabilization. All of the work occurs in a range of motion below shoulder height, which is valuable for people who have painful conditions such as shoulder impingement in which lifting the arm higher than the shoulder is often contraindicated.

Imagery

Imagine that you are swimming on your back and your arms are like large flippers, propelling the body through the water with each movement of the arms. Keep the movement smooth and integrated, with the body remaining stable. I always tell my students that *better stabilization produces better mobilization*. In this case, the focus of the movement is in the glenohumeral joint and the stabilization is in the trunk and scapulae.

☐ Maintain pelvic–lumbar and scapular stabilization.

☐ Set a smooth and even dynamic during both the concentric and eccentric phases of the arm movement.

☐ Keep the arms straight, without placing excessive force on the elbow.

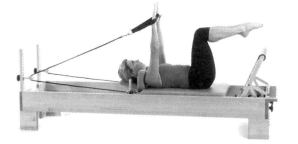

Inhale. Lie supine on the reformer in a neutral spine position, knees and hips at 90 degrees (tabletop position). Hold the arms perpendicular to the carriage, with the shoulders stable and the hands in the straps. Maintain slight tension in the straps, with the palms facing the knees.

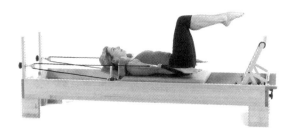

Exhale. Extend the shoulders, lowering the arms straight down toward the carriage. Pause when they reach the sides of the body, in line with the shoulders and parallel to the carriage.

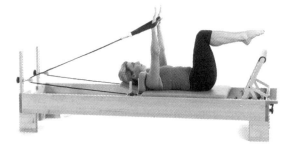

Inhale. Flex the shoulders, lifting the arms. Return to the start position.

Shoulder Adduction—Supine

This exercise is similar to the Reformer: Shoulder Extension—Supine, except that the shoulders adduct, and the arms move to the sides of the trunk. Emphasize the same points as in the shoulder extension exercise, including rhythmic coordination of the arms and scapulae, a neutral spine, trunk stabilization and scapular stabilization. In this exercise, the scapulae naturally tend to adduct, or squeeze together. Being in a supine position enables you to feel the scapulae against the carriage and dynamically stabilize them.

Imagery

Use the image of swimming on your back described in the previous exercise. The feeling as the arms, like large flippers, move toward the body should be one of propelling the body through water or soft gel.

☐ Maintain pelvic–lumbar stabilization.

☐ Avoid elevating and adducting the scapulae.

☐ Keep the arms straight, with the biceps activated, to avoid placing excessive force on the elbows.

Muscle Focus

• Latissimus dorsi

Objectives

• To strengthen the shoulder adductors
• To develop trunk and scapular stabilization

RESISTANCE

Light   Medium   Heavy

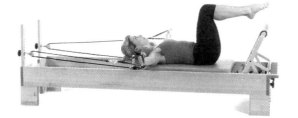

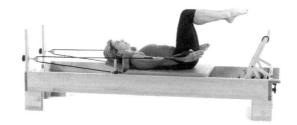

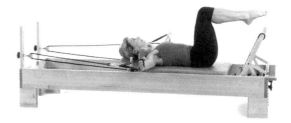

Inhale. Lie supine on the reformer in a neutral spine position, with legs in a tabletop position. Hold the arms out to the sides in a T-position, with the shoulders stable and the hands in the straps. Maintain slight tension in the straps, with the palms facing the sides of the body.

Exhale. Adduct the shoulders, and gently press the arms against the sides of the body.

Inhale. Abduct the shoulders, opening the arms. Return to the start position.

Muscle Focus

- Latissimus dorsi

Objectives

- To strengthen the shoulder extensors and adductors
- To develop trunk and scapular stabilization
- To improve shoulder mobility

RESISTANCE

Light | Medium | Heavy

Arm Circle Up—Supine

The circle is a combination of the Reformer: Shoulder Adduction—Supine and Reformer: Shoulder Extension—Supine exercises. The name can be misleading. Rather than tracing a true circle, the arms draw two semi-circles, created by joining the lines of movement of the adduction and extension exercises. Make the movement as large and defined as possible.

Imagery

The arm movement in the circles should be fluid and as large as possible, reaching each point of the semi-circle and rotating accordingly. The feeling should be like moving through gel, providing a sense of resistance throughout. There should be no difference in sensation or presentation between the concentric and eccentric phases.

> **VARIATION**
>
> This movement is also performed in reverse (arm circle down). Press the arms down toward the carriage to begin, then take them out to the sides to the T-position, and finally bring them back to the perpendicular position. Observe the same principles of maximizing the range of motion of the shoulder and using the movement pattern learned from the extension and abduction exercises, beginning, in this case, with extension.

☐ Do not raise the arms above shoulder height.

☐ Maintain flowing movement throughout.

☐ Define exact points that describe the shape of the arcs.

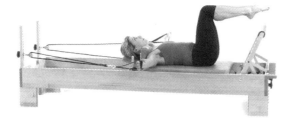

Inhale. Lie supine on the reformer in a neutral spine position, legs in a tabletop position. Hold the arms out to the sides in a T-position, keeping the shoulders stable, and place the hands in the straps. Maintain slight tension in the straps, with the palms facing the sides of the body.

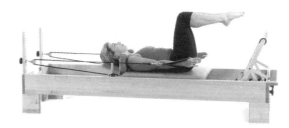

Exhale. Adduct the shoulders and gently press the arms against the sides of the body. Internally rotate the shoulders so that the palms face the carriage.

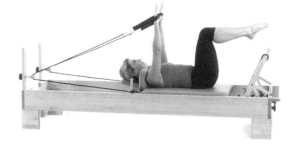

Inhale. Flex the shoulders, lifting the arms up to a position perpendicular to the carriage. Open the arms out to the T-position, returning to the start position.

Triceps—Supine

The motion in this exercise focuses solely on the triceps, isolating the movement of the elbow. The wrist must remain straight and firm, creating a line from the elbow through the fingers. The upper arms should press into the sides of the body throughout to assist in keeping the shoulders stable and maintaining good alignment. The movement commences with the elbows at a 90-degree angle and the fingers pointing straight up toward the ceiling. It ends with the elbows at 180 degrees, with the arms forming a straight line from the shoulders to the fingers. The upper arms remain parallel to the floor and do not push down onto the carriage. (Pushing down onto the carriage with the elbows, a common mistake, often results in adduction and elevation of the scapulae and thrusting the ribs forward.)

Imagery

Imagine pushing through water and propelling yourself with your forearms only, like an upside-down dog paddle.

☐ Hold the upper arms parallel to the carriage throughout the exercise.

☐ Press the elbows against the sides of the body and keep the upper arms still.

☐ Keep the wrists stable, in a neutral position (straight line with the arm).

Muscle Focus

- Triceps

Objectives

- To strengthen the elbow extensors
- To develop trunk and scapular stabilization

RESISTANCE

Light   Medium   Heavy

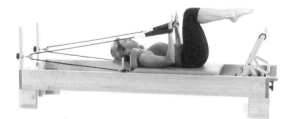

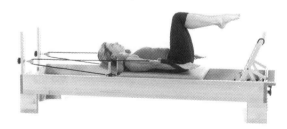

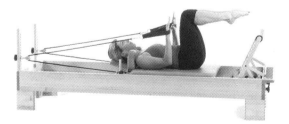

Inhale. Lie supine on the reformer in a neutral spine position, with the legs in a tabletop position. Place the arms by the sides of the body parallel to the floor, with the hands in the straps and the elbows at a 90-degree angle. Maintain slight tension in the straps, with the palms facing the foot bar.

Exhale. Extend the elbows, straighten the arms and press the hands down toward the carriage. Pause when the arms are in a straight line, parallel to the carriage.

Inhale. Flex the elbows, bending the arms (going beyond 90 degrees is optional).

Muscle Focus

- Latissimus dorsi

Objectives

- To strengthen the shoulder extensors
- To develop trunk and scapular stabilization

RESISTANCE

Light   Medium   Heavy

Chest Expansion—Seated

The key to this series is keeping the trunk upright and as close to neutral alignment as possible. Avoid the common tendency to round the upper body or, conversely, to thrust the ribs forward. As the arms move away from the foot bar, the shoulders extend beyond the centerline of the body. Precisely how far beyond the centerline the shoulders extend is dictated by strength, flexibility, and the ability to maintain correct trunk alignment. Once alignment is compromised, the exercise has exceeded its functional range of motion. Extending the shoulders beyond this point causes compensations, including scapular elevation and incorrect muscle recruitment.

Imagery

Many people visualize a horizontal back-and-forth motion of the arms in this exercise. I prefer to imagine the fingertips reaching down and drawing a line along the floor, while the head simultaneously reaches up toward the ceiling. This image gives more of a vertical feeling.

☐ Keep the trunk upright and stable.

☐ Focus on the fingertips reaching toward the floor.

☐ Avoid thrusting the ribs forward.

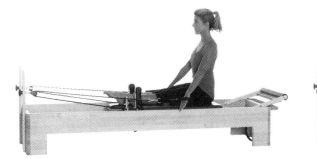

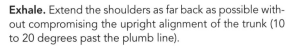

Inhale. Sit upright facing the back of the reformer at the edge of the carriage closest to the foot bar, with the legs straight and between the shoulder rests. Hold the straps with the palms facing back and fingertips reaching toward the floor. Keep the arms close to the sides of the body, approximately 20 to 30 degrees forward of the plumb line.

Exhale. Extend the shoulders as far back as possible without compromising the upright alignment of the trunk (10 to 20 degrees past the plumb line).

Inhale. Flex the shoulders, bringing the arms forward. Return to the start position.

Biceps—Seated

As with the Reformer: Chest Expansion—Seated, maintain a strong, balanced neutral spine position with correct upright alignment of the trunk. You should feel all the trunk stabilizers working. Avoid leaning back, which is a common mistake in this exercise.

The upper arms play a crucial role in the proper execution of this exercise. They are the stable foundation that remains immobile as the lower arms move. Straighten the arms directly forward and keep them absolutely stable and parallel to the floor. They should neither drop nor lift as they bend and straighten. Any deviation involves improper muscle recruitment and possible undesired elevation of the scapulae. This, in turn, compromises the isolated movement of the elbows and contraction of the biceps.

Imagery

The trunk and upper arm should create a stable platform for the lower arm to move on. The sensation should be like resting the upper arms on a table; the movement of the lower arms is completely disassociated from the upper arms. This image counters the tendency to lift the arms, which results in shoulder flexion as opposed to the desired isolated flexion of the elbows.

☐ Keep the upper arms parallel to the carriage and to each other throughout the exercise.

☐ Straighten the elbows completely after each repetition.

☐ Maintain the upright alignment of the trunk.

Muscle Focus

- Biceps

Objectives

- To strengthen the elbow flexors
- To develop trunk stabilization

RESISTANCE

Light   Medium   Heavy

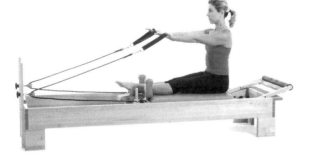

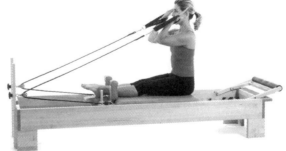

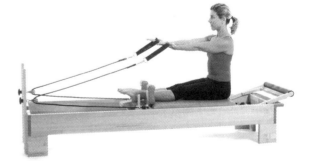

Inhale. Sit upright facing the back of the reformer at the edge of the carriage closest to the foot bar, with the legs straight and between the shoulder rests. Straighten the arms forward at shoulder height, parallel to the carriage, and hold the straps with the palms facing up.

Exhale. Flex the elbows, bending the arms to 90 degrees or beyond (as long as correct alignment can be maintained). Keep the upper arms stable.

Inhale. Extend the elbows, straightening the arms. Return to the start position.

Muscle Focus

- Posterior deltoid
- Rhomboids

Objectives

- To strengthen the shoulder horizontal abductors
- To strengthen the scapular adductors
- To develop trunk stabilization

RESISTANCE

Light   Medium   Heavy

Rhomboids—Seated

Although the name of this exercise singles out the rhomboids, the emphasis is initially on scapular stabilization and horizontal abduction of the shoulders. As in the Reformer: Biceps—Seated, focus on keeping the upper arms at a right angle to the body and parallel to the carriage with the elbows at a 90-degree angle. Horizontally abduct the shoulders just to the point where the scapulae are about to adduct, or retract (but do not retract them), and then bring the arms forward, returning the start position. Be aware of the rhomboids, which are located between the scapulae, and focus the energy there.

Imagery

The palms are like two spotlights shining beams of light toward the face. The more stable the arm position is, the more isolated the movement in the glenohumeral joint and eventually the more specific the scapular glide will be.

☐ Externally rotate the shoulders slightly to avoid internal rotation.

At a later stage, when good form and control have been achieved, you can add scapular adduction. The adduction occurs once you have reached the end range of humeral horizontal abduction. The scapular adduction should be viewed as an isolated motion of the scapulae and not part of the movement of the humerus. After the scapular adduction, the scapulae then abduct (protract) before the arms return to the start position.

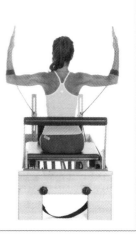

☐ Keep the humerus parallel to the floor throughout the movement.

☐ Avoid elevating the shoulders.

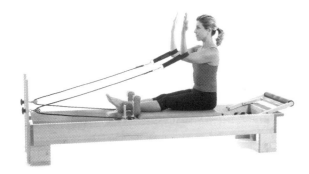

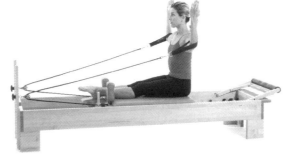

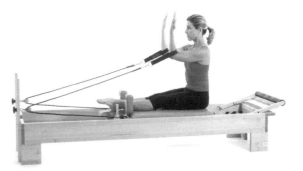

Inhale. Sit upright facing the back of the reformer at the edge of the carriage closest to the foot bar, with the legs straight and between the shoulder rests. Thread the arms through the straps, bend the elbows to a 90-degree angle and place the straps on the forearms close to the elbows. Make sure the upper arms are at shoulder height, parallel to both the carriage and to each other, with the palms facing the body.

Exhale. Horizontally abduct the shoulders, keeping the upper arms on a consistent horizontal plane and maintaining the 90-degree angle of the elbows.

Inhale. Horizontally adduct the shoulders, bringing the arms forward. Return to the start position.

Hug-a-Tree—Seated

The image of hugging a tree often results in rounding the arms and shoulders excessively, which is contrary to the goal of this exercise. As the shoulders are horizontally adducted, I advise focusing on the mid- and upper-back extensors, which prevents flexion and collapse of the upper thoracic spine. Elongating the arms out to the sides, rather than rounding them, encourages correct muscle recruitment, keeps the resistance engaged throughout the range of motion and creates a long lever arm, which makes the exercise more challenging. I cannot emphasize enough the importance of a strong upright position and a stable trunk. Focus the work in the chest, as opposed to the arms, and feel the wonderful stretch across the chest as the arms open.

Imagery

Imagine spreading your wings, like an eagle with a large wingspan. The tree image works well for the trunk of the body, which should feel like a strong, sturdy tree trunk.

☐ Keep the back and shoulders broad and the scapulae open (abducted).

☐ Keep the hands within your peripheral vision when the arms open.

☐ Externally rotate the shoulders slightly, feeling that you are leading the movement with the small finger.

Muscle Focus

• Pectorals

Objectives

• To strengthen the shoulder horizontal adductors

• To develop trunk stabilization

RESISTANCE

Light   Medium   Heavy

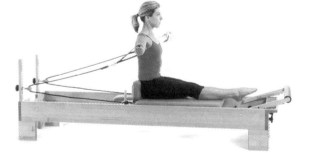 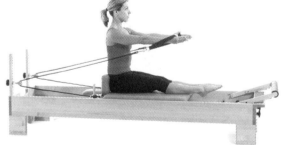 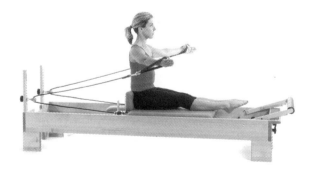

Inhale. Sit upright on the carriage facing the front of the reformer, with the back of the pelvis against the shoulder rests and the legs directly forward. Hold the arms out to the sides in a T-position, arms elongate with very slight flexion in the elbows.

Exhale. Horizontally adduct the shoulders until the arms are parallel to each other and in line with the shoulders.

Inhale. Horizontally abduct the shoulders, maximizing the eccentric contraction of the muscles of the chest as the arms return to a T-position, without moving the scapulae.

Muscle Focus
- Triceps

Objectives
- To strengthen the elbow extensors
- To develop trunk and scapular stabilization

RESISTANCE

Light | Medium | Heavy

Salute—Seated

Although the focus of this exercise is the triceps, the entire seated arm work series emphasizes trunk stabilization and correct positioning of the scapulae. In this exercise, in particular, there is a tendency to round the upper body and elevate the shoulders. A good indication of the correct height of the arms from the outset is for the hands to be alongside the temples and the ropes slightly above the shoulders, but not touching them. The fingers should face forward to guide the arms traveling on a diagonal line.

Imagery

Imagine the arms gliding along a ramp slightly above the horizon. Envisioning the horizon encourages a long, seemingly infinite line.

- ☐ Maintain scapular stabilization throughout the exercise.
- ☐ Keep the elbows lifted and reaching out to the sides when bent.
- ☐ Direct the fingers along the line of the movement.

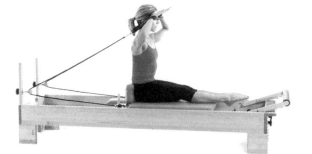 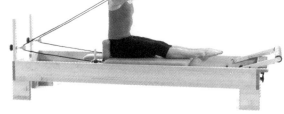 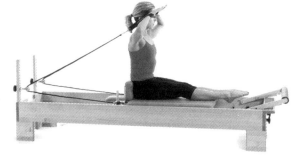

Inhale. Sit upright on the carriage facing the front of the reformer, with the back of the pelvis against the shoulder rests and the legs directly forward. Place the hands in the straps, alongside the temples, with the elbows out to the sides. The fingers face forward and slightly upward, in the direction of the movement.

Exhale. Extend the elbows, straightening the arms on a diagonal line, 20 to 30 degrees above horizontal.

Inhale. Flex the elbows, moving them out to the sides as you bend the arms. Return to the start position, with the fingers still facing forward.

Chest Expansion—Kneeling

This exercise is far more challenging than the seated version, the standing version on the cadillac or the version on the arm chair, primarily due to the element of instability in this version. It requires a very high degree of trunk stabilization, balance, control, and focus. The control is particularly required in the eccentric phase of the exercise, as the arms return to the start position. If this phase is done too quickly, the carriage will slide back toward the stopper rapidly and the body will likely lunge forward. Several factors encourage instability: the kneeling position itself, the body's high center of gravity in this position, a long lever arm (the trunk), and a small base of support.

This potential instability offers immediate feedback when and if the body is out of alignment. You only need to feel that you are being catapulted forward once for the body to quickly learn how to control the eccentric phase of the movement and stabilize the trunk. I avoid doing this particular exercise with pregnant women, due to their changing center of gravity, added weight, diminished balance and the obvious associated danger of falling.

Although a neutral spine is the ideal position, I often recommend a slight posterior tilt of the pelvis, which encourages abdominal activation. This in turn counters the tendency to flex at the hips, tilt the pelvis anteriorly, thrust the ribs forward, and hyperextend the back.

VARIATION

After the movement of the arms and the stabilization of the trunk have been mastered, at the point the shoulders are in full extension, you can add the head rotation only after the movement of the arms and stabilization of the trunk have been mastered and the exercise can be done without tension in the shoulders or neck.

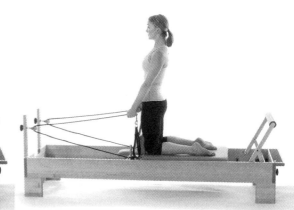

Muscle Focus

- Latissimus dorsi

Objectives

- To strengthen the shoulder extensors
- To strengthen the triceps
- To develop trunk stabilization

RESISTANCE

Light   Medium   Heavy

Imagery

The trunk should feel like the trunk of a tree; tall, upright and able to adapt to the subtle shifts as the arms move back and forth. Imagine the hands reaching down to the floor while the head simultaneously reaches up toward the ceiling.

☐ Keep the trunk upright and stable.

☐ Keep the hip flexors elongated, sensing the stretch through the thighs.

☐ Avoid thrusting the ribs forward.

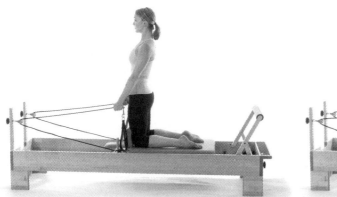

Inhale. Kneel facing the back of the reformer, with the knees against the shoulder rests and the body upright. Hold the ropes in the hands, just above the straps, with the palms facing each other. Place the arms in front of the body, approximately 20 to 30 degrees forward of the plumb line.

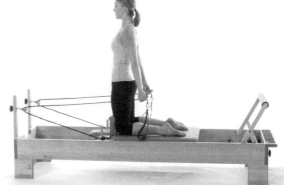

Exhale. Extend the shoulders, taking the arms back as far as possible without compromising the upright alignment of the trunk (10 to 20 degrees past the plumb line).

Inhale. Flex the shoulders, bringing the arms forward. Return to the start position.

191

Arm Circle Up—Kneeling

Muscle Focus

- Shoulder flexors (circle up)

Objectives

- To strengthen the shoulder flexors and the shoulder abductors
- To develop trunk and scapular stabilization

RESISTANCE

Light   Medium   Heavy

Few series of exercises challenge the upper body and the trunk as profoundly as the kneeling arm work series. I have given these exercises to athletes of many disciplines and they have all found them challenging and extremely beneficial. Swimmers in particular enjoy doing these exercises, as they address muscle patterns fundamental to swimming.

There is a tendency to overuse the quadriceps and often the legs fatigue more than the arms. As you learn to utilize the muscles of the core and the trunk becomes more stable, there will be less need to rely on the legs for support. As with the Reformer: Chest Expansion—Kneeling, maintain a slight posterior tilt of the pelvis and focus on elongating the hip flexors and thighs. Avoid elevating the arms higher than the flexibility of the shoulders allows, as this will result in scapular elevation and tension in the neck.

Imagery

In the initial phase, I like to imagine that I am lifting a large, light beach ball in each hand, as if to toss it high into the air. The arms rotate at the top, and the palms face front, small finger leading the way down to the sides of the body. This encourages a light and effortless feel in the arms.

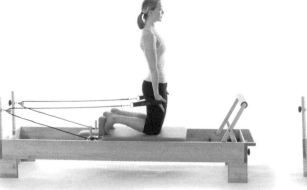

Inhale. Kneel facing the foot bar, with the feet against the shoulder rests and the trunk upright. Place the hands in the straps, with the palms facing forward and the arms by the sides of the body.

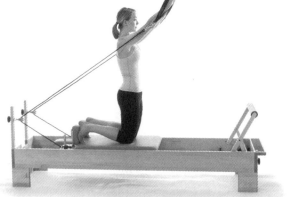

Exhale. Flex the shoulders, reaching the arms forward and upward, the palms continuing to face up.

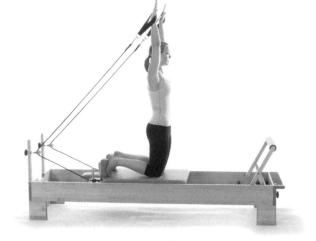

Inhale. Rotate the arms as they reach overhead so the palms face the front.

- [ ] Face the palms forward and then upward during shoulder flexion.

- [ ] Keep arms within peripheral vision as they circle around to the sides.

- [ ] Avoid elevating the scapulae as the arms rise above shoulder height.

VARIATION

This movement is also performed in reverse (called Arm Circle Down—Kneeling). Abduct the shoulders and reach the arms out to the sides and overhead, palms facing forward. When the arms are overhead, rotate the shoulders, so the palms face up, and then lower the arms to the start position. Maximize the range of motion of the shoulders. The reverse direction is more challenging in terms of scapular stabilization and the demand on the shoulder abductors; reduce the resistance, if necessary.

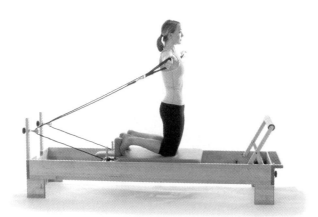

Still inhaling, circle the arms out to the side.

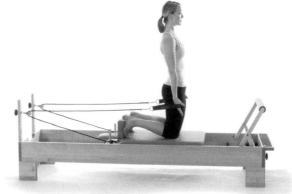

Bring the arms down, returning to the start position.

Muscle Focus

- Triceps

Objectives

- To strengthen the elbow extensors and shoulder abductors
- To develop trunk stabilization

RESISTANCE

Light   Medium   Heavy

Triceps—Kneeling

The focus of this exercise is the triceps and is similar to Reformer: Salute—Seated and the Arm Chair: Salute. But, given the unstable position, the high center of gravity, and the hands traveling upward rather than forward, it is a great deal more challenging. There is a strong tendency to round the upper body, elevate the shoulders, and reach the hands forward. All these negative patterns should be avoided.

The feel of this exercise should be extremely upright. There is a straight energy line traveling from the knees, through the trunk and finally through the straight arms as they straighten, hands reaching toward the ceiling.

Imagery

Imagine the hands shaving the back of the head as the arms straighten and bend. Think of the triangular shape created by the fingers as a spearhead, leading the movement, as the arms straighten.

☐ Maintain scapular stabilization throughout the exercise.

☐ Keep the elbows lifted and facing out.

☐ Direct the fingers along the line of movement.

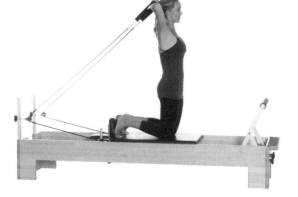

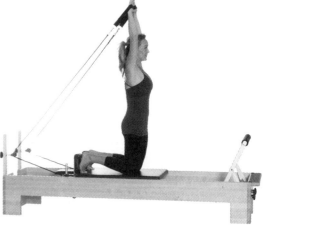

Inhale. Kneel facing the foot bar, with the feet against the shoulder rests and the trunk upright. Hold the straps with the hands behind the head, pressing the thumbs and index fingers together to create a triangle. The elbows remain wide, reaching out to the sides.

Exhale. Extend the elbows, straightening the arms and abducting the shoulders. Keep the fingers touching while reaching up to the ceiling.

Inhale. Flex the elbows, bending the arms. Return to the start position.

Biceps—Kneeling

This is an exercise I added to the original arm exercises created by Joseph Pilates. It is similar in many ways to the Cadillac: Biceps—Standing exercise in that both provide a profound stretch across the chest and top of the shoulders. The fully stretched position of the biceps is unique and very effective for developing strength and flexibility in the biceps specifically and the shoulder region in general. Men in particular are often tight in the biceps and across the chest, which tends to limit range of motion and interfere with normal function of the shoulders. I personally love this exercise, especially after cycling, surfing, or a long workday.

Imagery

I like to think of the body as a masthead, the figurine found at the front of those majestic old wooden boats. With each bend of the arms, the chest should open more, with a feeling of reaching the chest forward. It is important to keep the abdominals engaged so that the chest can open without the lower ribs thrusting forward.

☐ Keep the upper arms stable throughout the movement.

☐ Keep the arms parallel to each other.

☐ Maintain scapular stabilization.

Muscle Focus

- Biceps

Objectives

- To strengthen the elbow flexors
- To stretch the chest and anterior aspect of the shoulder
- To develop trunk stabilization

RESISTANCE

Light   Medium   Heavy

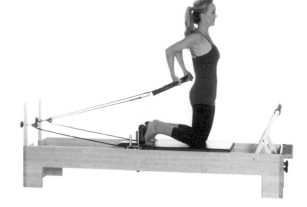

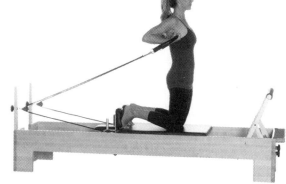

Inhale. Kneel facing the foot bar, with the feet against the shoulder rests and the trunk upright. Reach the arms back, extend the shoulders, and hold the straps.

Exhale. Flex the elbows, bending them while the upper arms remain absolutely still.

Inhale. Extend the elbows, straightening the arms. Return to the start position.

Muscle Focus

- Posterior deltoid and rhomboids

Objectives

- To strengthen the shoulder horizontal abductors
- To develop shoulder mobility and stability
- To increase abdominal control

RESISTANCE

Light   Medium   Heavy

Rowing Back I

The rowing series, which begins with this exercise, effectively integrates and displays all the wonderful elements of Pilates. Understanding this series will offer you insight into the intricacies of the method itself. Coordinated muscle activation is key, with the entire body working as an integrated unit. In fact, this series would fit quite comfortably into the full-body integration block, but due to the demands on the upper body I decided to include it in the arm work block. The combination of upper-body support and shoulder mobility, together with maximal stability of the trunk illuminates the principle of functional range of motion. Avoid neck tension and shoulder elevation, which often occur because of the enormous demands placed on the upper body.

Due to the complexity of the exercises in the rowing series, laying a good foundation before attempting them is highly recommended. Mastering related arm work exercises that are performed in a seated position on the reformer and the Mat Work: Roll-Up will assist in achieving this goal. Once the elements of these exercises have been learned and practiced, pay attention to flow. There should be a seamless flow of movement that both looks and feels wonderful. In the roll-down phase, the lower back imprints into the carriage, with a bias toward a posterior pelvic tilt.

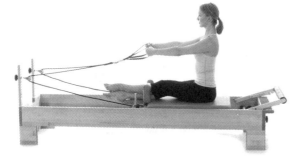 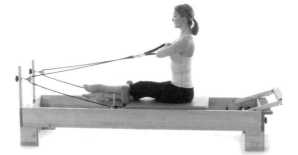 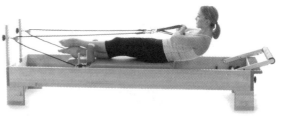

Exhale. Place the foot bar down. Sit upright on the carriage facing the back of the reformer, approximately one-third down the carriage. (Leave enough space on the carriage behind you to support the lower back when in the supine position). Keep the legs straight between the shoulder rests (you may need to cross them), the arms straight out in front, parallel to each other and to the floor. Hold the straps in the hands, with the hands facing each other.

Inhale. Flex the elbows, bending the arms and bringing the hands to the sternum, with the elbows wide.

Exhale. Roll down into a supine position, keeping the hands in front of the sternum and maintaining flexion of the trunk.

Imagery

Rowing a boat is a good visual image of the action in this exercise. I like to imagine a long, sleek boat gliding across smooth water, propelled by the long, dynamic strokes of the arms.

☐ Bring the hands to the chest before rolling down in the first phase of the exercise.

☐ Keep the carriage still when moving from the supine position with the arms in T-position to the forward flexion with the hands touching behind the back position.

☐ Circle the arms around to the front, keeping them as high as possible, as if swimming butterfly, before rolling the spine up to a sitting position.

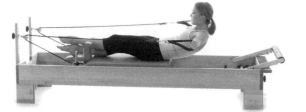

Inhale. Remain in the supine position. Internally rotate the shoulders and straighten the arms out to the sides, creating a T-position with the arms. Pause.

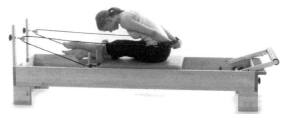

Exhale. Transfer the trunk into forward flexion over the legs, while reaching the arms behind the body and touching the hands together. Keep the carriage still and maintain tension on the straps throughout this phase.

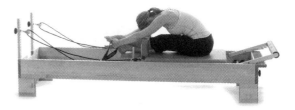

Inhale. Remain in forward flexion, stretching the hamstrings. Circle the arms around to the front over the legs, as if swimming the butterfly.

Exhale. Roll up the trunk, returning to the start position.

Muscle Focus

- Biceps

Objectives

- To strengthen the elbow flexors
- To develop abdominal and back control

RESISTANCE

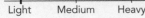

Light   Medium   Heavy

Rowing-Back II

The emphasis on full-body integration and flow continues in this exercise. In terms of arm work the focus is now directed to the biceps. The Reformer: Biceps—Seated is excellent preparation for this exercise, and I consider it a prerequisite. The elbows are held at a 90-degree angle for much of the exercise, with the biceps in an isometric contraction. Keeping this angle absolutely consistent adds greatly to the challenge of the exercise, together with the coordination of the entire body being involved in the movement.

Focus on the coordinated contraction of the abdominal muscles and the back extensors, particularly when lifting from supine into a sitting position. There is a tendency to throw the pelvis forward at this point, resulting in an anterior tilt of the pelvis and hyperlordosis, which can put strain on the lower back. In the classic form of this exercise, the trunk was held in extension throughout the movement. I prefer to roll down, reinforcing the familiar pattern of spinal articulation and reducing the possibility of straining the lower back.

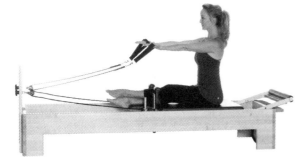

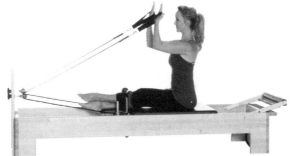

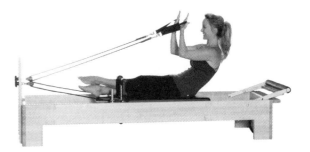

Exhale. Place the foot bar down. Sit upright on the carriage facing the back of the reformer, approximately one-third down the carriage. (Leave enough space on the carriage behind you to support the lower back when in the supine position). Keep the legs straight between the shoulder rests (you may need to cross them), the arms straight out in front at shoulder height, parallel to each other and to the floor. Hold the straps in the hands, with the hands facing upward.

Inhale. Flex the elbows, bending the arms to 90 degrees.

Exhale. Roll down into a supine position and lower the arms to the sides of the body, maintaining the 90-degree angle in the elbows.

Imagery

I enjoy feeling the undulating, circular motion of the entire trunk as it rolls down and then unwinds to roll up like a wave. Coordinating the arm movement with that of the trunk accentuates the rolling sensation and the strong connection between the movement of the trunk and the arms. Visualizing this flowing, rhythmic motion will assist in achieving the desired dynamic in this exercise.

☐ Keep the elbows at a 90-degree angle when rolling down to the supine position.

☐ Hold the elbows firmly by the sides of the body when supine.

☐ Begin the lift with slight lumbar flexion before transitioning into spinal extension.

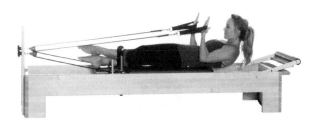

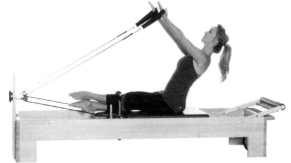

Inhale. Pause in the supine position, maintaining a stable trunk and arm position.

Exhale. Lift the body, initiating the movement by drawing in the abdominal muscles and deepening the spinal flexion. Extend the spine through coordinated contraction of the abdominals and back extensors to reach the upright sitting position. Simultaneously, reach the arms up on a diagonal and then forward to the start position. The arm motion should feel like it grows out of the movement of the trunk as it transitions from the supine position in spinal flexion to the upright sitting position.

Muscle Focus

- Deltoids
- Triceps

Objectives

- To strengthen the shoulder flexors and elbow extensors
- To develop trunk and scapular stabilization

RESISTANCE

Light   Medium   Heavy

Rowing Front I

In this exercise the trunk is upright and facing the foot bar. The trunk should feel as sturdy as the trunk of a huge tree, similar to Reformer: Hug-a-Tree—Seated exercise in the seated arm work series. I recommend being very familiar with the seated arm work series before embarking on the rowing exercises. The sensation of a strong, solid trunk is achieved by co-contracting the abdominal muscles and the back extensors.

The focus is on stillness of the trunk and mobility of the shoulders. Having the resistance pulling from behind makes the movement more challenging and gives the sensation that the body is being pulled backward.

If the hamstrings are tight and the back muscles are weak, the hip flexors will tend to work excessively and become fatigued. Sitting on a pad or small box to elevate the body is advisable; this takes the strain off the hamstrings and hip flexors and allows the focus to shift to the back extensors. It also allows you to establish the upright position of the trunk required in this exercise.

Avoid leaning back, and do not allow the arms to go behind the body at any point. This can be achieved by keeping the arms in your peripheral vision as they circle from overhead to the sides of the body.

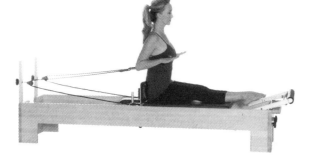
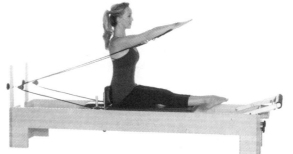
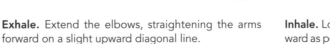

Inhale. Sit upright facing the foot bar, back of the pelvis against the shoulder rests and legs straight forward. Place the thumbs in the straps, with the rope running under the armpits. Bend the arms, with the hands opposite the sides of the chest, palms facing down and elbows reaching out to the sides.

Exhale. Extend the elbows, straightening the arms forward on a slight upward diagonal line.

Inhale. Lower the arms to the carriage, reaching as far forward as possible, and touch the carriage with the fingertips.

Imagery

Visualize laser beams shooting out from the fingertips as you take the arms through this multidirectional movement, maximizing the range in all directions. When in the start position, imagine that there is air under the arms, as if they are floating. This will allow the rope to pass comfortably under the arms.

☐ Stabilize the trunk and maintain an upright position throughout the exercise.

☐ Stabilize the scapulae prior to the movement.

☐ After straightening the arms on a slight diagonal and lowering them, reach as far forward as possible on the carriage to accentuate the feeling of length.

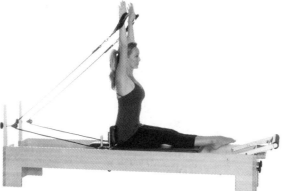 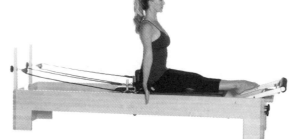 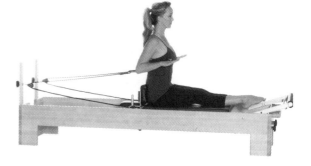

Exhale. Lift the arms overhead, internally rotating the shoulder so that the ropes pass the arms unobstructed.

Circle the arms around to the sides of the body, palms facing forward.

Inhale. Flex the elbows, bending and lifting the arms up. Return to the start position.

Rowing Front II

Muscle Focus

- Back extensors
- Deltoids

Objective

- To strengthen the back extensors, elbow extensors and shoulder flexors
- To stretch the hamstrings

RESISTANCE

Light   Medium   Heavy

This exercise is particularly valuable due to the profound involvement of the trunk and the coordination of movement of the trunk and arms required to do it well. Proper execution involves not only trunk strength and stability but also hamstring flexibility. The transition from flexion to extension of the trunk should be initiated from the lower back, with the energy flowing up through the trunk to the arms and then the fingers. By focusing on extending the spine and achieving a straight diagonal line with the trunk immediately prior to straightening the arms, you will likely avoid common mistakes such as shoulder elevation and inadequate extension of the trunk. I recommend pausing momentarily at the moment when the trunk and arms have created a powerful diagonal line, prior to sitting upright. Bringing the arms forward with the body as the trunk rounds into forward flexion is a small but very important movement that is often ignored. This places the arms in a strong position to then straighten on the diagonal line.

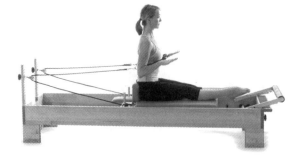

Inhale. Sit upright facing the foot bar, back of the pelvis against the shoulder rests and legs straight forward. Place the thumbs in the straps, with the rope running under the armpits. Bend the arms, with the hands opposite the sides of the chest, palms facing down and elbows pointing down.

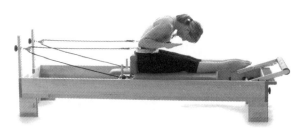

Exhale. Round the trunk into forward flexion over the thighs, keeping the arms close to the sides of the body and the hands directly under the shoulders.

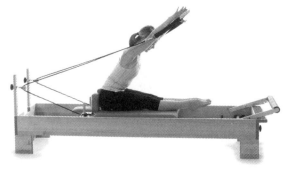

Inhale. Extend the back into a flat diagonal position. Follow this by straightening the arms on the same diagonal line, internally rotating the shoulders so that the ropes pass the arms unobstructed.

Imagery

Imagine a wave of energy, like an electrical current, moving sequentially up the back through the arms and fingers. Or think of colored ink rising up the back, like litmus paper changing color.

☐ Initiate the extension from the lumbar spine and then move through the mid and upper spine, before starting the arm movement.

☐ Pause in the diagonal straight back position before lifting to sitting upright.

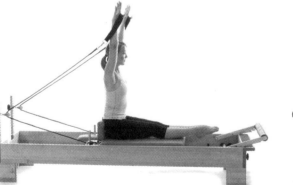

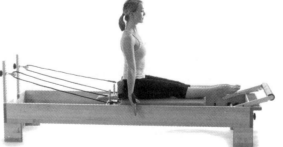

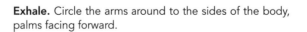

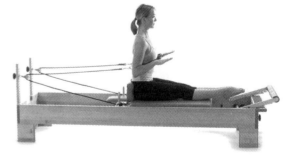

Continue to inhale. After a momentary pause, lift the body to the upright position, arms overhead, keeping the shoulders internally rotated.

Exhale. Circle the arms around to the sides of the body, palms facing forward.

Inhale. Flex the elbows, bending and lifting the arms up. Return to the start position.

Leg Work

This block of exercises supplements the foot work block. Like the footwork block, it provides an opportunity within the session for focused work on the legs and lower body. The specific agenda for this block depends on the goals of the individual. The workouts designed for a professional football player, a runner, a cyclist, a gymnast, a dancer, and someone who just wants to maintain good general fitness would be unique in some respects and similar in others. Each activity demands specialized skills which correlates with the recruitment of specific muscles and muscle groups. This block offers an opportunity to tailor the work to those muscles.

Typically we use this block to work the hip adductors and abductors (with emphasis on gluteus medius), which tend to be weak in relation to the larger muscles of the leg, the quadriceps and hamstrings. Exercises to develop the legs may involve resistance, balance, specific skills, or a combination of all three.

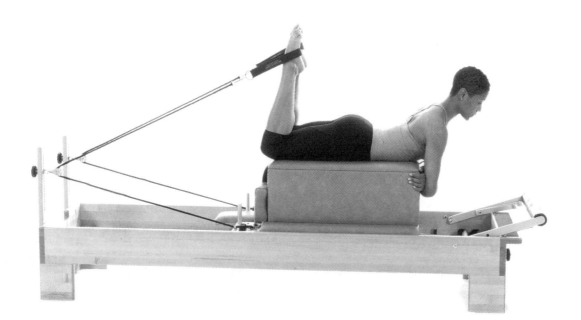

Side Split

Perhaps no other exercise demonstrates the concept of functional range of motion as well as this one does. The split demands an intricate balance of strength and flexibility. A lack of either strength or flexibility will limit the range of the movement and affect the integrity of the alignment.

Both phases require coordinated muscle activation of primarily the hip adductors, abdominals, and back extensors: The "out" phase involves an eccentric contraction of the hip adductors, and the "in" phase involves a concentric contraction of the same muscles. Although engagement of the ISS is assumed throughout the Pilates work, specific attention to the pelvic floor seems especially pertinent in the side split. The pelvic floor forms the foundation of the ISS, and it protects and supports the internal viscera, as the legs open out as wide as possible. The abdominal engagement prevents hyperlordosis and anterior tilting of the pelvis, which are particularly common at the point where the hips are in maximum abduction. The back extensors assist in maintaining upright alignment and avoiding posterior tilt of the pelvis. The beginning of concentric phase, as the legs begin to "pull in," is a very precarious moment in the exercise. Leaning forward must be avoided. The resistance should be challenging (meaning light). Note that if too much resistance is loaded the hip abductors will be recruited instead of the hip adductors.

Muscle Focus
- Hip adductors

Objectives
- To strengthen the hip adductors
- To develop pelvic lumbar stabilization

RESISTANCE

Light   Medium   Heavy

VARIATION

Initially, as you acquire control, it is best to be safe and place the foot in the middle of the carriage rather than against the shoulder rest. To prevent the foot from sliding I suggest placing a rubber pad under the outside portion of the foot that is on the carriage. Most of the weight will be on the instep of the foot. Progressively move the foot closer to the shoulder rest as you become more proficient.

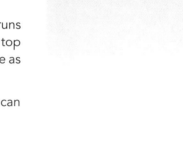

Imagery

I like the image of a puppet being lifted by a string that runs from the base of the pelvis, through the body and out the top of the head. There should be a sense of controlled release as the legs open and suction as they come together.

☐ Bias the pelvis toward a slight posterior tilt until you can achieve and maintain a neutral pelvic position.

☐ Keep the trunk upright throughout the exercise.

☐ Use an arm position that allows the arms and shoulders to relax.

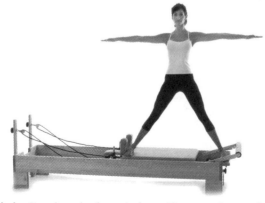

Exhale. Stand on the foot platform. Place one foot as far out as possible on the carriage (against the shoulder rest, if possible). Hold the arms in a T-position.

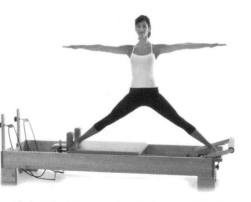

Inhale. Abduct the hips, opening the legs and allowing the carriage to move outward. Control the movement with the hip adductors. Pause at the end of the range of motion.

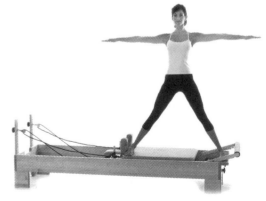

Exhale. Adduct the hips, bringing the legs toward each other. Return to the start position, pausing with the carriage against the stopper. After 5 repetitions the hip adductors will (and should) feel worked.

Muscle Focus
- Gluteus medius

Objectives
- To strengthen the hip abductors
- To develop pelvic lumbar stabilization

RESISTANCE

Light | Medium | Heavy

Skating

This is an excellent hip abductor exercise. Specific focus is placed on the gluteus medius, which is an important muscle for healthy hip function. The gluteus medius plays a prominent role in everyday movements such as walking, running, sitting down, and getting up.

It is important to distinguish between the standing leg and the working leg, as they perform very different functions. The standing leg creates a solid foundation from which to work. It is stabilizing in every sense of the word. The moving leg performs the action, relying on a stable platform established by the other leg to push off. Although the working leg creates the movement, an equal amount of attention must be allocated to the standing leg, which remains stable along with the pelvis. Avoid the common mistake of pushing with the standing leg at the same time as the working leg. This often indicates that the resistance is too high or the leg is weak, or both. Another indication that the resistance is too high is if the body lifts as the working leg straightens. Finally it is important to straighten the moving leg completely and not stop short of full extension. It is in the final 5 to 10 degrees of knee extension that the hip abductor works the hardest; also, the resistance at this point is the highest.

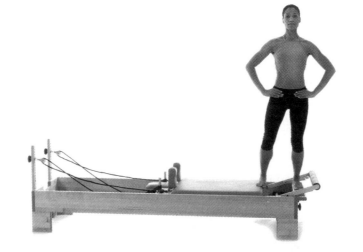

Inhale. Stand on the foot platform, then place one foot on the front edge of the carriage, keeping the weight entirely on the standing (outside) leg. Place the hands on the hips or behind the head, and keep the trunk upright. Bend the standing leg into a deep squat, keeping the weight off the moving (inside) leg at this point.

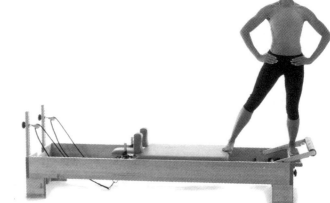

Exhale. Extend the inside knee, straightening the leg completely and pushing the carriage outward.

Imagery

I like to use the image of a sidekick in karate, powerful and directed, when performing the single-leg skating exercise. This is such a powerful image, which has particular relevance to me since I have been studying karate.

- ☐ Keep the weight on the standing leg and avoid pushing with it.

- ☐ Keep the trunk upright.

- ☐ Maintain a neutral and stable pelvis throughout.

- ☐ Straighten the working leg completely, and control its return to the start position.

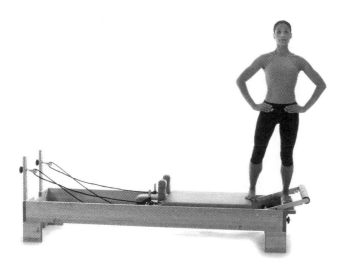

Inhale. Flex the inside knee, bending the leg. Return to the start position. Repeat several times before switching to the other leg.

Muscle Focus

• Hamstrings

Objective

• To strengthen the knee flexors and hip extensors

RESISTANCE

Light Medium Heavy

Hamstring Curl

As its name implies, this exercise focuses primarily on knee flexion. We add hip extension to the knee flexion, maximizing the work of the hamstrings. Engaging the hip extensors prior to bending the knee ensures stronger involvement of the hamstrings, being that they both flex the knee and extend the hip. Engaging the hip extensors also inhibits the action of the hip flexors, which often become involved when the knee bends, particularly if the rectus femoris is tight, and can pull the pelvis into anterior tilt and create hyperlordosis. This should be avoided. Recruitment of the abdominals also helps prevent hyperlordosis, and engagement of the back extensors counters rounding of the thoracic spine. The pelvis, together with the abdominals and the back extensors create a stable foundation for the exercise. Hugging the front of the box offers additional, welcome support.

Imagery

The image of the body as an archer's bow is a powerful one. This is the position the body should assume prior to the actual curl (knee bend). The bending of the knees can then be viewed as pulling the twine and placing tension on the bow. However, this image should not result in excessive extension of the back, particularly the lower back. Focus the extension in the mid- and upper back.

☐ Maintain hip extension throughout the exercise.

☐ Keep the mid- and upper back extended.

☐ Use the abdominals to protect the lower back and prevent hyperlordosis.

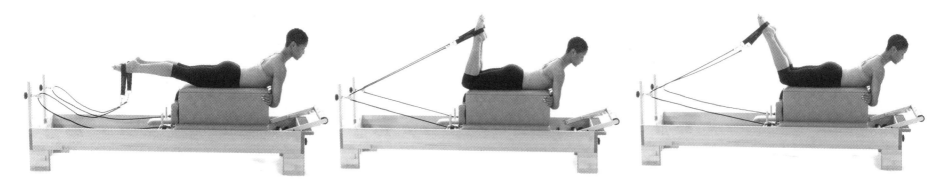

Inhale. Lie prone on the long box, facing the foot bar. Extend the mid- and upper back and engage the abdominals. Place the feet in the straps, with the hips extended and the legs straight and lifted slightly off the box. Hug the front of the box with the arms.

Exhale. Flex the knees, bending the legs and pressing the pubic symphysis into the box. Keep the hips extended throughout.

Inhale. Extend the knees, straightening the legs. Return to the start position.

Lateral Flexion and Rotation

Lateral flexion and rotation are important in both everyday activities and athletic pursuits. Yet, they are severely neglected in many fitness programs. When it comes to training the abdominals, the predominant action employed by many trainers is forward flexion, which is only a small part of the whole. Training the abdominals fully contributes significantly not only to the many actions these powerful muscles of the trunk initiate (for instance that illusive golf swing), but also to the spinal stabilization mechanism that protects the spine. Without spinal lateral flexion and rotation, the abdominals are not being trained to their full capacity. This may result in less than optimal performance and could eventually lead to ailments and injury.

Every program should include lateral flexion and rotation movements, at whatever level is appropriate. The muscles must be addressed in terms of both strength and flexibility. Often, in rotational activities, the arms and shoulders compensate for lack of rotation in the trunk; this results in compromised performance and excessive wear and tear on the body. When the power emanates from the trunk, from strong abdominal muscles working together with the other muscles of the trunk, the movement is infinitely more powerful. In Pilates we call it the power of the powerhouse!

Circular energy forms the basis of the imagery for lateral flexion. Often it is an arc rather than a full circle, but the shape is circular. When performing rotation the energy is more of a spiral. These circular and spiral energy trails promote smooth and flowing movement. When doing lateral flexion I like to visualize a circle, and, as I go through the range of motion, I try to touch every point on the circle. When doing rotation I view it as a spiral that gathers energy along the way, or a spring winding up. There is infinite energy to be found as the spiral unwinds.

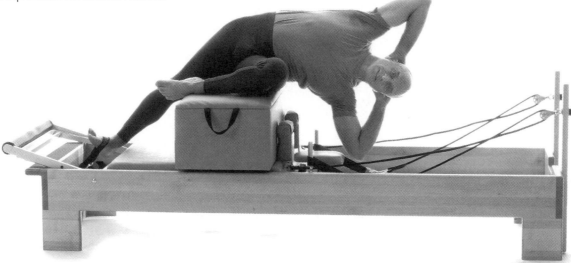

Muscle Focus
- Oblique abdominals

Objectives
- To stretch the oblique abdominal muscles
- To develop control of the oblique abdominal muscles

RESISTANCE

Light   Medium   Heavy

Tilt—Short Box

The tilt is part of the short box series. Although it is not a particularly challenging exercise, it prepares the body for more difficult exercises by teaching correct alignment and muscle recruitment for lateral flexion. An important aspect of this exercise is initiating the lateral motion from the region of the waist, while keeping the pelvis stable and your weight evenly distributed on the sit bones.

The movement works its way up from the pelvis through the spine; it should never start from the shoulders or elbows. Remember to keep the head aligned with the spine. Aim to achieve maximum range of motion, moving as far as possible to create a large arc shape, while keeping the pelvis anchored on the box. The lower body provides the foundation for this exercise and remains still throughout.

Imagery

The image of a young, green tree trunk being pulled over and springing back to an upright position illustrates the elongated, gentle curve that is desired (however, in this case the action begins from the base and not the top). The movement occurs in the sagittal plane, so the image of moving between two panes of glass is also helpful.

☐ Co-contract the abdominals and back extensors.

☐ Keep both sit bones in contact with the box throughout.

☐ Avoid thrusting the ribs forward and arching the back.

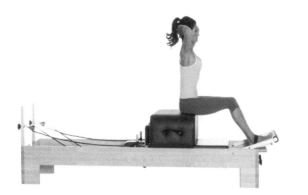 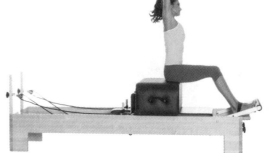 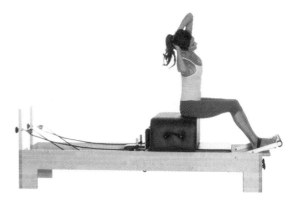

Exhale. Sit upright on the box, close to the front. Place the feet under the foot strap, toes resting on the foot bar (if possible), and firmly anchor them on the front end of the reformer, bend the knees, and interlace the fingers behind the head.

Inhale. Lower the trunk over to one side, reaching out and over, move from the waist and keep the pelvis stable.

Exhale. Lift the trunk, again moving from the waist, and return to the start position. Alternate sides with each repetition.

Twist—Short Box

Also from the short box series, this exercise has two distinct phases: first the trunk rotates around the longitudinal axis, and then the trunk glides diagonally back as one unit, hinging from the hips. This sequence is repeated in reverse as you return to the start position.

During the second phase, focus on a coordinated contraction of the abdominal muscles and the back extensors to prevent the common error of hyperextending the back. As in the Reformer: Tilt, the range of motion is dictated by the ability to keep the sit bones anchored on the box. The pelvis must move together with the trunk. Once the pelvis has reached its maximum range, the upper trunk should stop moving. Continuing to move the upper trunk once the pelvis has stopped potentially leads to hyperlordosis and excessive pressure on the lower back.

Imagery

Rotation around the longitudinal axis—in the initial and final phases—is key to executing this exercise correctly. I use the image of a revolving door. When the body has rotated and then lunges back on a diagonal path, I visualize the entire door being tilted on its side.

To do the Round-About, in lunge position, move through Reformer: Flat Back on a diagonal. Twist on opposite side and lift back to center. The transition to each side demands core control.

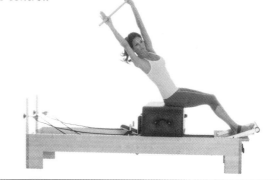

Muscle Focus

- Oblique abdominals

Objectives

- To strengthen the abdominal muscles, with special emphasis on the obliques
- To develop trunk stabilization

RESISTANCE

Light   Medium   Heavy

☐ Co-contract the abdominals and back extensors.

☐ Rotate around the longitudinal axis before gliding backward.

☐ Lift the trunk back onto the longitudinal axis before turning to face forward again.

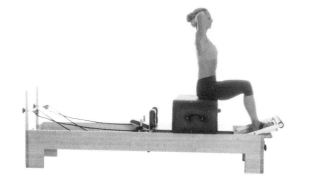

Exhale. Sit upright on the box, close to the front. Place the feet under the foot strap, toes resting on the footbar (if possible), and firmly anchor them on the front end of the reformer, bend the knees, and interlace the fingers behind the head.

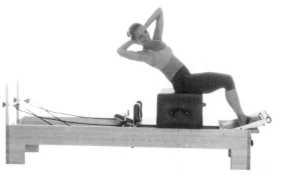

Inhale. Rotate around the longitudinal axis, focusing on elongation of the spine; then hinge from the hip joints, lowering the pelvis and trunk backward on a slight diagonal.

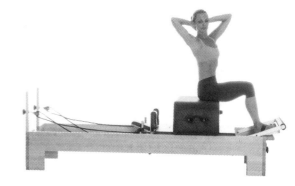

Exhale. Lift the trunk and return to the upright position while maintaining the rotation, and then face forward. Alternate sides with each repetition.

Muscle Focus

- Oblique abdominals

Objectives

- To strengthen the abdominal muscles, with special emphasis on the oblique muscles
- To develop trunk stabilization

RESISTANCE

Light	Medium	Heavy

Side Over—Short Box

I consider this to be the bread and butter of lateral flexion exercises—it is my favorite! The idea of an energy line that stretches from the feet through the leg and then the spine and out the top of the head is particularly pertinent in this movement. With the body in a straight, diagonally oriented start position, the movement is initiated in the region of the waist. As the trunk reaches out and over as if being stretch from the tip of the head and then pulled over like elastic, the energy line begins to arch while the pelvis and lower body remain stable.

Be mindful that the head is a continuation of the spine and extends the line of the body. When the body is in lateral flexion, avoid the common tendency to try and lift back up with the head, which creates tension in the neck; the head has nothing to do with the lift. Similarly, avoid pulling with the anchored leg to lift. The lift must come from the lateral flexors of the trunk. As with many of the lateral flexion exercises, co-contracting the abdominals and back extensors helps maintain the body alignment and keeps the movement in the coronal (frontal) plane. The abdominals prevent hyperextension and the back extensors prevent trunk flexion; working together they encourage activation of the correct muscles, the lateral flexors. Keep the pelvis anchored and as still as possible. Tipping the pelvis *slightly* forward or back may be necessary to achieve optimal activation of the oblique abdominals and to overcome compensations. In addition, be aware of the obliques on the underside of the body, which will prove important in achieving the elongated alignment of the spine.

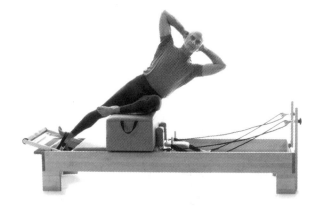

Exhale. Place the box in the short box position on the carriage. Sit sideways on the box and adjust for individual body height by placing the box closer to, or further from, the footbar. A guideline is that the anchored leg should be straight and able to reach the foot strap with you sitting comfortably on the box. Place the foot, dorsiflexed, under the foot strap with the leg straight in neutral hip alignment (minimize hip external rotation). Bend the other leg on top of the box in front of you. Interlace the fingers behind the head. Create a straight diagonal line running from the foot that is under the strap to the head.

Inhale. Lower the trunk over the box following a large arcing path. Keep the pelvis and both legs still.

Imagery

The Reformer: Tilt image of a tree trunk being pulled over and then allowed to return to its upright position offers an image of the correct dynamic and shape. Cultivating a sense of moving between two panes of glass is also appropriate for this exercise.

☐ Co-contract the abdominal muscles and the back extensors.

☐ Avoid lifting the trunk higher than the diagonal line established with the straight leg in the start position.

☐ Distribute the lateral flexion throughout the spine, creating an arc shape with the body.

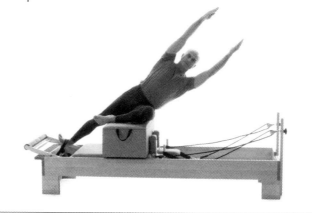

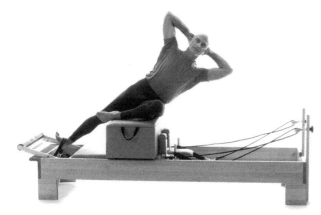

Exhale. Lift the trunk, returning to the straight diagonal line of the start position.

Muscle Focus

- Oblique abdominals

Objectives

- To increase spinal mobility
- To develop oblique abdominal control
- To enhance good shoulder mobility and stability

RESISTANCE

Light   Medium   Heavy

Mermaid

The mermaid has a beautiful flow and exemplifies the choreographic intricacy involved in Pilates. It can be viewed as a movement sequence with three distinct positions or parts. First, a stable position of the trunk is established at the outset. Second, the carriage is pushed out as far as possible and the trunk sinks toward the floor. The movement should feel as if it is emanating from under the arm, with the trunk moving as one stable unit, although in fact it is the shoulder abductors that create the movement. At this point the working arm should be parallel to the floor. Third, the body rotates around the shoulder. During this phase, the back extensors should remain engaged; there should be a feeling of disassociating the trunk from the pelvis and rotating the trunk around a pole. Although we attempt to keep the pelvis still, with both sit bones connected to the carriage, the pelvis will move and one sit bone will lift slightly, depending on the body's flexibility. At this point the shoulders are square, in line with each other and parallel to the floor.

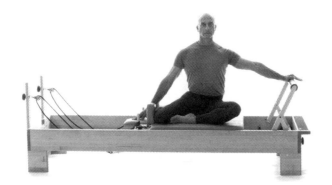

Exhale. Sit sideways on the carriage, with the leg closest to the foot bar bent in front of the pelvis and the other leg bent to the side so that the shin is against the shoulder rests. Place the hand of the arm closest to the foot bar on the foot bar, directly opposite the shoulder, and straighten the arm. Place the other arm down by the side, with the fingers reaching toward the headrest.

Inhale. Push the carriage away from the foot bar until the pushing arm is parallel to the floor and the trunk is nearly parallel. The trunk must move as one unit toward the carriage, and the head must remain aligned with the spine. Simultaneously, lift the breathing arm upward to form a diagonal line (no higher than the shoulder).

The return from the third rotated position back to position two should be precise and clear, with the trunk pivoting around the shoulder joint. Finally the return to the start position should be gradual; do not allow the supporting arm to bend or the shoulder to elevate. The carriage moves back toward the start position but does not need to reach the stopper. Each transition between positions should be accomplished with clarity and control. Avoid excessive movement with the upper arm. I call it the "breathing arm"; it should float weightlessly, responding to the breath and the movement of the trunk.

Imagery

Imagine the body as a spring being wound up and then unwinding with control and precision.

☐ Keep the supporting arm straight throughout.

☐ Pivot around the supporting shoulder during the rotation.

☐ Allow the breathing arm to move weightlessly with the movement of the trunk.

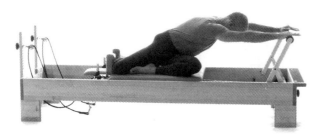

Exhale. Rotate the trunk, drawing in the abdominal muscles and pivoting around the shoulder, while bringing the breathing arm around to touch the foot bar. The trunk and shoulder girdle should now be square and parallel to the floor. Do not move the carriage during this transition.

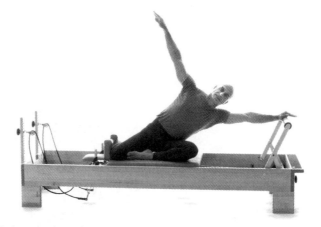

Inhale. Return to the previous position, pivoting around the shoulder again and lifting the breathing arm upward to form a diagonal line. Do not move the carriage.

Exhale. Lift the trunk and lower the breathing arm, while keeping the pushing arm straight and moving the carriage to return to the start position. It is not necessary for the carriage to reach the stopper.

Back Extension

I suppose I might be regarded as a back extension fanatic. There are many reasons I qualify for this title, the most apparent being that I virtually never forgo back extension in a session. I am all too aware that our modern lifestyle, coupled with the unavoidable gravitational pull and the natural inclination of the spine to fold forward, predisposes us to a forward-leaning posture and an eventual loss of range of spinal extension. As I approach my 60s, I experience daily the toll aging takes on spinal extension, as I have observed countless times with clients I have worked with.

Pilates places a great deal of focus on the abdominals and hence on spinal flexion, often at the expense of back extension; at the very least, the ratio of abdominal work to back extension work is often disproportionate. We must not forget that it is the extensors that hold us up, not the abdominals. Although the abdominals are certainly important in offering additional support, the extensors do the primary work.

It is also important to recognize that there are distinct regions in the back, and that different exercises target different regions and different muscles. Typically, when teaching fundamental level movements, I focus on bracing and stabilizing the lower back and concentrating the movement in the mid- and upper back. The main reason for this is that most people automatically extend from their lumbar region, because the natural curve of the lower spine is in the direction of extension. The upper back, which has a natural curve in the direction of flexion, is therefore often neglected. This results in a weakening of the mid- and upper back extensors, coupled with a tightening of their antagonists, the flexors of the chest region. These tendencies are exacerbated by a modern lifestyle; working on computers, driving, cycling, golfing, that encourages (or demands) forward leaning of the upper body, round shoulders and kyphotic posture. It takes time to become reacquainted with the often-neglected mid- and upper-back muscles, while learning to stabilize the lumbar region. To facilitate activation of the mid- and upper back, the program must be augmented by exercises to stretch the muscles of the chest and the abdominals—if the chest muscles are tight, thoracic extension and scapular retraction is restricted, and if the abdominals are tight, extension of the entire spine is restricted.

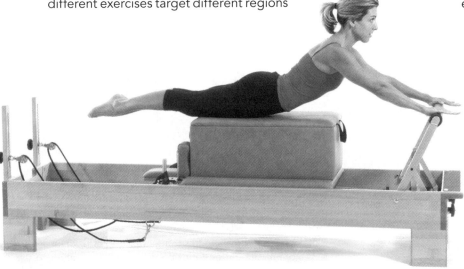

Once students of Pilates become accomplished in doing fundamental back extension exercises, they can move on to exercises with more extreme ranges of motion that require the participation of the lumbar extensors and even the hip extensors.

Three distinct images relate to extension exercises, and each results in the recruitment of different muscles and a different outcome.

The first is used when the goal is to emphasize the mid- and upper back, with the height of the extension being moderate. *Elongation* is the pertinent image; reaching out from the top of the head and relaxing the legs and gluteal muscles will help achieve this.

The second image is used when one of the primary goals is height. In this case I use the image of an *archer's bow* ready to unleash its power. This image works well for exercises that move in and out of extension, as well as those in which holding an arched, stable position is important, such as the Mat Work: Swan Dive.

The third image requires very intricate execution. The goal is seamless movement that utilizes the deep intervertebral muscles that are crucial to the integrity of movement and stabilization of the spine. *Spinal articulation in reverse direction* is used to meet this goal. Starting from the very tip of the head, the spine is articulated into extension. This is much more challenging than spinal articulation in flexion, such as in the pelvic curl.

Finally, I must emphasize the role of the breath. I use an inhale as the trunk extends in all the back extension exercises, on the mat and on the various apparatus, whether there is external resistance or not. This is for two reasons: first, conceptually the inhale assists in elevating the body, and second, certain muscles that assist in the inhalation process also assist in spinal extension. Therefore the inhale is favored for extension. However this does not mean that an exhale is never used during an extension. The prescribed breath pattern should be learned, but once an exercise is mastered, it should be possible to change the breath pattern around without compromising the quality of the movement.

Muscle Focus

- Back extensors

Objectives

- To strengthen the back extensors
- To develop scapular stabilization
- To develop abdominal control

RESISTANCE

Light   Medium   Heavy

Breaststroke Prep

This is an excellent back extensor exercise for people of all age groups and fitness levels. It uses relatively low resistance and has a large base of support, making it safe and user friendly. It works the arms and shoulders together with the back extensors, and the degree of extension can be easily moderated.

Imagery

The image of effortlessly gliding across a smooth surface, like ice or a very slippery floor, as you push away from the foot bar gives a flowing quality to the exercise. When doing the variation with added extension, the same gliding quality should be achieved; however, the energy lines will move both horizontally and vertically as the body arches.

☐ Engage the back extensors prior to moving the carriage.

☐ Keep the wrists firm and the fingers pointing forward.

☐ Keep the head

VARIATION

Once you have achieved good muscle activation and correct form in the start position and elongation phase, extend the trunk into a moderate arch while straightening the arms. You should reach the arched position of the trunk and the fully straightened position of the arms simultaneously. Then lower the body and bend the arms, returning to the start position.

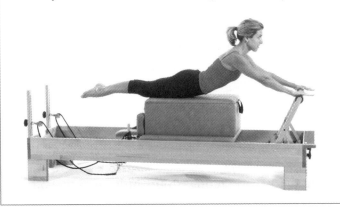

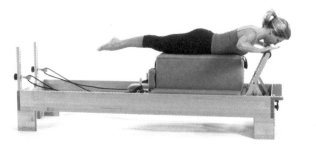

Exhale. Lie prone on the long box, facing the foot bar, with the sternum at the front edge. Place the hands on the foot bar, shoulder-width apart.

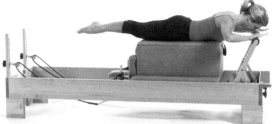

Direct the elbows out to the sides as if the arms were on a flat surface, and keep the body horizontal (parallel to the floor) with the back extensors and hip extensors engaged.

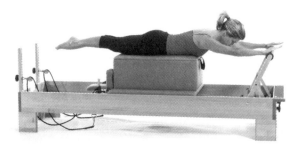

Inhale. Straighten the arms while elongating the entire body and moving horizontally.

Breaststroke

This exercise emphasizes coordinated movement of the shoulders and arms together with the back extensors. The movement emanates from the base of the spine, and the back and the arms should always follow, and not lead, the activation of the back extensors. The movement flows up the spine sequentially. The degree of extension should initially be moderate and evenly distributed throughout the back.

Following the extension of the back and straightening of the arms, the arms should remain straight and the back extended until the arms have circled around to the sides of the body; avoid bending the elbows during this phase. As the arms reach the sides of the body, the arms bend and the trunk is lowered. Keep the upper arms still and maximize shoulder external rotation as the elbows bend; the forearms should move as if sliding across a flat surface.

Everyone can benefit from this exercise. The height of the back extension should be determined by the specific objective. The mid- and upper back extensors work harder if the trunk is kept low and the movement has a horizontal orientation. The lower back is activated more when the trunk lifts into a higher arch. I often work people outside of their comfort zone. For instance, dancers love lifting into extreme hyperextension—this is within their comfort zone. Therefore, I keep them lower and emphasize even distribution of the extension throughout the back.

Imagery

I encourage the use of the image of swimming the breaststroke on the surface of the water or in a 1-inch-deep pool of water, keeping the movement of the arms almost two-dimensional in the coronal plane. This exercise promotes the concept of a strong horizontal component in back extension work keeping the trunk relatively low, the tendency being to immediately lift as high as possible.

☐ Move the arms as an extension of the trunk.

☐ Maintain external rotation of the shoulders as the elbows bend in the final phase.

☐ Focus on back extension without excessive hip extension; keep the legs parallel to the floor.

☐ Keep the palms facing down throughout.

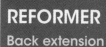
Muscle Focus

- Back extensors

Objectives

- To strengthen the back extensors, shoulder abductors, and elbow extensors

	RESISTANCE	
Light	Medium	Heavy

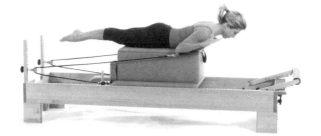

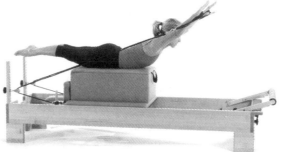

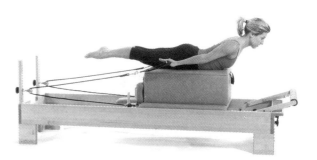

Exhale. Lie prone on the long box, facing the foot bar, with the sternum at the front edge. Place the thumbs in the straps so that the ropes run under the arms. The elbows are bent by the sides, facing outward, with the shoulders biased toward external rotation. Face the fingers forward, with the hands slightly higher than the elbows.

Inhale. Extend the trunk, then immediately straighten the arms forward and upward along a diagonal line.

Still inhaling, circle the arms around to the sides of the body while holding the trunk stable in extension.

Exhale. Bend the elbows, keeping them close by the sides of the body, hands higher than the elbows. Maintain external rotation of the shoulders and move the forearms as if they are gliding over a flat surface. Simultaneously lower the body, returning to the start position.

219

INTERMEDIATE

Muscle Focus
- Back extensors

Objectives
- To strengthen the back and shoulder extensors

RESISTANCE

Light — Medium — Heavy

Pulling Straps I

The pulling straps exercises highlight the back extensor complex and correct muscle activation, together with arm and shoulder work. Think of the Reformer: Breaststroke performed while facing in the opposite direction. Starting from the top of the head, the muscles are sequentially recruited toward the lower back. The back extension is accompanied by extension of the shoulders as the straps are pulled back—a powerful combination. As the extension occurs, the legs remain in a stable position, parallel to the floor. The degree of back extension depends on which area of the back you wish to target. The higher the arch, the more the lower back extensors will be activated. Keep the palms facing the reformer throughout, avoiding internal rotation of the shoulders and the temptation to round the chest. Focus first on arching the thoracic spine and opening the chest as the arms pull back,

followed, if you wish, by increasing the extension as the arms reach their end range.

Imagery

Being a surfer, I find it difficult to resist using the image of paddling a surfboard, which combines back, shoulder, and arm strength in a coordinated pattern. No exercise will better prepare surfers for that elusive perfect wave!

☐ Engage the back extensors from the outset.

☐ Keep the elbows straight and the palms facing the reformer.

☐ Press the hands against the thighs at the conclusion of the shoulder extension.

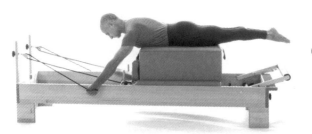

Exhale. Lie prone on the box, facing away from the foot bar, with the sternum at the edge of the box. Hold the ropes with the arms straight and approximately 20 degrees forward of a perpendicular line drawn down from the shoulders.

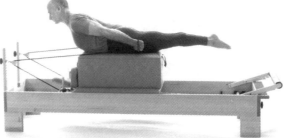

Inhale. Extend the trunk, arching the back, and pull the straps toward the sides of the thighs, with the palms facing the body.

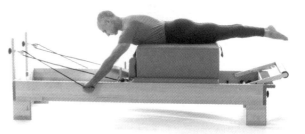

Exhale. Lower the body and bring the arms forward, returning to the start position.

Pulling Straps II

Like the Reformer: Pulling Straps I, this exercise emphasizes the importance of the back extensor complex and focuses on coordinated muscle activation of the back and the shoulders. However, in this case back extension is accompanied by shoulder adduction, rather than shoulder extension. This is a more complex and difficult movement, demanding tremendous strength of the back extensors, which serve as a platform for the arms to move on.

Both pulling straps exercises demand strong recruitment of the latissimus dorsi, which extends the shoulders in the first exercise, and adducts the shoulders in this one. Yet the latissimus dorsi is also a strong internal rotator of the shoulder, an action that is not desired in either exercise. This action of the latissimus dorsi is neutralized by the shoulder external rotators, which function as synergists in both these pulling strap exercises, countering the tendency to internally rotate the shoulders. The close relationship of the shoulder external rotators and the back extensors, particularly the mid- and upper extensors, is highlighted in this exercise. By keeping the palms facing the floor recruitment of these muscles, shoulder external rotators and mid- and upper-back extensors, is encouraged. Move the arms along a horizontal plane.

In addition the posterior aspect of the shoulder, particularly the posterior deltoid, must work very hard in keeping the arms lifted and able to move along a horizontal plane. It may be necessary to work with very light resistance in order to achieve this.

Imagery

Imagine pulling the body forward along two rails or cables, one on either side of the body, with the arms never rising above shoulder level or dropping below shoulder level. Although the motion is primarily horizontal, and the horizontal energy line is very powerful, a vertical energy line appears as the trunk lifts into extension.

☐ Maintain external rotation of the shoulders.

☐ Hold the arms at the same height as the body throughout the exercise.

☐ Pause with the arms in the T-position after each repetition.

☐ Keep the hands facing down throughout.

Muscle Focus
- Back extensors

Objectives
- To strengthen the back extensors
- To strengthen the shoulder adductors and horizontal abductors

RESISTANCE

Light   Medium   Heavy

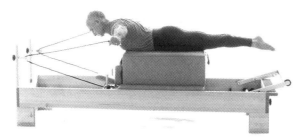

Exhale. Lie prone on the box, facing away from the foot bar, with the sternum at the edge of the box. Hold the ropes with the arms in a T-position, parallel to the floor and with the palms facing the floor.

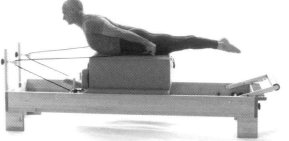

Inhale. Extend the back and pull the arms to the sides of the thighs, with the palms continuing to face the floor. Lead the movement of the arms with the small finger.

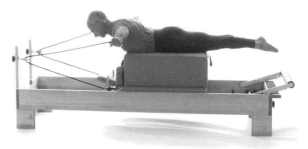

Exhale. Lower the body, moving the arms forward along a horizontal plane parallel to the floor. Return to the start position.

6

Cadillac

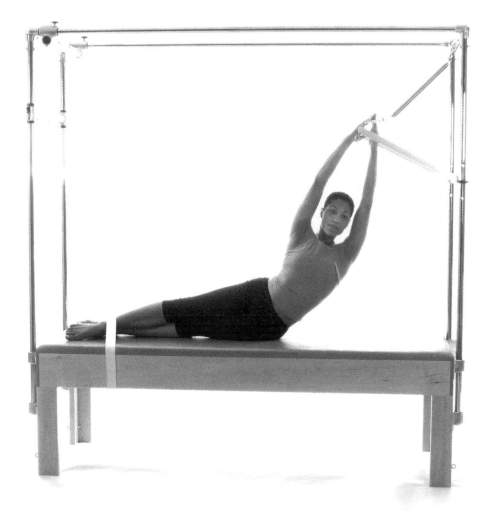

Much has been written about Joseph Pilates' work with the ill, the sickly, and the injured. He helped rehabilitate many of them and in turn was inspired by them. When viewing the cadillac (also called the *trap* or *trap table*), it is clear that the inspiration for this piece of apparatus was a hospital bed.

Like all the Pilates apparatus, the cadillac is unique and versatile, with infinite applications. The foot work on the cadillac, for instance, highlights the hamstrings in terms of both flexibility and strength. This is quite different from the foot work on the reformer and it offers many advantages, as long as you maintain the correct position and are careful not to compromise alignment. The hamstrings are engaged and typically in a state of stretch, from the outset, and the stretch increases as the work progresses.

The cadillac's structure also permits hanging exercises, opening up tremendous possibilities for the upper and lower body. These exercises develop balance, coordination, flexibility, and strength through acrobatic-type movements, which offer myriad benefits as well and are a lot of fun to do.

The fact that the cadillac does not move, but instead provides a stable base of support, is an advantage for people who lack balance and stability, such as the elderly and injured. In addition, it is relatively high off the ground, making it is easier for those with limited mobility to mount and dismount. These characteristics also make it comfortable for the teacher to work closely with students and provide physical support.

The cadillac facilitates ranges of motion that surpass even those of the reformer, particularly in the leg spring work, which can be performed while supine, side-lying, prone, and standing and while facing in all directions. The cadillac is a three-dimensional piece of apparatus in every sense of the word. Finally, just as the reformer offers stretches for the legs that cannot be duplicated on the other apparatus, the cadillac offers unique stretches for the upper body that can only be performed on the cadillac. Enjoy this intriguing piece of equipment—it always makes me feel like a kid again, spending hours on my favorite jungle gym!

Parallel Heels and Toes

The foot work on the cadillac duplicates that done on the reformer and all the same cues and directives apply. Although the foot positions are identical, the positioning of the legs is different: On the reformer the legs move horizontally, on the same plane as the trunk; on the cadillac they move on a vertical line perpendicular to the trunk. This translates to approximately 90 degrees of hip flexion on the cadillac, when the legs are straight. People with tight hamstrings who are unable to maintain the recommended position may lie with head facing the opposite direction and rather than the hip joints being directly under the crossbar of the foot bar they can be further back. This will decrease the angle of hip flexion as well as the stretch on the hamstrings significantly and allow correct alignment. The same benefits will still be reaped in this position.

The more limited range of knee flexion on the cadillac (as compared with the reformer) can be seen as an advantage, as this smaller degree of knee flexion is in fact the "power range" of the knee when jumping. Potentially damaging forces on the knee are avoided, and we are training in a more functional range of motion.

While the heels position amplifies the stretch and work felt in the hip extensors, the toes position generates greater resistance. Maintaining plantarflexion in the feet is important in order to keep the resistance constant. The stretch felt in the back of the legs is not as profound in the toe positions as in the heel positions, yet the sense of elongation up the back of the legs remains as prominent.

Imagery

Imagine that the legs are like pillars, holding up the ceiling of a large building. You lift the ceiling a little higher with each extension of the knees and then lower it as the knees bend. You should feel tremendous power in the legs.

☐ Bend the knees as far as possible without tucking the pelvis.

Muscle Focus
- Hamstrings
- Quadriceps

Objectives
- To strengthen the hip extensors and knee extensors
- To improve hamstring flexibility
- To develop pelvic–lumbar stabilization

RESISTANCE

Light Medium Heavy

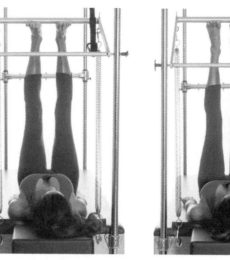
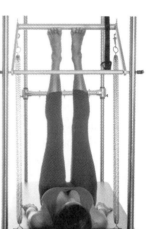

Front view of parallel heels position.

Front view of parallel toes position.

☐ Keep the hip extensors engaged throughout the movement.

☐ Straighten the legs with each repetition, fully extending the knees.

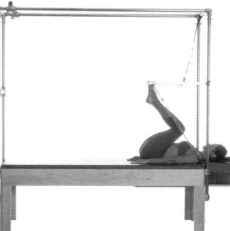
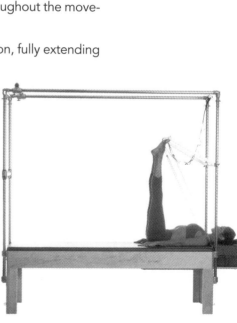

Inhale. Lie supine, arms by the sides of the body, knees bent, legs parallel with either heels or toes on the bar.

Exhale. Straighten the knees and extend the hips.
Inhale. Bend the knees and flex the hips.

225

Muscle Focus
- Hamstrings
- Quadriceps

Objectives
- To strengthen the hip extensors and adductors, and knee extensors
- To improve hamstring flexibility
- To develop pelvic–lumbar stabilization

RESISTANCE

Light   Medium   Heavy

V-Position Toes

Create the modest V-position by simply bringing the heels together from the parallel position. In this position the restriction of the thighs on the chest is not as great. The thighs hug the side of the chest as the knees bend, therefore the knee flexion can be slightly greater than in the parallel positions.

It is important to keep the heels actively pressing together throughout. This will in turn engage the hip external rotators and adductors. Maintaining plantarflexion in the feet is important in order to keep the resistance constant. Although the foot bar is typically narrower on the cadillac than on the reformer, it is still important to try to keep all the toes engaged with the foot bar, even the small toe.

An advantage of the cadillac is that the position for foot work, while engaging the internal support system (ISS), minimizes the possibility of hyperlordosis and, in fact, stretches the lower back. However, you must avoid the common mistake of allowing the pelvis to curl up (tilt posteriorly), lifting the sacrum from the mat. The sacrum, and pelvis as a whole, should serve as an anchor, a stable platform from which the legs can move. Compromising the position of the pelvis will in turn reduce the impact of the foot work exercises, in particular the profound work of the hamstrings.

Imagery

The image of a frog leaping works well in this position. Keep the shape of the V quite moderate; resist opening the legs too wide although the temptation is great.

- ☐ Bend the knees as far as possible without tucking the pelvis.

- ☐ Keep the heels pressing together.

- ☐ Maintain plantar flexion throughout the movement (in the toes position).

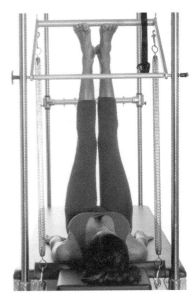

Front view of toes in the V-position.

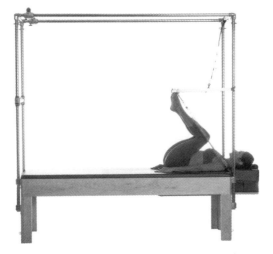

Inhale. Lie supine, arms by the sides of the body, knees bent, toes on the foot bar, feet in small V-position with the heels together.

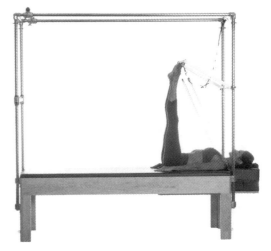

Exhale. Straighten the knees and extend the hips.
Inhale. Bend the knees and flex the hips.

Wide V-Position Heels and Toes

In the two wide V-positions the degree of hip external rotation remains the same as the V-position except that now the legs are apart. In this position the knees can bend much further without restriction and a tremendous stretch for the hips can be achieved. However, remember to still keep the sacrum anchored.

The heel position has two options. The first option, which is the preferred one, demands flexibility of the calf muscles and the Achilles tendon. The heels are placed on the bar and the toes are placed under the respective sidebars. If the stretch is too intense in this position, use the second option. Simply place the heels on the bar and maintain moderate dorsiflexion with the feet. The toes wide V-position provides the deepest stretch of all the positions for the hip joint. Maintain plantar flexion throughout the movement to ensure consistent resistance.

Imagery

The image of a frog leaping used in the V-position works well here too. In this position the legs do open out wide, so as long as the sacrum is anchored you can maximize and enjoy the stretch.

Muscle Focus
- Hamstrings
- Quadriceps

Objectives
- To strengthen the hip extensors, hip adductors, and knee extensors
- To improve hamstring flexibility
- To develop pelvic–lumbar stabilization

RESISTANCE

Light — Medium — Heavy

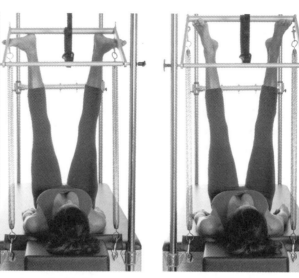

Front view of wide V-position heels.

Front view of wide V-position toes.

☐ Bend the knees as far as possible without tucking the pelvis.

☐ Keep the heels pressing in the bar (in the heels position).

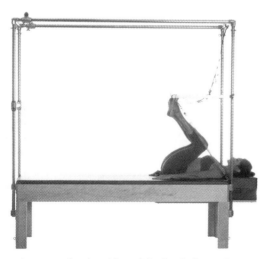

Inhale. Lie supine, arms by the sides of the body, knees bent, toes on the foot bar, feet in wide V-position with the heels or toes on the bar.

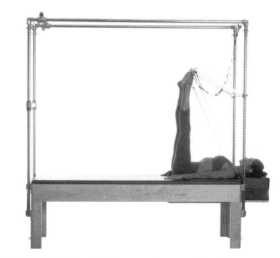

Exhale. Straighten the knees and extend the hips.

Inhale. Bend the knees and flex the hips.

227

Muscle Focus

- Foot plantarflexors

Objectives

- To strengthen the foot stabilizers and plantarflexors
- To stretch the foot plantarflexors and hamstrings

RESISTANCE

Light	Medium	Heavy

Calf Raise

The calf raise exercise takes advantage of a full stretch up the back of the legs that can often be felt all the way through the trunk and even up to the neck. The stretch on the cadillac is more intense than on the reformer because of the upright position of the legs. Another advantage of being in this position is the opportunity to actually look at the feet during the exercise. The visual feedback assists in observing and correcting alignment.

Imagery

I try to imagine lightness in the feet, as if I were tossing a ball into the air with the feet and then catching the ball as it lands lightly on the feet.

- ☐ Use the full range of motion of the ankle and foot.
- ☐ Actively dorsiflex the feet, relying not only on the pull of the springs.
- ☐ Keep the knees straight.

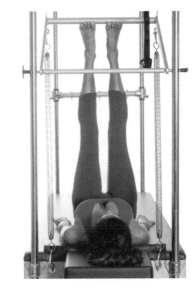

Front view of feet on the calf raise start position.

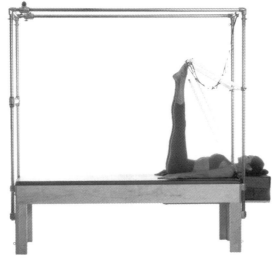

Exhale. Lie supine, arms by the sides of the body, toes on the bar, legs parallel and hip-width apart, knees straight, and feet plantarflexed.

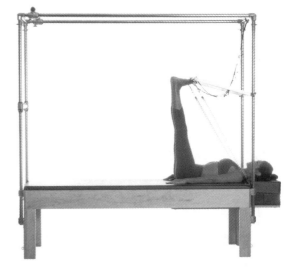

Inhale. Dorsiflex both feet.

Exhale. Plantarflex both feet, alternately performing one full cycle while exhaling and one full cycle while inhaling.

Prance

When performing the prance exercise on the cadillac, the same flow and smooth transitions that are required on the Reformer: Prance should prevail. The anchored position of the pelvis helps stabilize it, reducing the tendency to tilt the pelvis from side to side.

Imagery

I try to imagine lightness in the feet, as if I were tossing a ball into the air with the feet and then catching the ball as it lands lightly on the feet.

☐ Use the full range of motion of the ankle and foot.

☐ Actively dorsiflex the one foot while maximizing the plantar flexion for the other.

☐ Transition through full plantarflexion after each repetition.

Muscle Focus
- Foot plantarflexors

Objectives
- To strengthen the foot stabilizers and plantarflexors
- To stretch the foot plantarflexors and hamstrings

RESISTANCE

Light   Medium   Heavy

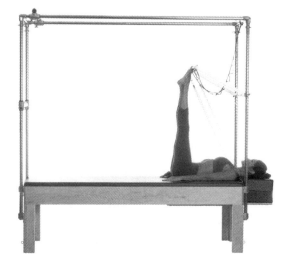
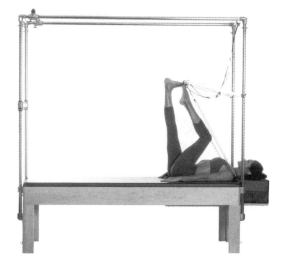
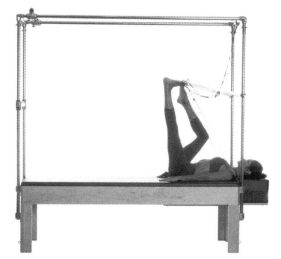

Exhale. Lie supine, arms by the sides of the body, toes on the bar, legs parallel and hip-width apart, knees straight and the feet plantarflexed.

Inhale. One foot plantarflexes as the other knee bends and the foot dorsiflexes. Straighten the bent leg and plantarflex the foot so that both legs are straight and both feet plantarflexed before transitioning to the other leg. Repeat on the other side.

Exhale. One foot plantarflexes as the other knee bends and the foot dorsiflexes.

Alternate; one full cycle while exhaling and one full cycle while inhaling.

Muscle Focus

- Hamstrings
- Quadriceps

Objectives

- To strengthen the hip extensors and knee extensors
- To improve flexibility of the hamstrings
- To develop pelvic–lumbar stabilization

RESISTANCE

Light   Medium   Heavy

Single-Leg Heel

The single-leg position places the body in optimal alignment to stretch the hamstrings of the working leg and to stretch the hip flexors of the supporting leg. The interplay between strength and flexibility of the working leg underscores the principle of *balance* in Pilates. In this heel position, you can readily feel the stretch up the back of the leg and the work of the hip extensors. The supporting leg should lie flat on the mat aligned with the hip joint. There is a tendency for the supporting leg to "float" laterally and the knee to bend, especially if the hip flexors are tight. If this tendency cannot be controlled, bend the supporting leg and place the foot firmly on the mat. This releases the stretch on the hip flexors of the supporting leg and the hip extensors of the working leg.

Imagery

Energy lines offer a profound image for this position, with one line shooting upward vertically from the hip joint of the working leg through the leg and out through the foot.

The other shoots horizontally from the hip joint of the supporting leg, through the leg and out through the toes, and in the opposite direction through the trunk and out through the head. This image helps maintain optimum alignment.

- ☐ Keep the pelvis stable.

- ☐ Bend the supporting leg if the hamstrings and hip flexors are tight.

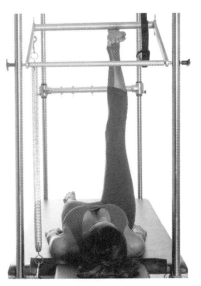

Front view of knee and hip extended with heel on the bar.

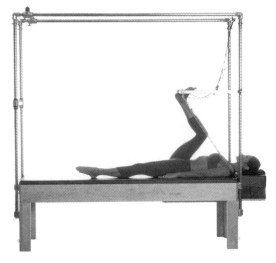

Lie supine, arms by the sides of the body. Place the heel of one leg on the bar, and bend the knee. The other (supporting) leg remains straight and anchored on the mat.

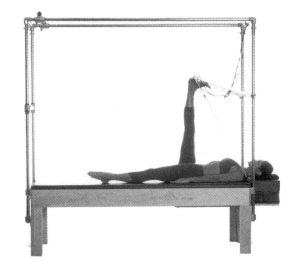

Exhale. Straighten the knee and extend the hip.

Inhale. Bend the knee and flex the hip. Repeat the sequence with the other leg.

Single-Leg Toes

In the toes position, the resistance increases slightly because the springs are being stretched more. The foot plantarflexors, as well as the muscles that control supination and pronation, play a very prominent role in this version. As with the heel version, there is a tendency for the supporting leg to "float" laterally and the knee to bend. If this tendency cannot be controlled, bend the supporting leg and place the foot firmly on the mat.

Imagery

Energy lines offer a profound image for this position, with one line shooting upward vertically from the hip joint of the working leg through the leg and out through the foot. The other shoots horizontally from the hip joint of the supporting leg, through the leg and out through the toes, and in the opposite direction through the trunk and out through the head. This image helps maintain optimum alignment.

☐ Keep the pelvis stable.

☐ Bend the supporting leg if the hamstrings are tight.

☐ Maintain plantarflexion throughout the movement.

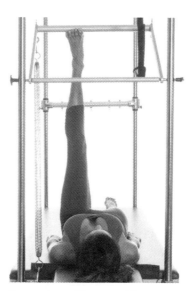

Front view of knee and hip extended with toes on the bar.

Muscle Focus

- Hamstrings
- Quadriceps

Objectives

- To strengthen the hip extensors and knee extensors
- To improve ankle control
- To develop pelvic–lumbar stabilization

RESISTANCE

Light · Medium · Heavy

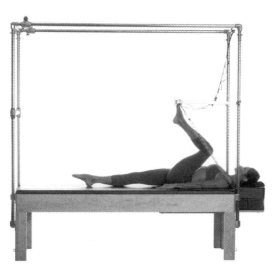

Lie supine, arms by the sides of the body. Place the toes of one leg on the bar, and bend the knee. The other (supporting) leg remains straight and anchored on the mat.

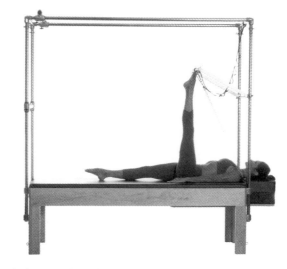

Exhale. Straighten the knee and extend the hip.

Inhale. Bend the knee and flex the hip. Repeat with the sequence with the other leg.

231

Muscle Focus
- Abdominal muscles

Objectives
- To strengthen the abdominal muscles
- To stretch the back muscles
- To develop trunk stabilization

RESISTANCE

Light   Medium   Heavy

Roll-Up

This is essentially a spring-assisted roll-up, much like the Mat Work: Roll-Up. This exercise is often helpful for people who are experiencing difficulty performing the roll-up on the mat correctly, and it is also an excellent option to include in a warm up on the cadillac. The springs help the abdominal muscles, providing an extra boost in facilitating the recruitment of the correct muscles in the correct sequence. The result is good form. The assistance of the springs also helps release excess tension, which may be hampering proper execution of this exercise, from the muscles, particularly from the hip flexors and the muscles of the lower back.

Imagery

As with most of the spring-assisted exercises, you should work with the springs as if they were an integral part of your body and musculature, rather than an external force. Think of them as an extension of the abdominal muscles or an extra abdominal muscle.

☐ The movement begins with the abdominals, which stabilize the trunk as the head and shoulder girdle begin to flex. The hip flexors are then activated to lift the trunk and pelvis into flexion.

☐ The abdominals initially act to stabilize the trunk and deepen abdominal hollowing. Then they work with the hip flexors to lift the trunk and pelvis into flexion.

☐ Keep the knees soft while elongating the legs.

☐ Engage the adductors throughout the exercise.

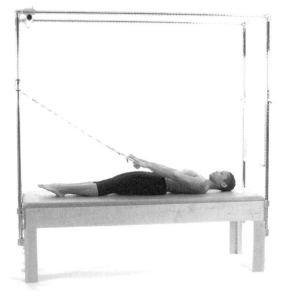

Exhale. Lie supine with the legs straight. Hold the roll-up bar with the hands shoulder-width apart, placing the body far enough back on the bed of the cadillac that there is tension in the springs.

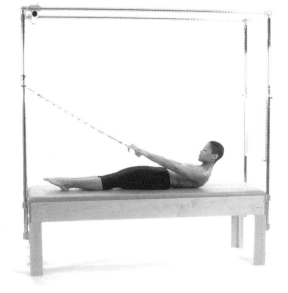

Inhale. Lift the head and shoulder girdle into spinal flexion establishing the C curve.

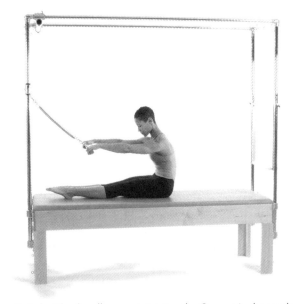

Exhale. Slowly roll up, maintaining the C curve in the trunk.

Inhale, pausing at the point where the shoulders are above the hip joints.

Exhale. Roll back down through each vertebra to the start position.

Mini Roll-Up

This exercise is in essence a spring-assisted Mat Work: Chest Lift. I view the springs as an extension of the abdominal muscles, supplementing their strength. The springs assist the abdominals in performing their function, making it easier to overcome compensations and achieve perfect form. The assistance in this case relates largely to the abdominal muscles stabilizing and allowing the release of redundant tension in the lower back extensors, which often prevents the trunk from achieving adequate forward flexion and the abdominals from fully contracting. Note that the trunk should remain in forward flexion throughout, and the feeling should be similar to that of the Mat Work: Rolling Like a Ball exercise in that the round shape of the body remains constant. The movement occurs between the base of the scapulae and the sacrum, peeling the spine off the mat, vertebra by vertebra, and then lowering back down.

Imagery

Think of a wheel or ball rolling backward and forward in a small arc. Focus on deepening the hollow abdominal bowl with each roll.

- ☐ Focus on maintaining spinal flexion.

- ☐ Keep the shoulders relaxed.

- ☐ Maintain a neutral pelvis throughout the exercise, if possible. (Allow a slight posterior tilt of the pelvis, particularly when hyperlordosis is present, if it helps achieve the desired goals.)

Muscle Focus
- Abdominals

Objective
- To strengthen the abdominal muscles
- To stretch the muscles of the lower back
- To teach the use of neutral pelvis during abdominal work

RESISTANCE

Light   Medium   Heavy

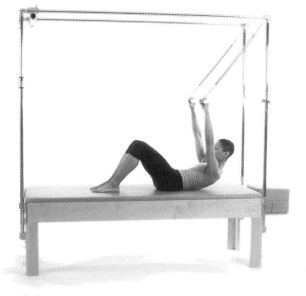

Inhale. Lie in a supine position with the knees bent and the feet anchored on the mat, hip-width apart. Hold the push-through bar with an overhand grip, hands placed in line with the shoulders. Raise the head and shoulder girdle into spinal flexion.

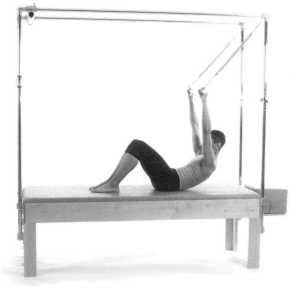

Exhale. Slowly roll up, maintaining the C curve of the trunk. The shoulders should be directly under the push-through bar at this point.

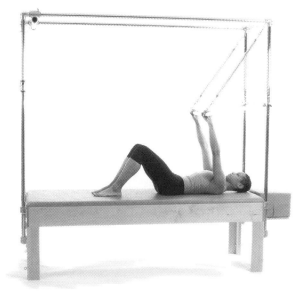

Inhale. Lower to the start position. Repeat 5 to 10 times before lowering to a supine position.

Muscle Focus
- Abdominals

Objectives
- To strengthen the abdominal muscles
- To strengthen the arms and stretch the shoulders

RESISTANCE

Light	Medium	Heavy

Roll-Up—Top Loaded

The sequence of this exercise is similar to the spring-assisted Cadillac: Roll-Up, however, this top-loaded version includes a transition from spinal flexion through spinal extension and into an upright seated position. It includes an arm movement to strengthen the arms, stretch the shoulders, and challenge the upright alignment of the trunk. (There is a tendency to thrust the ribs forward when in upright alignment, particularly during the arm movement, which should be avoided.) During the flexion of the elbows, accentuate shoulder external rotation and abduction of the scapulae.

Imagery

I always feel a sense of pushing the ceiling up and supporting it with my arms, like pillars holding up a building. When the elbows bend, imagine that they are being pulled out to the sides by strong springs. As the elbows draw back in and straighten, imagine that they are working against the pull of the imaginary springs, again pushing the ceiling up.

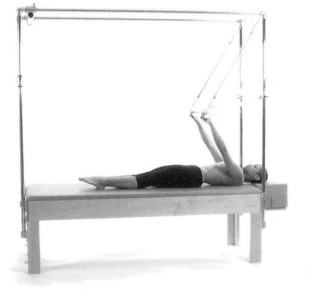

Exhale. Lie supine with the legs straight. Hold the push-through bar with the arms at an angle of approximately 45 degrees to the body. The head is beyond the edge of the cadillac on the headrest. (If your cadillac does not have a built-in headrest, you can make one by placing a stool with a cushion on top at the head of the apparatus.)

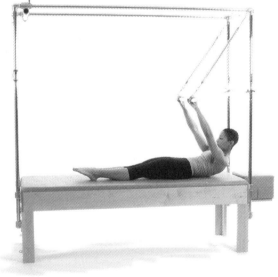

Inhale. Raise the head and shoulder girdle into spinal flexion.

Exhale. Slowly roll up, articulating the spine. Extend the trunk to a seated perpendicular position and reach the arms overhead, pushing the push-through bar up.

- Position the body on the cadillac so that when the trunk reaches the final seated position with the arms overhead it will be perpendicular to the mat.

- Co-contract the abdominals and back extensors to stabilize the trunk when sitting upright.

- Maintain slight shoulder external rotation while bending the elbows.

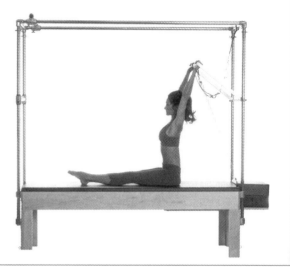

VARIATION

This exercise can be done by loading the springs from the bottom rather than the top (remember to use the safety strap!), in which case the springs resist rather than assist the motion, generating an increased challenge for the abdominals, back extensors, arms, and shoulders. This version is called the Roll-Up—Bottom-Loaded.

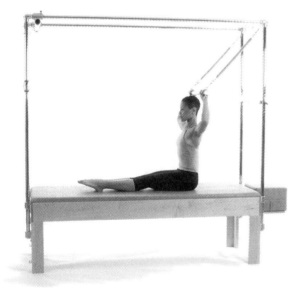

Inhale. Bend the elbows out to the sides and slightly forward (external shoulder rotation), abducting the scapulae, then straighten the elbows.

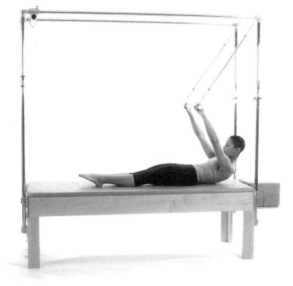

Exhale. Roll down to the start position.

Mini Roll-Up—Oblique

Muscle Focus

- Oblique abdominals

Objectives

- To strengthen the abdominal muscles, with an emphasis on the oblique abdominals
- To stretch the muscles of the lumbar region
- To establish the use of a neutral pelvis during abdominal work

RESISTANCE

Light Medium Heavy

This exercise uses the same form and positioning as the Cadillac: Mini Roll-Up, but it is made more challenging by adding a rotational component to the spinal flexion. Because of the rotation of the trunk, the pelvis is inclined to tilt laterally and lift on one side; resist this by stabilizing the pelvis and keeping the feet evenly weighted. Also, the shoulders tend to elevate. Switching to an underhand grip on the bar assists in maintaining scapular stabilization and relaxed shoulders. Avoid allowing the ribs to flare on one side of the trunk (typically the side you are rotating to), resulting in a swivel (lateral flexion) rather than a true rotation of the trunk. To counteract this, draw the ribs in on the side you are rotating toward, which helps recruit the internal oblique. Finally, avoid the temptation to pull up with the arm by bending the elbow. The arm should remain straight and function simply as a connecting rod between the trunk and the push-through bar.

Imagery

Consciously think of generating the movement from the abdominal region, rather than from the arms or feet. Also think of keeping the distance between the lower ribs and the iliac crests on both sides equal. This helps to produce rotation rather than swiveling.

- ☐ Engage the internal and external oblique abdominals on both sides of the body.
- ☐ Maintain flexion of the spine throughout.
- ☐ Keep the holding arm straight and the shoulders relaxed.

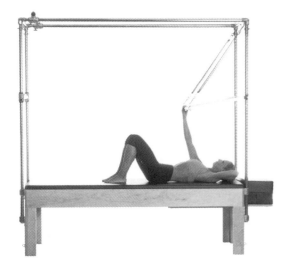

Inhale. Lie supine with the knees bent and the feet anchored on the mat, hip-width apart. Hold the push-through bar with an underhand grip, hands shoulder-width apart. Place one hand behind the head.

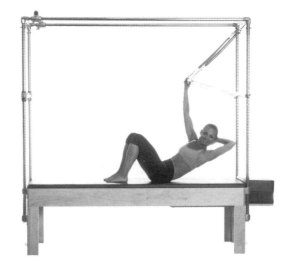

Exhale. Raise the head and shoulder girdle into spinal flexion, and rotate the trunk away from the arm holding the push-through bar. Roll up, while keeping the C-curve position and maintaining rotation of the trunk.

Inhale. Lower to the start position, maintaining rotation of the trunk. Repeat 5 to 10 times before returning to center and lowering to the supine position.

Teaser

The teaser is performed in various forms on the mat, reformer, barrel, and the cadillac. The support provided by the springs in the very demanding cadillac exercise supplements the abdominal muscles and back extensors, facilitating refinement of the movement and muscle recruitment. The push-through bar can be used to assist in all the cadillac versions of the teaser, from the most basic to the most advanced. Use two springs for a lot of assistance, one spring to make it more challenging, and no springs for the greatest degree of challenge and only minimal assistance.

The start position should be based on being able to align the arms with the trunk to form a straight diagonal line when in the V-sit position. I suggest starting with the shoulders directly under the push-through bar when supine.

Imagery

The fact that you are hanging from a spring-loaded bar allows the feeling of weightlessness; of floating up and slowly rolling down. We strive for this quality of movement in the teaser, whether it is performed on the mat, the reformer, the step barrel, or the cadillac.

☐ Articulate through the spine during the roll-up and roll-down phases.

☐ Extend the back fully in the final V-position.

☐ Keep the legs as high as possible, yet at a height you can sustain throughout the exercise.

Muscle Focus

- Abdominals
- Back extensors

Objectives

- To strengthen the abdominals and back extensors
- To develop hip flexor control
- To develop trunk stabilization

RESISTANCE

Light — Medium — Heavy

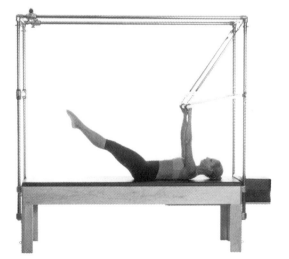

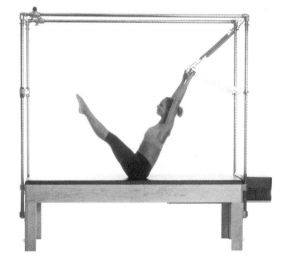

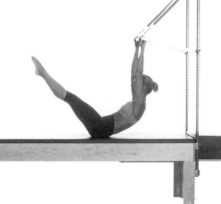

Exhale. Lie supine, holding the push-through bar. Position the shoulders directly below the hands. Keep the legs straight at an angle of approximately 45 degrees.

Inhale. Roll up from the head through the spine. Transition from spinal flexion to extension, creating a V shape with the body, with the arms overhead and diagonally aligned with the trunk.

Exhale. Roll down through the spine to the start position, keeping the legs still.

Muscle Focus

- Hip adductors

Objective

- To strengthen the hip adductors and hip extensors
- To develop pelvic–lumbar stabilization

RESISTANCE

Light   Medium   Heavy

Frog

Hip exercises performed on the cadillac have several advantages over the same exercises done on the reformer. First, lying on the cadillac promotes a feeling of stability. Second, the height of the cadillac makes mounting and dismounting easier than on the reformer. Finally, on the cadillac each leg uses a separate spring, which facilitates the legs working individually, whereas on the reformer the dominant side may take more of the load. This advantage can be used to address any imbalances that may exist in the legs, and throughout the body.

Although the cadillac version of the frog is similar to the version done on the reformer, the muscle action is slightly different because of the angle of resistance. In broad terms, a greater load is placed on the hip extensors. Consider the movement of the heels following a horizontal path, as opposed to the diagonal path they follow on the reformer.

Imagery

The image of the jumping frog used for the Reformer: Frog is a good starting point, but the frog on the cadillac has a distinctly different feel. I visualize pushing away from a wall, with the feet remaining in one place while the body moves. This translates into the feet remaining on a consistent horizontal plane and creates the feeling of internal resistance.

☐ Maintain a neutral spine throughout the movement.

☐ Keep the feet traveling along a consistent horizontal plane.

☐ Initiate the movement with the hamstrings and adductors.

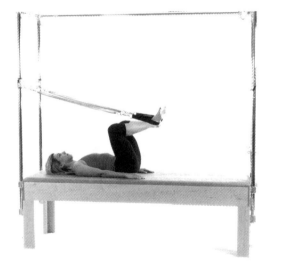

Inhale. Lie supine, feet in the straps, heels together, feet dorsiflexed in a V-position, and knees bent. Place the arms palms down on the cadillac or hold the poles, and relax the shoulders.

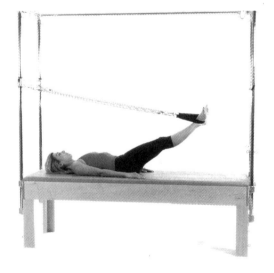

Exhale. Straighten the knees, squeezing the heels together.

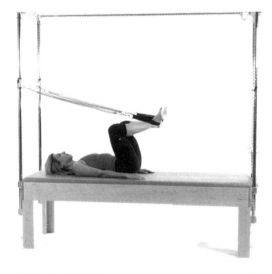

Inhale. Bend the knees, returning to the start position.

Hip Circle

Like the hip work on the reformer, this exercise highlights the principles of hip disassociation and hip joint mobility. On the cadillac, however, the primary emphasis shifts from the hip adductors to the hip extensors because of the angle of resistance. In addition, as in the Cadillac: Frog, each leg has an individual spring and therefore works independently, preventing a dominant side from overpowering a weaker side and doing more of the work, as is sometimes the case on the reformer. This is an advantage, particularly when a significant imbalance is present.

Imagery

As on the reformer, you should work on drawing two back-to-back D shapes (or semicircles) in the air, increasing the size as your control improves. When moving down the centerline on the cadillac, I imagine the legs not only squeezing together, to highlight the adductor work, but also pressing down, as if pressing against a big ball or balloon.

☐ Maximize hip disassociation.

☐ Maintain external rotation of the hip joints.

☐ Keep the size of the circles within a range that can be comfortably controlled.

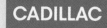

Muscle Focus

- Hamstrings
- Hip adductors

Objectives

- To strengthen the hip extensors
- To develop hip adductor control
- To improve hip disassociation

RESISTANCE

Light   Medium   Heavy

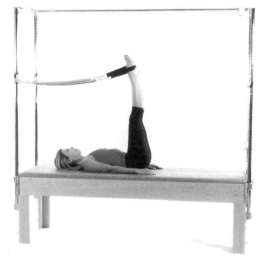

Inhale. Lie supine, with the feet in the straps the legs straight and together, perpendicular to the mat. Externally rotate the hips and plantarflex the feet. Place the arms at the sides or hold the poles, and relax the shoulders.

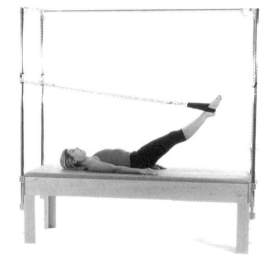

Exhale. Extend the hips, pressing the legs down the centerline and squeezing them together.

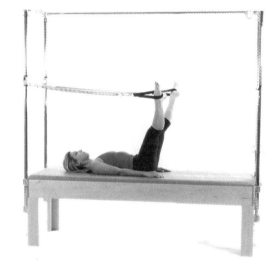

Inhale. Circle the legs around to the sides and return to the start position. Repeat 5 to 10 times and then reverse the direction.

239

Muscle Focus

- Hamstrings

Objectives

- To strengthen the hamstrings
- To develop hip disassociation
- To develop pelvic–lumbar stabilization

RESISTANCE

Light	Medium	Heavy

Walking

The emphasis in this exercise shifts from the hip extensors *and* adductors worked in the frog and circles to the hip extensors only. Because the action of the hamstrings is the primary focus, the hips change from an externally rotated position to a parallel one. This facilitates a more balanced recruitment of the hamstrings.

Two types of movement occur simultaneously. The first is the continuous switching of the legs, up and down a few inches in opposition to one another; the second is the descent of both legs toward the mat of the cadillac (opening the hip joints) and subsequent ascent to the perpendicular position (90-degree angle in the hip joints). Although neither type of movement is particularly daunting on its own, accomplishing both at the same time demands great coordination and can be quite challenging. The small, vigorous fluttering of the legs continues without interruption as the large-scale, gradual lowering and lifting takes place.

Imagery

Rather than thinking of this as walking, I prefer to imagine flutter kicks, as if swimming. The movement should be small and contained, as opposed to the larger movement of actual walking.

- ☐ Keep the leg switches small.
- ☐ Keep tension in the springs throughout the exercise.
- ☐ Maintain a stable pelvis.

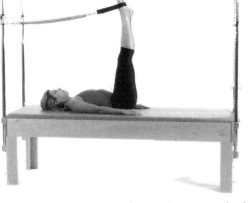

Inhale. Lie supine, with the feet in the straps, the legs straight, parallel and together perpendicular to the bed. Place the arms by the sides of the body or hold the poles, and relax the shoulders.

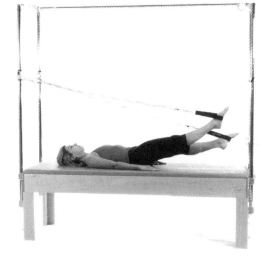

Exhale. Alternately switch the legs up and down in a small scissor-like motion, while simultaneously extending the hips and pressing the legs down toward the mat over the course of a count of 5 counts.

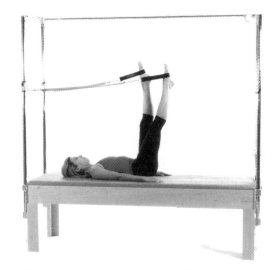

Inhale. Continuing the same scissor-like motion, flex the hips and lift the legs upward until they are perpendicular to the mat over the course of a count of 5 counts while resisting the springs. Return to the start position.

Bicycle

The coordination required for this exercise can be challenging. Focus on making a large cycling motion with the legs. The movement should be fluid, with a sense of elongation, and the hip extensors should be recruited throughout. Maintaining a parallel position of the legs helps engage the hamstrings. Keep the knee of the leg that is pressing down toward the bed slightly bent and stable to help promote a strong contraction of the hamstrings, which act as both a knee flexor and hip extensor.

During this large movement of the hip and knee joints, the pelvis must remain anchored and provide a stable platform for the legs.

Imagery

The image I often use is of a penny-farthing bicycle, one of those old-fashioned bicycles with a large front wheel and a small back one. The small wheel (the pelvis) stabilizes the bicycle, while the big wheel (the legs) provides the movement.

VARIATION

You can reverse the direction, which changes the muscle action and coordination substantially, making it essentially a different exercise (known as "Bicycle—Reverse"). Feel the hip extensors stretching as they contract eccentrically.

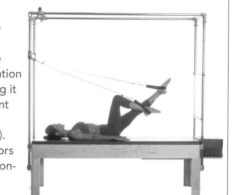

☐ Straighten both legs, establishing an L-position, with one leg close to the bed and the other perpendicular to it, before switching.

☐ Maintain pelvic stabilization and spring tension throughout the exercise.

CADILLAC
Hip work
INTERMEDIATE

Muscle Focus
- Hamstrings

Objectives
- To strengthen the hip extensors
- To develop hip disassociation
- To develop pelvic–lumbar stabilization

RESISTANCE

Light — Medium — Heavy

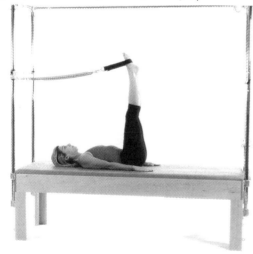

Inhale. Lie supine, with the feet in the straps. Legs should be straight and together in a parallel position, at an angle of approximately 90 degrees to the mat. Place the arms by the sides of the body or hold the poles, and relax the shoulders.

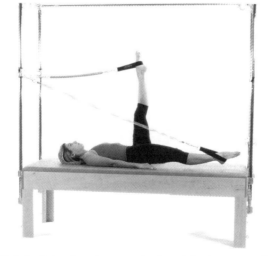

Exhale. Extend one leg, pressing it straight down toward the bed.

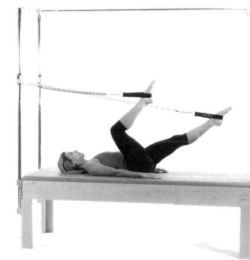

Inhale. Bend the extended leg in toward the chest, sliding the toes on or slightly above the bed and then straighten the leg towards the ceiling. Simultaneously extend the other leg straight down toward the bed of the cadillac, keeping tension in both springs throughout. After 10 repetitions, reverse the direction.

241

Muscle Focus
- Abdominals
- Back extensors
- Hamstrings

Objectives
- To develop abdominal control
- To increase spinal mobility
- To improve flexibility of the hamstrings and calves

RESISTANCE

Light   Medium   Heavy

Monkey

This exercise, which focuses on spinal articulation and hamstring flexibility, serves as an excellent preparation for the next exercise in the series, the Cadillac: Tower. It also reinforces the deep pike position, which is used in many of the flexion exercises on all the apparatus, particularly on the wunda chair (chapter 7). Use the abdominals to create the spinal flexion, followed by the back extensors, which help magnify the hamstring stretch. The arms are used only for support, like rods connecting the trunk and the push-through bar.

Imagery

The top phase of this exercise is reminiscent of a springboard diver's body folding into a tight pike position in the air. This powerful image encourages the correct muscle recruitment and the dynamic of this exercise, which in turn establishes a solid foundation for all the exercises that use a similar position.

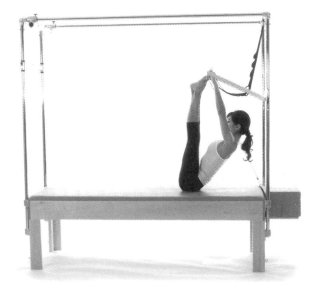

Inhale. Lie supine, with the head on the headrest, facing the push-through bar. (If your cadillac does not have a built-in headrest, you can make one by placing a stool with a cushion on top at the head of the apparatus.) Bend the knees and place the toes on the bar so that the hips are directly under the feet, which are plantarflexed. Grasp the bar, with the hands slightly wider apart than the feet. Strive to anchor the sacrum.

Exhale. Roll up through the spine into a pike position while straightening the knees and maintaining plantarflexion of the feet.

- [ ] Engage the abdominal muscles to lift the trunk into flexion.

- [ ] Maintain plantarflexion while articulating up and down through the spine.

- [ ] Hold the kegs straight when dorsiflexing the feet.

- [ ] Keep the shoulders relaxed and the scapulae stabilized.

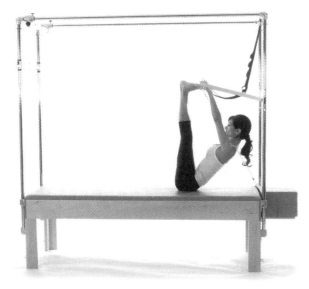

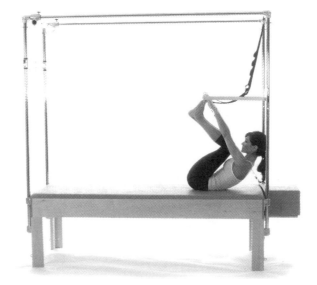

Inhale. Dorsiflex and plantarflex the feet once, maintaining the pike position and keeping the shoulders relaxed.

Exhale. Bend the knees and roll down to the start position.

Muscle Focus

- Abdominals
- Hamstrings

Objectives

- To develop spinal articulation
- To improve flexibility of the hamstrings and lower back muscles

RESISTANCE

Light   Medium   Heavy

Tower

This exercise addresses spinal articulation as well as back and hamstring flexibility. It is a wonderfully satisfying and enjoyable exercise, however it must be approached with caution because of the loading of weight on the spine. Push away from the poles with straight arms, as this helps alleviate excessive pressure on the spine, particularly the cervical region. In addition, activate the back extensors together with the abdominals to support the trunk, especially when rolling up onto the shoulders. This helps prevent sinking into the back and neck, which could potentially result in excessive pressure on the spine. Maximize the stretch of the hamstrings and calves, particularly when the feet are dorsiflexed during the final phase. When rolling down, focus on the eccentric contraction of the back extensors and aim to anchor the sacrum on the mat at the end of the movement.

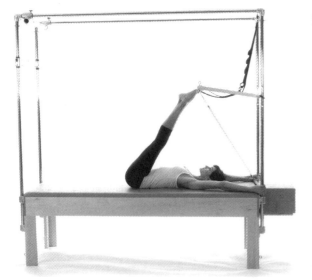

Exhale. Lie supine, and reach the arms straight overhead to hold the poles. Place the toes on the push-through bar, with the feet dorsiflexed and the legs straight and parallel.

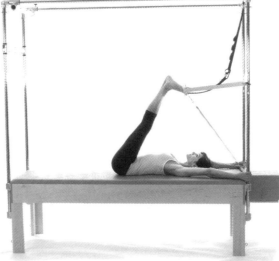

Inhale. Plantarflex the feet.

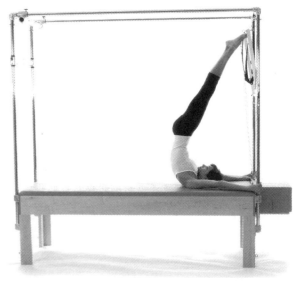

Exhale. Roll up, articulating the spine, onto the shoulder girdle.

Imagery

The image of an accordion opening and closing captures the rhythm of the opening, folding, and reopening of the body in this exercise. Although the physical positions clearly differ from those of an accordion, the dynamic of the movement is similar.

☐ Initiate the spinal articulation with activation of the abdominals and deep flexion of the spine.

☐ Maintain hip extensor and back extensor engagement when up on the shoulders.

☐ Bend the knees moderately at the top, without sinking into the spine and shoulders.

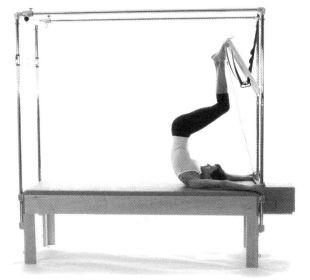 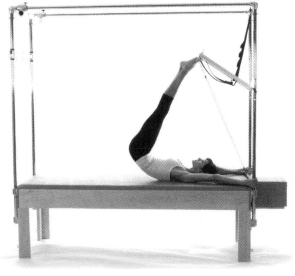

Inhale. Bend and straighten the knees, keeping the hip extensors engaged.

Exhale. Roll down through the spine to the start position, anchoring the sacrum in the final phase.

Muscle Focus

- Abdominal muscles
- Back extensors

Objectives

- To develop abdominal muscle control
- To develop back extensor control
- To develop shoulder extensor control
- To improve flexibility of the hamstrings

RESISTANCE

Light   Medium   Heavy

Push-Through—Sitting Forward

This exercise demonstrates very well the transition of the trunk from spinal flexion to spinal extension and vice versa. It includes extension of the shoulders together with spinal flexion, a muscle recruitment pattern that appears in many Pilates exercises. Along with the profound work of the spinal flexors, it offers the benefit of a hamstring stretch in concert with spinal extension when the push-through bar is pushed forward. It truly is a full body integration exercise in every sense.

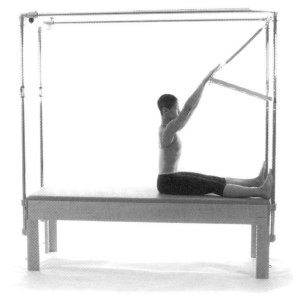

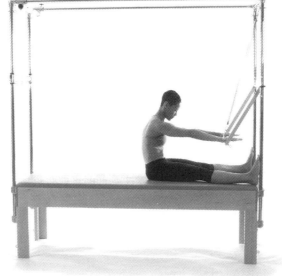

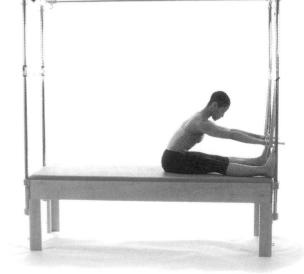

Inhale. Sit upright, facing the push-through bar, and press the feet against the poles. Grasp the bar, with the arms straight and shoulder-width apart.

Exhale. Round the trunk. Press the push-through bar down and then forward, reaching the body over the legs.

Inhale. Extend the spine, flattening the back on a diagonal.

Imagery

The backward and forward motion of the trunk and the use of the push-through bar for control remind me of rowing a boat.

☐ Keep the arms straight throughout the exercise.

☐ Differentiate between the movement of the trunk and that of the arms.

☐ Press the heels against the upright poles of the cadillac throughout the exercise.

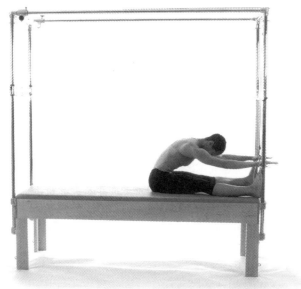

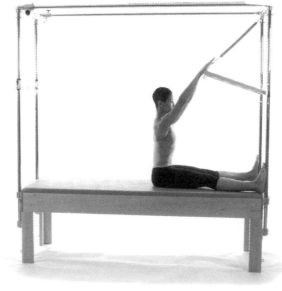

Exhale. Draw the trunk back into spinal flexion.

Inhale. Control the push-through bar while bringing it back and up, maintaining flexion of the trunk. Then extend the spine to the start position, sitting upright.

Muscle Focus

- Abdominal muscles
- Back extensors

Objectives

- To improve spinal artic-ulation
- To improve shoulder flexibility
- To develop trunk stabi-lization

RESISTANCE

Light   Medium   Heavy

Cat Stretch

I perform this exercise when I want to spoil myself, because it feels so good! The cat stretch fortifies the neutral alignment of the spine, both in an upright position and then in the more demanding forward-leaning position. The exercise requires trunk stability as well as shoulder stability and flexibility. The shoulder-stretch position is challenging, so limit the stretch to the range in which you can comfortably maintain stability of the shoulders and trunk. Be careful not to hyperextend the back and place excessive stress on the lumbar spine and the shoulders.

When rolling down at the beginning of the exercise and rolling up at the end, articulate the spine and keep the body as close to the plumb line as possible.

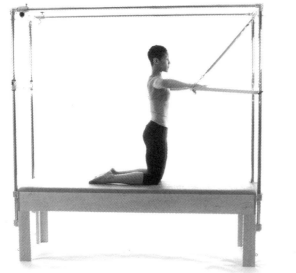

Inhale. Kneel facing the push-through bar. Hold the bar, with hands shoulder-width apart and the arms bent, elbows reaching out to the sides.

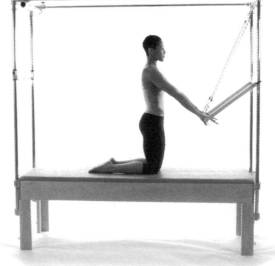

Continue inhaling and press the arms down, straightening the elbows.

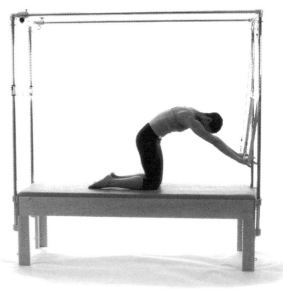

Exhale. Roll down, articulating through the spine.

248

Imagery

The name says it all—stretch like a cat! A cat exemplifies immaculate spinal articulation and the quality of luxurious stretching. Of course, it is important to establish control before you try to reach the more extreme ranges of catlike movement, but the image helps.

☐ Maintain abdominal support throughout the movement.

☐ Avoid thrusting the ribs forward during the shoulder stretch.

☐ Maintain scapular stability during the shoulder stretch.

☐ Align the spine in a neutral position in the initial phase and during the leaning-forward shoulder stretch.

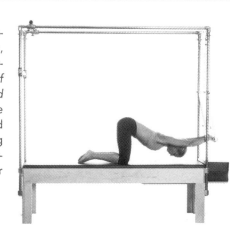

VARIATION

When in the neutral spine position, with the trunk parallel to the floor, *if you feel secure and stable*, press the trunk down toward the bed, stretching the shoulders further into shoulder flexion.

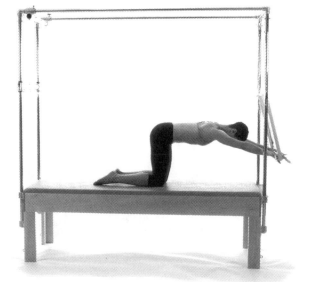

Inhale. Extend the trunk forward into a neutral spine position, parallel to the floor. Elongate the spine, maintaining the neutral position and stabilizing the shoulders.

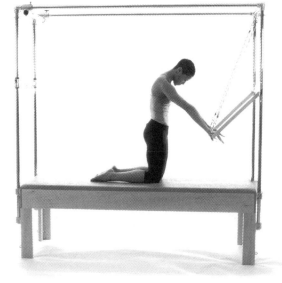

Exhale. Draw back into spinal flexion, articulating the spine as you return to the upright position. Bend the elbows and lift the arms to the start position.

Muscle Focus

- Latissimus dorsi

Objectives

- To strengthen shoulder extensors and elbow extensors
- To develop trunk stabilization

RESISTANCE

Light   Medium   Heavy

Chest Expansion—Standing

Relatively few exercises from the classic repertoire are performed in a standing upright position; therefore, the ones that are should be fully utilized and integrated into a comprehensive program. They are very valuable, and I regard them as gems of the Pilates repertoire. The standing arm work exercises are no exception; they offer unique and far-reaching benefits. The standing position not only develops arm and shoulder strength, flexibility, and control, but also demands core strength and good posture and alignment. To intensify the impact, increase challenge, and develop balance, these exercises can be performed on an unstable surface, such as a balance board or rotating disc, or while standing on one leg.

Note that the distance from the cadillac is crucial—the further away you stand, the more tension there is, and vice versa, the closer you stand to the cadillac the less tension there is. Adjust accordingly.

Imagery

On the reformer, this exercise is done in a seated, kneeling, or supine position. On the arm chair, it is done while seated, and on the ped-a-pul standing, leaning against the pole. Each position offers unique benefits and lends itself to different imagery, although the imagery from one can certainly be used for the others. I like to visualize the body as a statue (think of Michelangelo's *David*, although even he has some alignment issues!) with one moving part, the glenohumeral joint. Feel the solidity of the structure and the intricate, controlled movement of the shoulder.

- ☐ Reach the arms down, as if touching the fingertips to the floor.
- ☐ Minimize scapular movement.
- ☐ Engage the stabilizers of the trunk, maintaining correct alignment.
- ☐ Increase upper back extensor activation as the shoulders extend.

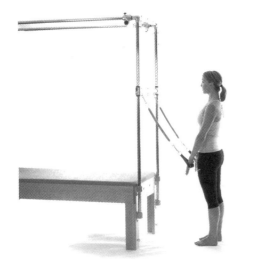

Inhale. Stand approximately 24 inches (60 centimeters) away from the cadillac, facing the apparatus, with the crossbar a little above shoulder height. Hold the handles, with the palms facing back and slight tension in the springs.

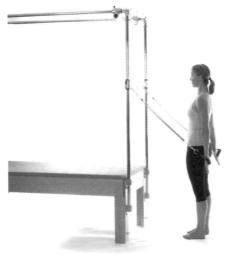

Exhale. Extend the shoulders, pressing the arms back while maintaining the upright alignment of the body.

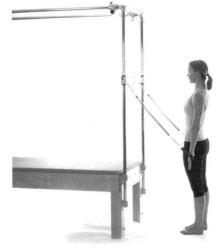

Inhale. Flex the shoulders, keeping tension in the springs, and slowly return the arms to the start position.

Hug-a-Tree—Standing

This exercise is similar to the Reformer: Hug-a-Tree and Arm Chair Hug-a-Tree and, as with those exercises, trunk stabilization is crucial. When standing, however, stabilization is taken a step further by integrating the element of balance, and this makes the work particularly fascinating, functional, and challenging. Few exercises are better for discovering your *center*.

As with the Cadillac: Chest Expansion—Standing, the further you stand from the apparatus, the greater the resistance; adjust the distance accordingly.

Lean forward just enough to counteract the backward pull of the springs, but not enough to rely on the springs for support. Recruiting the ISS, particularly the abdominals, is vital in maintaining ideal alignment; it is the essence of successful execution of this exercise as well as the entire standing arm work series.

Imagery

The image I offer here is a large bird spreading its wings. The arms spread like wings to achieve the largest span possible, moving in and out gracefully. There are few sensations as wonderful as feeling that you are soaring like an eagle, centered and stable.

☐ Keep the back broad and the scapulae stabilized.

☐ Lean slightly forward throughout, while maintaining ideal posture and alignment.

☐ Keep the arms elongated, with the elbows soft and the fingers reaching out.

Muscle Focus
- Pectoralis major

Objectives
- To strengthen and increase flexibility of the shoulder horizontal adductors
- To develop trunk and scapular stabilization

RESISTANCE

Light   Medium   Heavy

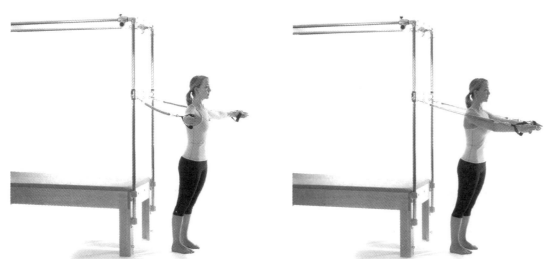

Inhale. Stand approximately 12 inches (30 centimeters) away from the cadillac, with the back to the apparatus and the crossbar a little above shoulder height. Lean slightly forward with the body and engage the abdominal muscles. Reach the arms out to the sides, and hold the handles with either an open grip or a fist grip. (I prefer the open-handed grip.) Bend the elbows are slightly, with the hands facing forward, and some tension in the springs.

Exhale. Bring the arms toward each other until they are parallel and in line with the shoulders.

Inhale. Return to the start position, maintaining tension in the springs. During this eccentric contraction of the shoulder horizontal adductors, keep the scapulae still and maximize the stretch across the front of the chest.

Muscle Focus

- Shoulder extensors
- Shoulder horizontal adductors

Objectives

- To develop scapular stabilization
- To strengthen the shoulders
- To develop shoulder flexibility
- To develop trunk stabilization

RESISTANCE

Light   Medium   Heavy

Arm Circle—Standing

The arm circle highlights control and range of motion of the shoulder complex. It is an extension of the Cadillac: Hug-a-Tree—Standing, performed in the same unique, balanced position, but after the horizontal adduction of the shoulders the arms circle overhead and back around to the T-position. The Arm Chair: Circle exercise (chapter 9), which I recommend learning as a preparation to this exercise, is similar, however the cadillac relies on the body's ability to support itself without the external support of a chair. This is the essence of progression in many Pilates exercises: The movements become more challenging as a higher level of stabilization and internal support is required.

Imagery

Imagine the arms moving through a thick gel—not thick enough to create tension, but sufficient to provide a sense of consistent resistance at every point of the circle.

☐ Face the palms forward in the first phase of the exercise, and then rotate the shoulders so the hands face the floor when the arms are directly in front and prepare to move overhead.

☐ Keep the circles within peripheral vision.

☐ Avoid elevating the scapulae as the arms rise above shoulder height.

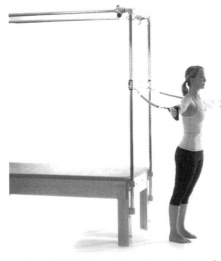

Inhale. Stand approximately 12 inches (30 centimeters) away from the cadillac, with the back to the apparatus and the crossbar a little above shoulder height. Lean slightly forward with the body and engage the abdominal muscles. Reach the arms out to the sides, and hold the handles with either an open grip or a fist grip. Bend the elbows slightly, with the hands facing forward and some tension in the springs.

Exhale. Bring the arms toward each other until they are parallel and in line with the shoulders. Palms are facing each other, as in the Cadillac: Hug-a-Tree.

Inhale. Rotate the arms, so that the palms face the floor, and lift the arms overhead. Keeping the scapulae stable, circle the arms out to the sides to the T-position, with the palms facing forward (start position).

Arm Punch—Standing

Besides the obvious element of developing arm strength, this movement also develops core strength. It demands tremendous trunk stabilization because of the natural tendency to rotate the trunk with each punch.

Imagery

As the name indicates, the movement should feel like a punch. Imagine a precise point in front of you, in line with the shoulder; envision the hand reaching this target with every punch.

- ☐ Focus the movement in the arms, while the trunk and shoulder girdle remain still.

- ☐ Face the fingers toward the direction of the movement throughout the exercise (if using a fist then the fist should be directed forward throughout).

- ☐ Move the arms along a horizontal line.

VARIATION

Once a high degree of stabilization has been achieved, you can add a rotation of the trunk to the straightening of each arm. This rotation increases the power of the punch significantly, as the action emanates from the very powerful rotators of the trunk rather than from the arm.

Muscle Focus

- Triceps
- Pectoralis major

Objectives

- To strengthen the elbow extensors and shoulder horizontal adductors
- To develop core strength

RESISTANCE

Light   Medium   Heavy

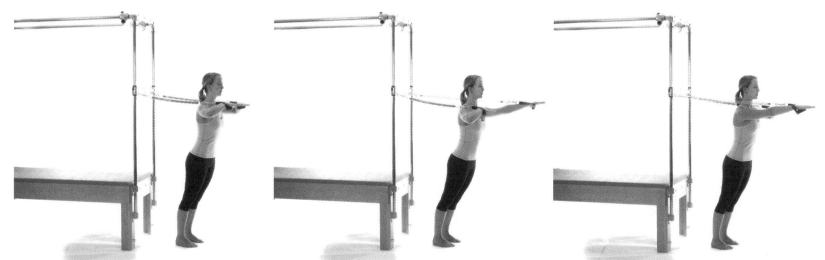

Inhale. Stand approximately 12 inches (30 centimeters) away from the cadillac, with the back to the apparatus and the crossbar a little above shoulder height. Lean slightly forward, placing the hands directly in front of the shoulders. Bend the elbows out to the sides, while holding the handles with the palms facing downward and the fingers forward. There should be tension in the springs from the outset.

Exhale. Straighten one arm forward, then bend it as you simultaneously straighten the other arm; the hands pass each other on their respective paths midway through the movement.

Inhale. Repeat the cycle, performing two to four punches with each breath.

Muscle Focus

- Biceps

Objectives

- To strengthen the elbow flexors
- To stretch the anterior aspect of the shoulder and the chest

RESISTANCE

Light   Medium   Heavy

Biceps—Standing

Although this movement is essentially a standard biceps curl, the positioning of the arms and trunk offer certain advantages. If you have been working the shoulder horizontal adductors in the Cadillac: Hug-a-Tree—Standing, Cadillac: Arm Circle—Standing, and Cadillac: Arm Punch—Standing, you will feel a significant stretch across the chest when you perform this exercise. In addition, the long head of the biceps is held in a fully stretched position, which enhances flexibility and provides a unique angle for developing strength of the biceps.

Imagery

The position of the body can be likened to the figurehead of an old ship. With each bend of the arms, the chest should open more. The feeling should be one of reaching the chest forward (without thrusting the ribs and hyperextending the back).

- ☐ Maintain constant and consistent shoulder extension.
- ☐ Keep the upper arms still and the scapulae stable throughout the movement.
- ☐ Keep the elbows parallel to each other.

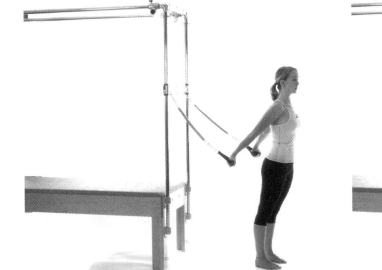 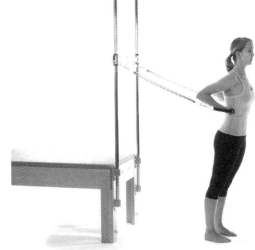 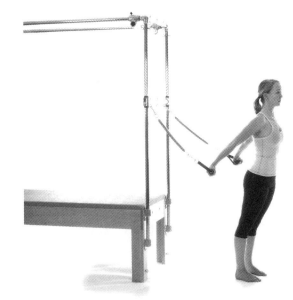

Inhale. Stand approximately 4 feet (1.2 meters) away from the cadillac, with the back to the apparatus and the crossbar a little above shoulder height. Lean slightly forward and reach the arms behind the body, parallel to each other and straight. Hold the handles firmly with a fist grip, and place the shoulders in a neutral position.

Exhale. Bend the elbows, keeping the upper arms still and the elbows at the same height and pointing backward, as in the start position.

Inhale. Straighten the arms, returning to the start position.

Squat

In addition to the obvious challenge for the legs, the squat presents an even greater challenge for the upper body. The trunk is held in an upright position throughout the movement, which encourages neutral alignment and makes the exercise more functional and less risky; the conventional squat position can place excessive load on the lower back. The isometric contraction of the biceps along with the squat action of the legs develops biceps strength, leg strength, and core strength, particularly the back extensors.

Because of the profound biceps work and the general body position, I have included this exercise in the standing arm work series. However, it addresses many areas of the body and could comfortably fit into the leg work, hip work, or full-body integration blocks. It is a valuable addition to any program.

Imagery

Maintain good alignment of the trunk by imagining that you are leaning backward against a wall as your body slides up and down the smooth surface. To make sure the legs are properly aligned to accommodate the smooth gliding movement of the trunk, picture each leg gliding between two vertical panes of glass.

☐ Keep the trunk upright in a neutral spine position.

☐ Hold the upper arms stable and parallel to each other and to the floor throughout.

☐ Maintain correct tracking of the legs, with the knees aligned over (but not in front of) the feet as they bend and straighten.

Muscle Focus

- Biceps
- Quadriceps

Objective

- To strengthen the elbow flexors and knee extensors
- To develop knee control
- To improve alignment and develop trunk stabilization

RESISTANCE

Light   Medium   Heavy

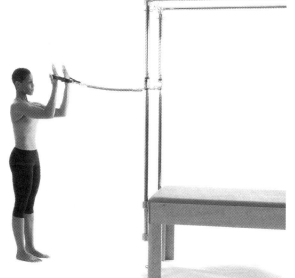

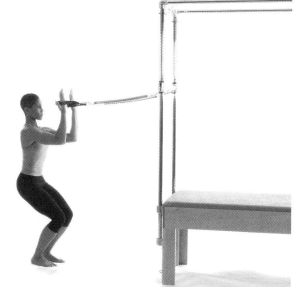

Exhale. Stand facing the cadillac with the legs parallel. Extend the arms in front of the body at shoulder height, hold the straps with slight tension in the springs, and bend the elbows to a 90-degree angle.

Inhale. Bend the knees into a squat, keeping the heels on the floor, the arms stable and the trunk upright.

Exhale. Straighten the knees, continuing to maintain the stable arm position, and return to the start position. Perform 5 to 10 squats, straightening the arms only after the final repetition.

Muscle Focus

- Oblique abdominal muscles

Objectives

- To stretch the oblique abdominals and lower and mid-back muscles
- To develop control of the oblique abdominals

RESISTANCE

Light · Medium · Heavy

Butterfly

This complex movement with a beautiful name combines lateral flexion with rotation, while taking advantage of the resistance and the element of balance. The movement pattern has two distinct phases: lateral flexion, followed by rotation. This pattern can be found in several advanced Pilates exercises, including the Mat Work: Twist, as well as in many athletic activities, including golf, volleyball, and baseball.

In the first phase, the movement is pure lateral flexion of the trunk with no arm movement. The arms maintain an exact T-position, resisting the backward pull of the springs. This is followed by the rotation of the trunk; only at the point of maximum rotation do the arms circle around to reach the "backward" T-position, facing the cadillac. The movement pattern is then reversed to return to the start position.

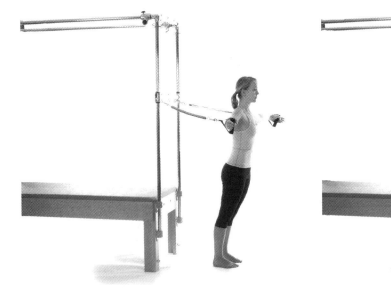

Exhale. Stand approximately 1 foot (30 centimeters) away from the cadillac, with the back to the apparatus and the crossbar a little above shoulder height. Lean forward, with the hands in the straps, arms in a T-position. palms facing forward and slight tension in the springs.

Inhale. Reach over to one side, laterally flexing the trunk.

Exhale. Rotate and round the upper body to face the cadillac, bringing the top arm up and over (with the spring going over the head) and the other arm down and across, to create a T-position again, this time facing toward the cadillac. The arms continue pulling the springs out to the sides and back.

Imagery

The feeling of this movement is like a spring being wound up and then carefully unwound, similar to the dynamic of the Reformer: Mermaid. These two challenging exercises are closely related; finding the connection between them may prove valuable in mastering them both. Another image I like to use is that of the name of the exercise, a butterfly.

As the arms reach out to the sides throughout the exercise, they should feel like wings.

☐ Keep the pelvis facing forward as long as possible before allowing it to adapt to the rotation of the trunk.

☐ Maintain constant tension in the springs.

☐ Keep the arms as wide as possible throughout.

Inhale. Unwind and return to lateral flexion, following the exact path of the body and arms in reverse.

Exhale. Lift the trunk to return to the start position.

Side Lift

Muscle Focus

- Oblique abdominal muscles

Objectives

- To strengthen the lateral flexors (upper side)
- To stretch the lateral flexors (lower side)

RESISTANCE

Light   Medium   Heavy

This exercise is not from the classic Pilates repertoire, but it has evolved from the traditional work. It has a wonderful flow, and besides being a valuable exercise for developing the lateral flexors of the trunk, it is beautiful to watch and exhilarating to perform.

Although the body is ideally in a straight line, it may be necessary to place the legs slightly forward of the centerline, which in turn emphasizes activation of the oblique abdominal muscles. This is helpful when the back extensors, particularly the quadratus lumborum, tend to overpower the abdominal muscles. The same result can be achieved by tipping the upper side of the pelvis slightly back.

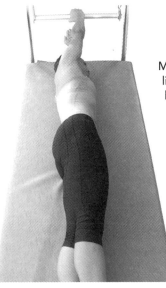

Maintain as close to a straight line as possible with the body, without compromising balanced muscle activation.

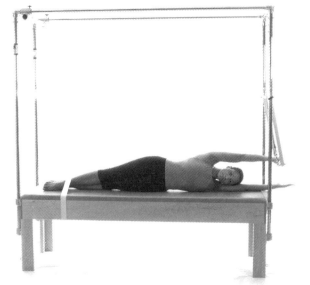

Exhale. Lie on one side, with the legs straight and the top leg in front of the bottom leg. Place the feet under the foot strap. The bottom arm is straight overhead with the head resting on the shoulder. The top arm is also straight overhead, holding the push-through bar.

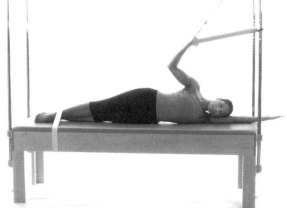

Inhale. Bend the top arm, bringing the push-through bar to the inside of the cadillac frame.

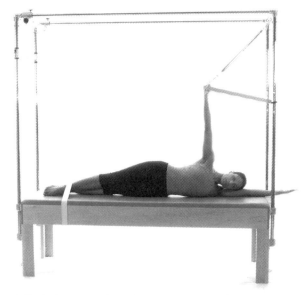

Still inhaling, straighten the top arm upward.

People tend to try to lift the body by pulling up with the arm holding the push-through bar. Avoid this by keeping the top arm straight and focusing on lifting from the waist. Complete the movement by lifting the bottom arm to the push-through bar and touching it (or reaching as close to it as possible). This provides a dramatic stretch to the underside of the body and works the lateral flexors on the upper side intensely. The lateral flexors on the underside should work throughout the exercise to help create a girdle of support around the midsection and provide stability.

Imagery

This movement always reminds me of dance choreography. I like to imagine flying through the air after a leap, reaching out and up. If only we could fly!

☐ Keep the arm holding the push-through bar straight when lifting into lateral flexion.

☐ Engage the abdominal muscles throughout the exercise.

☐ Move up and down in the coronal plane, as if between two panes of glass.

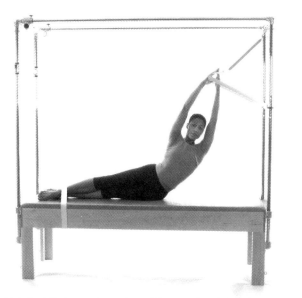

Exhale. Lift the trunk into lateral flexion, then lift the bottom arm to touch the push-through bar.

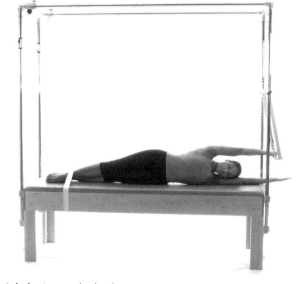

Inhale. Lower the body.

Exhale. Bend the upper arm and then straighten it overhead. Return to the start position.

Muscle Focus

- Oblique abdominal muscles

Objectives

- To develop abdominal control
- To improve oblique flexibility
- To stretch the shoulder adductors

RESISTANCE

Light   Medium   Heavy

Side Reach

Few exercises feel as good as this one. It provides a focused stretch to the side of the trunk and the underarm. Maintaining a good anchor with the legs and pelvis in order to maximize the stretch is vital. This is a unique position; because the pelvic–lumbar region remains in flexion to reinforce the anchoring of the pelvis, while the upper trunk flexes laterally on one side and extends laterally on the other, displaying the control we strive for in each segment of the spine and in the body as a whole.

Imagery

The movement should be a sweeping action out to the side and back, like a large hand-held fan opening and closing.

I also like to think of the side of the body and arm as a rubber band being stretched by an external force attached to the arm; when the force is removed, the body and arm recoil back to the center.

☐ Maintain pelvic–lumbar stabilization when reaching the arm back.

☐ Press both heels against the upright poles, particularly the one on the reaching side.

☐ Turn the palm of the free hand toward the ceiling while reaching back.

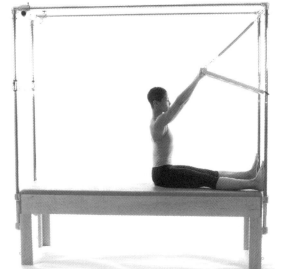 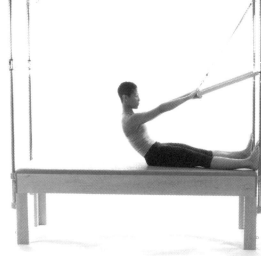 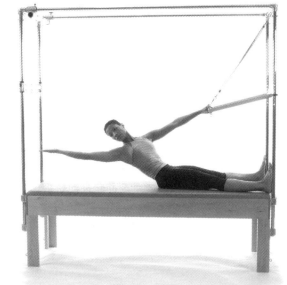

Inhale. Sit upright, facing the push-through bar. Place the feet against the upright poles and the hands on the push-through bar, shoulder-width apart. Keep the arms straight.

Exhale. Round the trunk, hanging back on the push-through bar and pressing the feet into the upright poles.

Inhale. While maintaining lumbar flexion, release one hand and sweep it out to the side and as far back as possible, palm up, to maximize the stretch.

Exhale. Return to the previous position, placing the hand back on the bar and deepening the spinal flexion.

Inhale. Extend the spine to the upright sitting position. Return to the start position.

Prone I

Prone I is the foundation movement of a wonderful series of back extension exercises on the cadillac. It teaches the fundamental principle of distributing the extension throughout the spine, as opposed to focusing it in one area. This is achieved by recruiting the abdominal muscles in concert with the spinal extensors, which assists in protecting the lower back from excessive pressure. It also reinforces coordination of scapular stabilization with spinal extension. Note that the supporting musculature should remain engaged throughout, including between the repetitions.

Imagery

The image of an archer's bow being stretched and then released works well to create the powerful, arching shape of the body. The energy is never completely released; the power is held within the musculature at all times, available on demand.

☐ Glide the scapulae down the back prior to the movement.

☐ Engage the abdominal muscles throughout the movement.

☐ Press down on the push-through bar continuously, with the arms straight.

Muscle Focus
- Back extensors

Objectives
- To strengthen the back extensors
- To develop control of the shoulder girdle and abdominal muscles

RESISTANCE

Light   Medium   Heavy

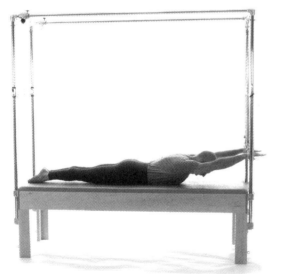

Exhale. Lie prone, holding the push-through bar with the arms straight overhead (forward).

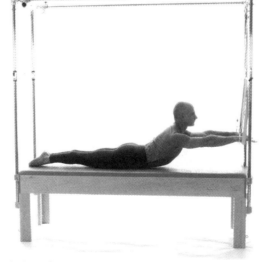

Inhale. Lift the trunk into spinal extension, pressing the arms down gently on the push-through bar.

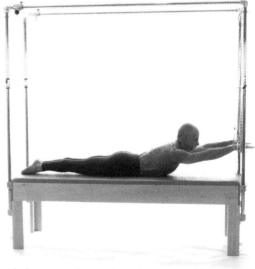

Exhale. Lower the trunk to the start position.

Muscle Focus

- Back extensors

Objectives

- To strengthen the back extensors
- To develop control of the shoulder and abdominal muscles
- To improve flexibility in the shoulder region

RESISTANCE

Light   Medium   Heavy

Prone II

Few exercises integrate spinal extension with the strength and flexibility of the shoulder girdle as beautifully and intricately as Prone II. Although the shoulder stretch and the back extension are linked, they should be regarded as two separate movements. Stretching the shoulders as far as possible before extending the back is important. Then when the trunk reaches full extension, the effort is transferred largely to the back extensors, not relying on the arms or the push-through bar to maintain the elevation of the trunk.

When you reverse the movement, again maximize the stretch of the shoulders before bringing the push-through bar down and lowering the trunk to the start position.

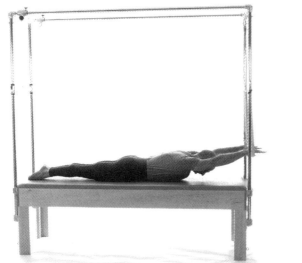

Exhale. Lie prone, holding the push-through bar with the arms straight overhead (forward).

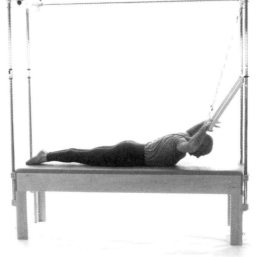

Inhale. Bend the elbows out to the sides, bringing the arms back and behind the head. Begin straightening the arms upward.

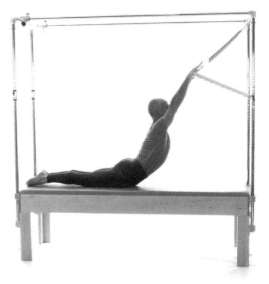

Exhale. When they can move no farther, lift the trunk and continue straightening the arms until the elbows and back are fully extended.

Imagery

The image of stretching and releasing an archer's bow used in Cadillac: Prone I works well in this exercise, yet here it is taken even further as the body reaches a higher, more extreme bow shape. After the full back extension, as you begin to lower the trunk, you should feel like you are hanging from the shoulders.

☐ Achieve maximum stretch of the shoulders before lifting the trunk into extension.

☐ In the second part of the exercise, lower the trunk as far as possible and stretch the shoulders, before bringing the arms through to complete the movement.

☐ Engage the abdominal muscles throughout the movement.

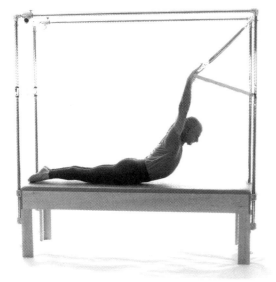

Inhale. Lower the trunk, keeping the arms straight and reaching up.

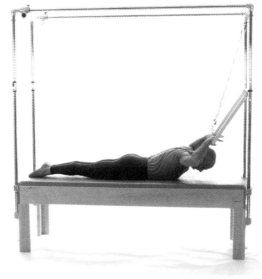

Exhale. Bend the elbows and lower the trunk, bringing the push-through bar down, then straighten the arms directly overhead (forward) to return to the start position.

Muscle Focus

- Back extensors

Objectives

- To strengthen the back extensors
- To stretch the chest muscles
- To develop hip extensor control

RESISTANCE

| Light | Medium | Heavy |

Hanging Back

This exercise is impressive to watch and even more fun to do. Although categorized as an advanced exercise, it is within the reach of many people, even those who may not believe they can perform such a challenging movement. It encapsulates several fundamental concepts, such as spinal articulation, distribution of forces in back extension, scapular stabilization, abdominal support and the relationship between back extension and hip extension.

I like to focus this movement in the mid-back, between and just below the scapulae. When you reach the plank position with the body straight and parallel to the floor, maintain pelvic–lumbar stabilization and then maximize thoracic extension. When the thoracic spine is fully extended, add lumbar extension, and finally hip extension to provide the finishing touches to the movement.

The arms serve simply as rods or levers connecting the body to the crossbars. The shoulders, however, fulfill an important role; good shoulder function is critical to successful execution of this exercise.

The head follows the line of the spine. Avoid the tendency to throw the head back too far when in the hanging-back position, hyperextending the cervical spine. This will inevitably result in neck tension. Instead, you should feel like the crown of the head is reaching down toward the mat, completing the gentle, arcing shape.

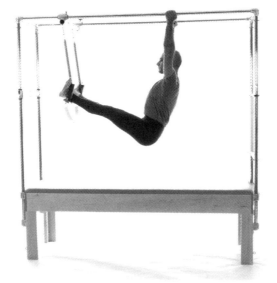

Inhale. Hold onto the crossbars of the cadillac with straight arms. Place the feet on the trapeze swing, dorsiflexed and externally rotated, so they wrap around the springs (for safety). Hold the spine in as close to a neutral position as possible while you hang.

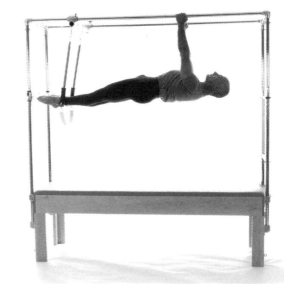

Exhale. Roll up, articulating through the spine, into a plank position so that the body hangs parallel to the bed in neutral alignment. (Plantar-flexing the feet is optional at this point.)

Imagery

Visualizing energy lines works well for this exercise. In the cradle-hanging start position there is an energy line running through the legs and another running through the trunk. They meet at the pelvis to create a V shape. In the hanging-back position, one long energy line runs from the feet to the pelvis, then is gently bent to arc through the trunk and head, tracing the arch shape of the body.

☐ Reach the tailbone toward the bed of the cadillac when hanging in the start position.

☐ Stabilize the scapulae in the hanging position before starting the movement.

☐ Draw in the abdominals, creating deep spinal flexion, to initiate the movement.

☐ Achieve maximum extension in the mid- and upper back before using lumbar and hip extension to complete the movement.

☐ Reach the crown of the head toward the mat in the final position.

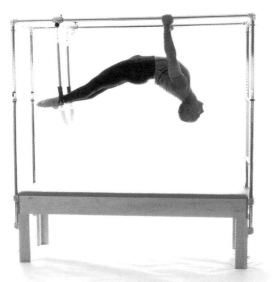

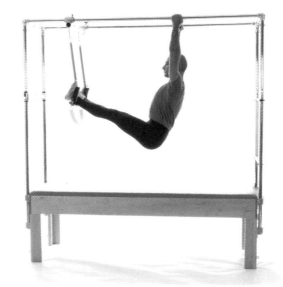

Inhale. Extend the spine further, maximizing thoracic extension. Add lumbar and hip extension, pivoting from the shoulders and keeping the arms straight.

Exhale. Return to the plank position, and then articulate the spine down to the V-shape start position.

7

Wunda Chair

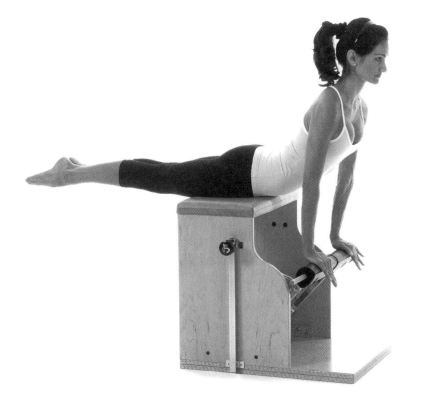

I have a special

sentiment for the wunda chair (also known simply as *the chair*). The genius of its design never ceases to amaze me. This unassuming box with four springs offers infinite possibilities. Displayed proudly by Joseph Pilates in what may have been the original infomercial, it was arguably the first piece of home gym equipment. Yet even today there are few if any pieces of equipment that can rival the wunda chair's capacity: hundreds of exercises for every part of the body and every fitness level. And, to cap it all, the original wunda chair could double as a piece of furniture.

The chair is not easy to use and it often proves quite unforgiving. It readily highlights imbalances and weaknesses in a way that is unique and specific to the chair. However, it also provides tremendous possibilities for dealing with those very same imbalances and weaknesses. Well suited for improving general fitness and enhancing athletic performance, the chair is in many ways more functional than other exercise equipment, even other Pilates apparatus. When doing the foot work on the chair, for instance, the body is in an upright position, demanding greater activation of the trunk stabilizers than the reformer or cadillac. Being upright also more closely simulates everyday movements, making the exercises functional. The wunda chair is extremely useful for pregnant women because it enables them to do the foot work in a sitting rather than supine position.

However, because of its design, the wunda chair does not readily accommodate full ranges of motion; the movements performed on it are typically short in range. For this reason, it may prove advantageous to use pads or a small box to elevate the body during the foot work and increase the range of motion of the joints. Also, the chair offers far fewer possibilities for developing flexion of the limbs than for developing extension. As long as you are aware of these possible shortcomings, the wunda chair is simply a must-have item.

I had the privilege of being introduced to the wonders of the chair by one of the greatest Pilates teachers to grace our community, Kathy Stanford Grant. Although I had worked on it prior to meeting Kathy, it was this insightful teacher that truly opened my eyes to the uniqueness of the chair. Kathy was among Mr. Pilates' early students, and one of only two people to receive a teacher's certification from him. (The other is Lolita San Miguel, also a teacher of great distinction and one I am honored to call a friend. Her accomplishments are many and she is acknowledged as a Living Treasure of Puerto Rico.) Kathy may have been singularly responsible for the rebirth of the wunda chair, bringing it from relative obscurity to center stage in the early '90s. Today it is possibly one of the most popular pieces of apparatus, both in Pilates studios and in gym environments, where it is frequently used for large group classes.

I recall as if it were yesterday the day I met Kathy and naively volunteered to perform several moves on the chair. I had some experience on this apparatus and had been doing Pilates for about 12 years. Kathy, who was small in stature and large in presence, honed in on every compensation pattern, protection mechanism, tension, and imbalance present in my body. This was an epiphany. I recognized a depth of work that I had previously ignored. I had relied on a strong body and athletic skill to perform choreography well—but that was only the outside of the movement. My humbling experience on the chair taught me the meaning of moving from within and set my teaching on a new and exciting path. I had to go back to square one, learning and exploring every movement anew. The experience also taught me to use what I call "MRI vision" (beyond X-ray vision!) to see deeply into other people's bodies and to detect where a movement is coming from even before it happens. This enhanced awareness taught me to move differently, to cue differently, to teach differently, and to anticipate more profound results. I often think of my dear mentor Kathy and the gift of insightfulness that she gave me.

Parallel Heels and Toes

The foot work on the wunda chair duplicates that of the reformer and the cadillac in terms of the foot positions, which are identical. However, the positions of the trunk and legs are quite different—on the wunda chair, the trunk is upright and the legs push down toward the floor. Interestingly, each of these three apparatus allows the legs to move in a different direction when doing the foot work—horizontal (reformer), upward (cadillac), and downward (wunda chair.) Each direction has its unique benefits, and the diverse muscle actions provide a broad range of potentially positive outcomes.

The dynamic of the leg movement on the wunda chair is like a pumping action, with a relatively short range of motion compared to the full-range knee extension on the reformer and cadillac. Feeling the quadriceps more prominently is common on the wunda chair; I refer to this as having "wunda chair legs," a delightful, wobbly sensation often experienced upon completing the foot work.

Imagery

On the cadillac the feeling is like supporting the ceiling, with the legs as pillars; on the reformer it is like propelling yourself

Muscle Focus
- Quadriceps
- Hamstrings

Objectives
- To strengthen the knee extensors
- To develop hip extensor control
- To develop trunk and pelvic stabilization

RESISTANCE

Light   Medium   Heavy

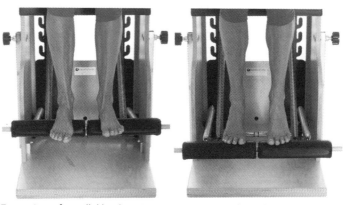

Front view of parallel heel position.   Front view of parallel toes position.

on a horizontal line by pushing against a wall. On the wunda chair the feeling is like pressing against the floor, becoming taller with each leg extension, to the point of feeling levitated above the chair.

- ☐ Maintain a stable, upright trunk throughout.
- ☐ Push down through the heels when in the heels position.
- ☐ Maintain plantarflexion when in the toes position.

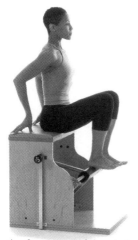

Inhale. Sit upright on the front part of the chair, hands resting on the fingertips near the rear of the platform, elbows bent and reaching back. Place the feet on the pedal, legs parallel, either on the heels or toes. Start the movement with the thighs parallel to the floor or slightly higher.

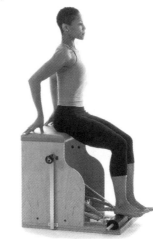

Exhale. Press down with the legs, lowering the pedal until it is about to touch the base.

Inhale. Lift the legs, raising the pedal to the start position.

Muscle Focus
- Quadriceps
- Hamstrings

Objectives
- To strengthen the knee extensors
- To develop hip extensor control
- To develop trunk and pelvic stabilization

RESISTANCE

| Light | Medium | Heavy |

V-Position Toes

As with the other apparatus, create the modest V-position by simply bringing the heels together from the parallel position. It is important to keep the heels actively pressing together throughout. This will in turn engage the hip external rotators and adductors. The range of motion may be even smaller than the parallel position due to the outer thighs pressing against the chair. Maintain plantarflexion in the feet in order to keep the resistance constant, as there is a tendency to drop the heels which in turn releases the tension in the springs. Keep all the toes pressing into the foot bar.

Imagery

The image of a frog leaping is an excellent one for this position. The fact that the body is upright makes the image feel all the more real.

☐ Maintain a stable, upright trunk.

☐ Keep the elbows slightly bent and facing back.

☐ Maintain plantarflexion throughout.

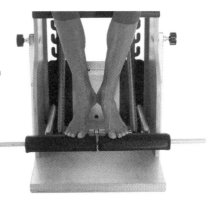

Front view of V-position toes, heels pressing together.

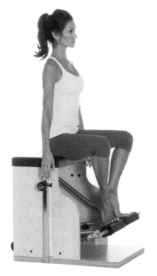

Inhale. Sit upright on the front part of the chair, arms by the sides of the body, fingers reaching toward the floor. Place the toes on the pedal, heels pressing together creating a V-position. Start the movement with the thighs parallel to the floor or slightly higher.

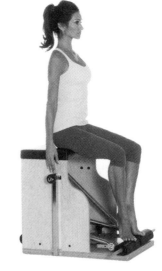

Exhale. Press down with the legs, lowering the pedal until it is about to touch the base.

Inhale. Lift the legs, raising the pedal to the start position.

Wide V-Position Heels and Toes

The wide V-positions on the wunda chair will not be as wide as the reformer or Cadillac due to the foot bar being narrower. However the same benefits the hip external rotators and the hip adductors can be reaped.

Imagery

I like to use the concept of energy lines in this position. There is a feeling of pressing down into the ground with the legs and at the same time reaching up with the trunk through the tip of the head. I sometimes reach the arms overhead, which conjures up an image of being able to support the world on your shoulders.

☐ Maintain a stable, upright trunk.

☐ Keep the elbows slightly bent and facing back.

☐ Maintain plantarflexion throughout.

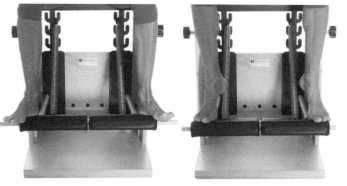

Front view of wide V-position heels.

Front view of wide V-position toes.

WUNDA CHAIR
Foot work
FUNDAMENTAL

Muscle Focus
- Quadriceps
- Hamstrings

Objectives
- To strengthen the knee extensors
- To develop hip extensor control
- To develop trunk and pelvic stabilization

RESISTANCE

Light　　Medium　　Heavy

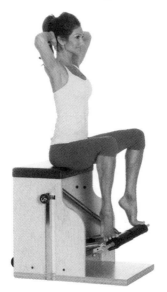

Inhale. Sit upright on the front part of the chair, hands resting on the fingertips near the rear of the platform, elbows bent and reaching back. Place the heels or toes on each end of the pedal, hips externally rotated the same degree as the V-position, but now with the legs apart. Start the movement with the thighs parallel to the floor or slightly higher.

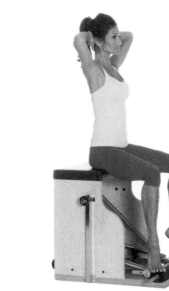

Exhale. Press down with the legs, lowering the pedal until it is about to touch the base.

Inhale. Lift the legs, raising the pedal to the starting position.

271

Muscle Focus

- Foot plantarflexors (calf)

Objectives

- To strengthen the calves
- To stretch the calves and hip flexors

RESISTANCE

Light   Medium   Heavy

Calf Raise

This position exemplifies the concept of multidimensional, full-body integration. Although the calf of the moving leg is the focus of the exercise, trunk stability is being challenged, the hip flexors and calf of the opposite leg are being stretched and even the shoulder stabilizers are being activated. This exercise is exceptional for highlighting correct foot alignment as well as pelvic and trunk alignment.

Imagery

The diagonal position of the body in this exercise reminds me of a ski jumper flying down the ramp. Add to this powerful image the completely isolated movement of the foot, as if pressing down on an accelerator pedal of a car.

- ☐ Maintain a level pelvis.

- ☐ Keep the legs parallel rather than externally rotated, with the back heel pressing into the floor.

- ☐ Utilize the full range of motion of the ankle, moving from full plantarflexion to full dorsiflexion.

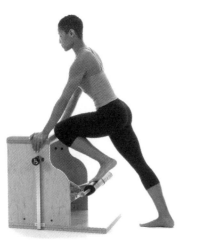 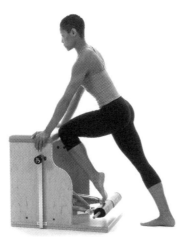 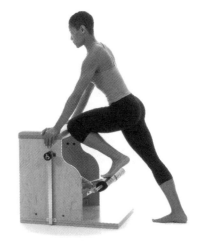

Inhale. Stand facing the chair, with the trunk stable on a diagonal line, and place the hands firmly on the front section of the platform, holding onto it from the sides. Place the toes of one foot on the pedal and press the pedal partly down. Set the leg, just below the knee, firmly onto the front edge of the platform. The back leg is straight and quite far back from the chair, and the heel presses into the floor, creating a long diagonal line with the trunk.

Exhale. Plantarflex the foot, lowering the pedal.

Inhale. Dorsiflex the foot, raising the pedal.

Single-Leg Heel and Toes

All of the advantages and benefits of doing single-leg work on the other apparatus are magnified on the wunda chair. Stabilization is challenging in the sitting position and every possible weakness, imbalance, and compensation is brought to the fore. Few pieces of apparatus, if any, are as valuable as the wunda chair for developing and improving leg function, while stabilizing with the trunk.

Imagery

I find the movement similar to kick-starting a motorcycle (something I have done many times, but you may be too young to have had experience with older motorbikes and to appreciate this image) while keeping the rest of the body stable.

☐ Maintain equal weight on both sit bones.

☐ Keep the trunk stable, avoiding rotation as the leg presses down.

☐ Keep the supporting leg absolutely still.

Muscle Focus
- Quadriceps
- Hamstrings

Objectives
- To strengthen the knee extensors
- To develop hip extensor control
- To develop trunk and pelvic stabilization

RESISTANCE

Light —— Medium —— Heavy

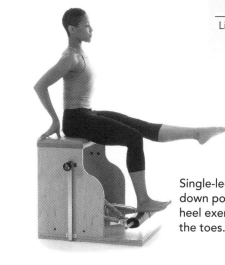

VARIATION

If holding one leg parallel to the floor proves difficult, bend the knee of this leg. If this is still too challenging and you are unable to stabilize the body or hold the leg in the air, rest the leg on a large ball approximately 65 centimeters in size or on the reformer box.

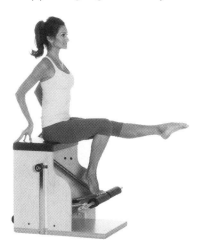

Single-leg heel exercise, down position. Typically, the heel exercise is done before the toes.

Inhale. Sit upright on the front part of the chair, hands resting on the fingertips near the rear of the platform, with elbows bent and reaching back. Place one foot on the pedal in either the single-leg heel or the single-leg toes position. Hold the opposite leg directly forward, parallel to the floor. Start the movement with the thigh of the moving leg parallel to the floor or slightly higher.

Exhale. Press down with the leg, lowering the pedal until it is about to touch the base.

Inhale. Lift the leg, raising the pedal to the start position.

Muscle Focus
- Abdominal muscles

Objectives
- To develop abdominal control
- To develop scapular stabilization
- To increase lumbar flexibility

RESISTANCE

Light | Medium | Heavy

Standing Pike

The movement of this exercise is similar to the Mat Work: Roll-Down described in chapter 2, but it has the advantage of support provided by the spring. This alleviates potential strain on the spine during the roll-down, particularly when it is done with straight legs. This fundamental version of the pike exercise lays the foundation for the abdominal exercises that follow, which are progressively more advanced and challenging and are all performed in a similar pike position. The pike position relies on deep flexion of the trunk and sound shoulder stabilization.

Imagery

All versions and variations of the pike exercise (there are many, on all the apparatus) demand spinal flexion and focus around the image of folding the body in two, bringing the thighs and pelvis toward the trunk and head. A perfect image is a springboard diver in mid-flight, tucked into a powerful pike position.

☐ Aim for maximum lumbar flexion.

☐ Stabilize the scapulae.

☐ Keep the knees straight and the legs vertical.

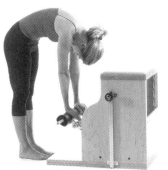 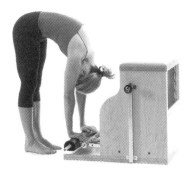 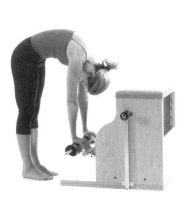 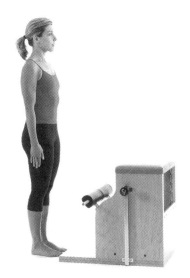

Exhale. Stand facing and close to the front of the chair, with the legs parallel. Roll down, placing the hands on the pedal, with the shoulders aligned over the hands.

Inhale. Roll down, pressing the pedal toward the floor.

Exhale. Roll up, increasing the spinal flexion and raising the pedal. Keep a little tension in the spring before rolling down again. Repeat 5 to 10 times.

On the final exhalation, roll up all the way to the standing start position.

Cat Stretch

This stretch is one of a series of abdominal exercises, including the Wunda Chair: Standing Pike and the Wunda Chair: Full Pike, that focuses on deep spinal flexion. However, this exercise incorporates spinal extension and demonstrates the fine interplay between spinal flexion and extension. During the spinal extension, reach the head toward the floor and aim for 180-degree flexion of the shoulders, creating as close to a straight line as possible with the trunk and arms. At the same time, try to keep the hips over the knees so that the thighs remain vertical. This helps ensure that the movement occurs in the spine, as opposed to the whole body rocking back and forth, and encourages a deep, hollow, round shape of the trunk as the pedal is lifted.

Imagery

The name says it all—the shape, the intricate articulation of the spine, the flexibility, and the control—there is no better image to strive for than a cat stretching.

☐ Align the hips over the knees throughout the movement.

☐ Keep the head aligned with the spine.

☐ Reach the head down toward the pedal during the spinal extension.

Muscle Focus
- Abdominal muscles
- Back extensors

Objectives
- To develop abdominal and back extensor control
- To stretch the lower back
- To develop scapular stabilization

RESISTANCE

Light   Medium   Heavy

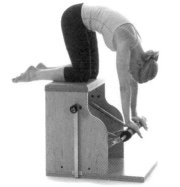

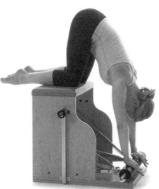

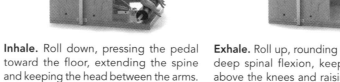

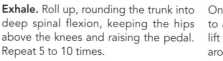

Exhale. Kneel on the chair, close to the front edge and facing the pedal, with the body upright and the hips over the knees. Roll down, placing the hands on the pedal, with the shoulders aligned over the hands.

Inhale. Roll down, pressing the pedal toward the floor, extending the spine and keeping the head between the arms.

Exhale. Roll up, rounding the trunk into deep spinal flexion, keeping the hips above the knees and raising the pedal. Repeat 5 to 10 times.

On a final exhale, roll up all the way to an upright kneeling position, then lift the arms overhead and circle them around to the sides of the body, returning to the start position.

275

Muscle Focus

- Abdominal muscles
- Serratus anterior

Objectives

- To develop abdominal control
- To develop scapular stabilization
- To strengthen the shoulder girdle

RESISTANCE

Light   Medium   Heavy

Full Pike

Few exercises exemplify masterful muscle coordination and integration better than the full pike. And few exercises can be as humbling for even the fittest and strongest among us. You must try it to understand how profound it is. Viewing from the sidelines, it is impossible to appreciate its full intensity; but those who attempt the full pike will never be quite the same. This exercise can guide you to discover the sensation of working deep into the abdominals. The abdominal work is profound and produces a degree of muscle activation few other experiences can match. It must be performed on a relatively light spring; otherwise there is a tendency to rely on the lift of the spring rather than the profound work of the abdominals. Layered on top of the abdominal work is the intense shoulder work, which can be likened to performing a handstand. The influence gymnastics has had on the development of the Pilates repertoire is evident in the full pike. This is a personal favorite!

Imagery

In this exercise, the sensation should be of floating upward—levitating—a feeling that can be achieved only when all components, both mental and physical, are in place and aligned.

☐ Maximize lumbar flexion.

☐ Keep the shoulders over the hands and the head aligned with the spine, the crown of the head reaching down toward the chair.

☐ Maintain stable plantarflexion of the feet.

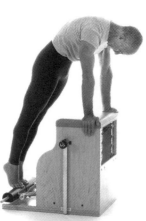

Inhale. Stand on the pedal, facing the chair. Place the hands on the back portion of the platform, holding it from the sides. Align the shoulders directly over the hands. Keep the scapulae stable and round the trunk, establishing a solid pike position.

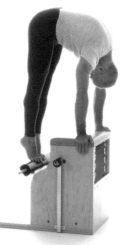

Exhale. Draw deeper into spinal flexion, raising the pedal to the top of its range.

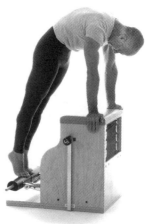

Inhale. Lower the pedal (not quite to the floor), maintaining the pike position.

Torso Press Sit

With the legs stable and still, and the trunk a solid integrated unit, the movement in this exercise occurs at the hip joint. Control of the hip flexors is important, but the focus of the effort should be on the abdominals and back extensors working in a co-contraction mode to keep the trunk stable. This exercise demands a high level of precision and coordination of muscle activation. It serves as a good preparation for advanced abdominal exercises, such as the many versions of the teaser on the various apparatus (although some people find this exercise more demanding than the teaser). Because of the arm position, the torso press offers a significant stretch for the shoulders and the chest that many people will benefit from.

Imagery

I liken this position to a drawbridge, initially lying flat and then hinging in the center; one segment lifting as a solid unit, the remainder of the bridge remaining still (the legs).

☐ Keep the legs stable and parallel to the floor.

VARIATION

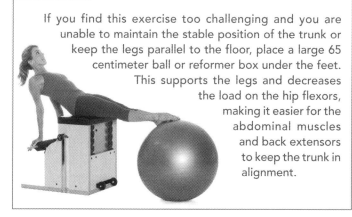

If you find this exercise too challenging and you are unable to maintain the stable position of the trunk or keep the legs parallel to the floor, place a large 65 centimeter ball or reformer box under the feet. This supports the legs and decreases the load on the hip flexors, making it easier for the abdominal muscles and back extensors to keep the trunk in alignment.

☐ Maintain co-contraction of the abdominal muscles and back extensors throughout the movement.

☐ Align the head with the spine.

☐ Maintain shoulder stability with the shoulders externally rotated.

Muscle Focus
- Abdominals
- Back extensors

Objectives
- To strengthen the abdominal muscles and back extensors
- To stretch the shoulders and chest
- To develop hip flexor control

RESISTANCE

Light — Medium — Heavy

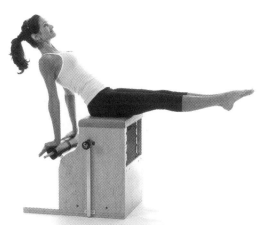

Exhale. Sit on the chair facing forward. Place the hands on the pedal with the fingers facing backward and the shoulders aligned over the hands. Hold the legs directly forward, parallel to the floor, with the trunk in a neutral spine position on a diagonal line.

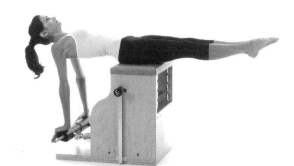

Inhale. Lower the trunk to a flat supine position parallel to the floor, pressing the pedal down.

Exhale. Lift the trunk, raising the pedal to the start position.

Muscle Focus

- Triceps
- Biceps

Objectives

- To strengthen the elbow extensors and shoulder flexors
- To develop trunk stabilization
- To emphasize scapular depression

RESISTANCE

Light	Medium	Heavy

Triceps—Seated

This exercise teaches the fundamentals of what are commonly called *dips*. I cannot overemphasize the importance of good trunk alignment and stability, in addition to excellent scapular stabilization. The movement is a combination of shoulder flexion, highlighting the long head of the biceps, and elbow extension, with a focus on the triceps.

I like to lead into this exercise with shoulder shrugs, allowing the shoulders to lift toward the ears and then pressing them down to engage the scapular depressors, particularly the lower trapezius. This is done with arms straight throughout.(Note that in terms of muscle action this is the opposite of a typical shrug, in which the shoulders are actively lifted and the upper trapezius is engaged.) Once trunk and scapular stabilization has been established, setting the stage for the movement, the triceps exercise can commence.

Imagery

Visualize lifting the body off the ground rather than merely straightening the arms. The involvement of the back extensors and the image of the scapulae gliding down the back are vital to the success of this movement.

- ☐ Keep the elbows parallel to each other and reaching back.
- ☐ Maintain scapular stabilization.
- ☐ Maintain an upright and stable trunk.

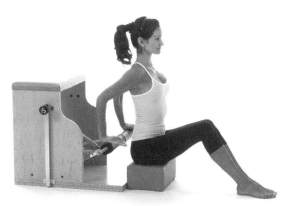 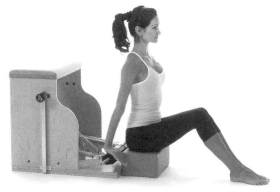 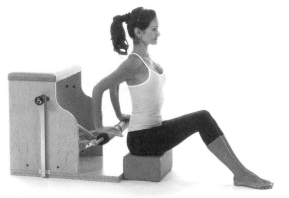

Inhale. Sit upright on a small box approximately 6-12 inches (15-30 centimeters) high facing away from the front of the chair, with legs together, knees bent and feet placed firmly on the floor. Place the hands on the pedal with the fingers facing the body and the elbows bent and reaching back.

Exhale. Straighten the elbows, pushing the pedal down.

Inhale. Bend the elbows, raising the pedal.

Triceps—Prone

This exercise resembles the classic push-up and can teach its correct and precise execution, which is seldom seen. Two areas should be highlighted. The first is the pelvic–lumbar region, which is supported by the chair platform and is therefore less likely to collapse, compared to during a typical push-up. The other area is the scapulae, which tend to adduct, elevate, and wing. Proper placement of the scapulae is often ignored in the push-up; it should not be neglected in whatever position the push-up is performed. The trunk and scapulae must remain stable, requiring that the movement occur in the arms alone, with only slight adaptation of the scapulae.

I recommend initially doing this exercise with the arms parallel and bringing the elbows close to the sides when raising the pedal. This is equivalent to a triceps-driven push-up.

Imagery

Although it is the pedal that is lowered and lifted, the sense should be that the entire body is being lowered and lifted, as one integrated and stable unit.

INTERMEDIATE

Muscle Focus
- Triceps

Objectives
- To strengthen the elbow extensors
- To develop trunk and scapular stabilization

RESISTANCE

Light   Medium   Heavy

VARIATION

The exercise can also be performed with the elbows reaching out to the sides as the pedal rises, in which case it resembles more a pectorals-driven push-up.

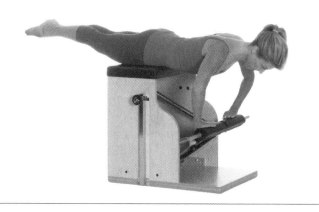

☐ Keep the body stable and parallel to the floor.

☐ Avoid adducting and elevating the scapulae.

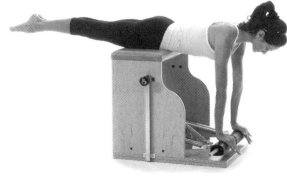

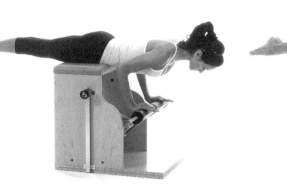

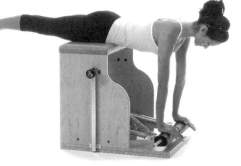

Exhale. Lie prone on the chair, with the legs straight and together and the hands on the pedal. Align the hands directly under the shoulders and straighten the arms. The entire body is parallel to the floor.

Inhale. Bend the elbows, bringing them straight up to the sides and raising the pedal.

Exhale. Straighten the elbows, pressing the pedal down.

Muscle Focus

- Triceps
- Biceps

Objectives

- To strengthen the elbow extensors and shoulder flexors
- To develop trunk and scapular stabilization

RESISTANCE

Light　　Medium　　Heavy

Backward-Facing Dip

The similarity of these dips to the triceps dip commonly seen in a gym ends with the name. The placement of the body in the backward-facing dip amplifies the intensity of the exercise, requiring tremendous strength as well as body control, awareness, and muscle integration. As in the Wunda Chair: Triceps—Seated (an excellent preparation for this exercise), good trunk alignment and stability, and excellent scapular stabilization are important. The movement combines shoulder flexion highlighting the anterior deltoid and long head of the biceps and elbow extension, focusing on the triceps. The movement should commence with the shoulder flexors and then follow with the elbow extensors.

The body must remain perpendicular and in line with the pedal, holding true to the plumb line. Leaning back with the body and bringing the shoulders over the handles makes it much easier, yet sacrifices some of the key benefits of the exercise. When performed correctly, the exercise not only develops tremendous upper body strength but also improves trunk and scapular stabilization, and back extensor control.

As in the milder Wunda Chair: Triceps—Seated exercise, scapular depression should precede the actual movement to counter scapular elevation. The height of the handles should be set so that ideally the upper arms are parallel to the floor when starting, however this will depend on the flexibility of the shoulders. Some wunda chairs do not have side handles, in which case this particular exercise is not possible.

Imagery

Ideally, this exercise should appear and feel effortless, as if the force is being generated under the pedal as opposed to in the arms, and the body is levitating.

- ☐ Keep the elbows facing back and parallel to each other.
- ☐ Maintain scapular stabilization.
- ☐ Maintain an upright, stable trunk.

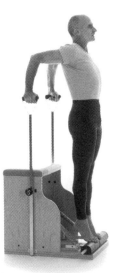

Inhale. Stand upright on the pedal facing away from the chair and place the hands on the handles with the elbows reaching back.

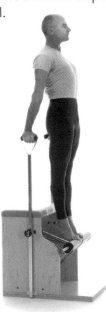

Exhale. Flex the shoulders and extend the elbows completely, pushing down into the handles and elevating the body and the pedal.

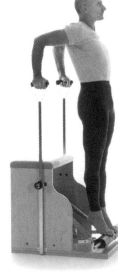

Inhale. Bend the elbows, lowering the body and the pedal to the start position (not quite touching the floor).

Hamstring Curl

This hamstring curl exercise is very focused and effective, with the body in a stable and comfortable position. The back is not in danger of being pulled into hyperextension, as is the case with some other hamstring curl exercises performed in a prone position. Another advantage is the ability to perform this hamstring curl unilaterally, exercising each leg independently. This is of great benefit when a significant imbalance in the strength of the hamstrings is present (one side is often dominant).

The range of motion of this curl is limited; it works the flexors of the knee from approximately 120 degrees to 70 degrees of knee flexion. Only the top section of the pedal's arc is utilized in this exercise, as this entails pure knee flexion. The bottom part of the arc, in which the pedal would be pressed down to the base, requires hip extension, which is not the objective of this exercise and therefore is not used.

Imagery

When pulling the heels toward the sit bones visualize a rubber band connecting each heel to the opposite sit bone. This image ensures the precise direction of pull. When you have maximized the knee flexion (before starting to extend the

Muscle Focus
- Hamstrings

Objectives
- To develop knee flexor strength
- To develop pelvic–lumbar stabilization

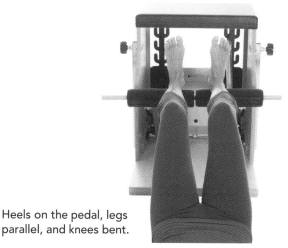

Heels on the pedal, legs parallel, and knees bent.

RESISTANCE

Light — Medium — Heavy

hips), straighten the knees and lift the pedal slowly, resisting the pull of the imaginary rubber band as you return to the start position. Never fully release the tension.

- ☐ Maintain a neutral pelvis.
- ☐ Isolate the knee flexion.
- ☐ Keep the feet stable.

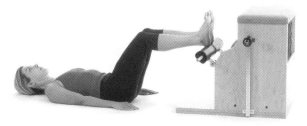

Inhale. Lie supine on the floor. Place the heels on the pedal, feet in a neutral position, with the legs parallel and the knees bent at approximately a 120-degree angle.

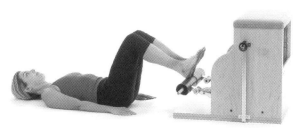

Exhale. Bend the knees, drawing the pedal halfway down and toward you.

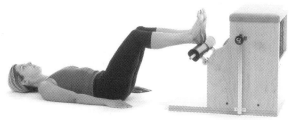

Inhale. Raise the pedal, returning to the start position.

Muscle Focus

- Hamstrings
- Quadriceps

Objectives

- To develop hip extensor control
- To develop knee extensor control
- To develop balance

RESISTANCE

Light   Medium   Heavy

Leg Press—Standing

This exercise is important in teaching functional movement of the leg, improving balance, and perfecting muscle recruitment patterns pertaining to knee and hip extension. The combination of supporting with the standing leg, aligning the pelvis and trunk, and moving with the pressing leg enhances the ability to disassociate the action of the leg from the rest of the body and highlights the value of functional movement.

The alignment of the body is key to activating the correct muscles and ensuring a successful outcome. In order to challenge the hip extensors, the standing leg must be sufficiently far back from the chair and the initiation must occur in the hip extensors rather than in the knee extensors. Avoid the tendency to stand too close to the chair and lean forward; this transforms the movement, placing the focus on the quadriceps, and eliminates much of the challenge.

Imagery

Visualize climbing a vertical staircase while keeping the body perfectly upright. The sensation should be like doing the moonwalk, but moving in a vertical rather than horizontal direction.

- ☐ Initiate the movement with the hamstrings.
- ☐ Maintain plantarflexion with the pressing foot throughout the movement.
- ☐ Maintain upright posture; avoid leaning forward.

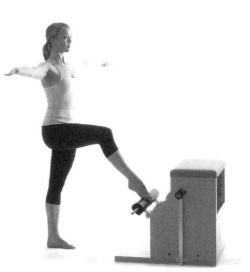

Inhale. Stand upright, 12 to 24 inches (30 to 60 centimeters) from the front of the chair. Place one foot on the pedal in a plantarflexed position. Hold arms out to the sides in a T-position.

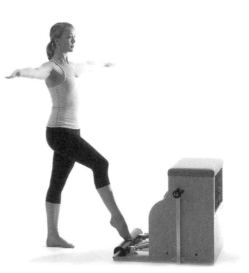

Exhale. Extend the hip, pressing the pedal down.

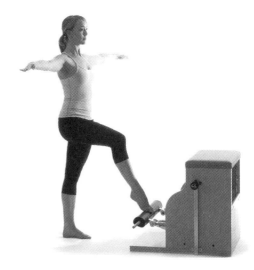

Inhale. Lift the leg, controlling the pedal as it returns to the start position.

Forward Lunge

The forward lunge is another favorite of mine. I have helped many athletes improve their running, leaping, jumping, and overall performance with this exercise. It is a great equalizer—no matter how strong the legs are, the exercise will not be successful without certain essentials being in place: correct muscle activation patterns, pelvic–lumbar stabilization, balance, full body integration, and an optimal strength ratio between the hip extensors, hip abductors, and knee extensors.

Sequencing the muscle activation is key, starting with the hip extensors as the body moves upward and the pedal rises, followed by the hip abductors as the back foot lifts off the pedal, and finally the quadriceps as the knee straightens completely. Of paramount importance is maintaining ideal vertical alignment. The tendency to lean forward, using the strength of the quadriceps from the outset, should be avoided. The adaptations and variations for select populations and activities are endless, once the basic movement has been mastered.

Imagery

This exercise is about levitation. You should feel a sensation of rising from the start position, as if a force under the pedal is propelling you upward or a string from the sky is lifting you up.

☐ Activate the muscles sequentially: hip extensors, hip abductors, then knee extensors.

☐ Maintain a stable, level pelvis throughout the exercise (particularly as the foot lifts off the pedal).

☐ Move on a vertical line, avoiding leaning forward.

Muscle Focus

- Hamstrings
- Hip abductors
- Quadriceps

Objectives

- To strengthen the hip extensors, hip abductors and knee extensors
- To develop pelvic-lumbar stabilization
- To increase awareness and control of optimal alignment

RESISTANCE

| Light | Medium | Heavy |

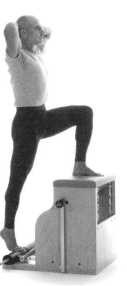

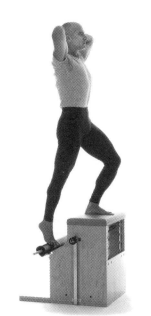

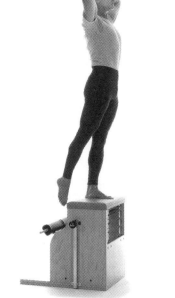

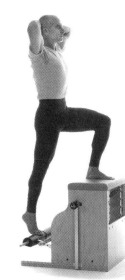

Inhale. Stand facing the chair, holding the sides of the platform for support. Place one foot on the pedal, plantarflexed, and press the pedal down. Place the other foot on the platform of the chair and align the knee above the ankle. Stand upright with the hip joints directly over the pedal and the hands behind the head or reaching out to the sides.

Exhale. Extend the hip, pressing down onto the platform of the chair and straightening the leg as the pedal rises.

Continue straightening the leg and lift the back foot off the pedal, completing the knee extension.

Inhale. Bend the knee, place the foot back on the pedal and lower down to the point that the thigh is approximately parallel to the floor (place pads under the pedal to prevent the pedal going too low and the angle of the knee being much less than 90 degrees, which will occur if you are short).

Repeat 5 times on the same leg before switching to the other side.

Muscle Focus

- Oblique abdominals

Objectives

- To develop control of the lateral flexors (particularly the oblique abdominals)
- To stretch the lateral flexors

RESISTANCE

Light   Medium   Heavy

Side Over

This is an excellent exercise for teaching precise lateral flexion and correct alignment, thereby laying a foundation to later perform the same movement in more challenging positions on other pieces of apparatus. By adding small increments of spring tension, the exercise can be made less challenging, if necessary. By the same token, decreasing the spring tension will make the exercise more challenging. From a teacher's perspective, the student's body is in an ideal position for cueing and offering input and corrections.

Imagery

Imagine the movement as being two-dimensional, occurring between two panes of glass preventing you from leaning forward or backward.

☐ Lift no higher than the diagonal line created by the straight leg and trunk.

☐ Keep the legs and pelvis stable, with the foot of the straight leg anchored on the floor.

☐ Move from the waist area.

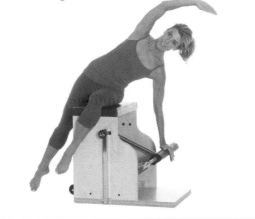

VARIATION

To increase both the load and the stretch of the lateral muscles of the trunk and underarm, reach the top arm overhead with the shoulder internally rotated, and the palm facing up toward the ceiling.

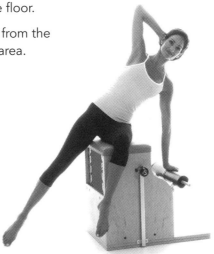

Exhale. Sit sideways on the chair, hooking the lower leg on the side of the chair and keeping the other leg straight and in line with the body. Establish a long diagonal bodyline, with the foot touching the floor. Place the lower hand on the pedal and the other hand behind the head.

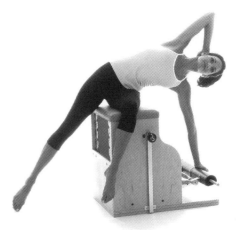

Inhale. Laterally flex the trunk, lowering the pedal.

Exhale. Lift the trunk, raising the pedal and returning to the start position.

Basic Swan

As with the Wunda Chair: Side Over, this exercise can be made easier by adding small increments of spring tension or more challenging by reducing the spring tension. This adjustability is invaluable when dealing with back problems because you can regulate how much muscle activation should be present as well as the range of motion of the trunk. The springs can move the body through a predetermined range of motion via almost-passive movement as neuromuscular patterns are reeducated, and then the muscles can be progressively challenged (by decreasing the tension) as improvement takes place.

This exercise is valuable for teaching the crucial role of the abdominal muscles during spinal extension and the skill of load distribution through the spine when executing back extension exercises. Often, as soon as the abdominal muscles are activated there is a tendency to draw the trunk into flexion. As a result, when the trunk is then lifted, the majority of the extension occurs in the lumbar spine, placing excessive load on this region. This is completely contrary to the effect we are striving for. Correct abdominal activation should provide support for the spine and, together with the back extensors, assist in creating a long, evenly distributed arc through the trunk.

VARIATION

To reduce the challenge, place the feet on a box or ball so that the alignment is still horizontal and parallel to the floor, but the feet are supported. If this still proves too challenging, the feet can be placed on the floor with the knees bent and thighs pressing against the back of the chair.

Muscle Focus

- Back extensors

Objectives

- To strengthen the back extensors
- To develop scapular stabilization
- To emphasize abdominal control

RESISTANCE

Light   Medium   Heavy

Imagery

Visualize a reverse articulation of the spine, starting with the head and moving down the spine, drawing the trunk into extension. This tends to distribute the work throughout the back and establishes a gentle arc shape, rather than excessive hyperextension in the lumbar region.

☐ Maintain abdominal muscle engagement throughout.

☐ Keep the legs parallel to the floor.

☐ Press the hands back into the pedal, extending the shoulders, as the body lifts.

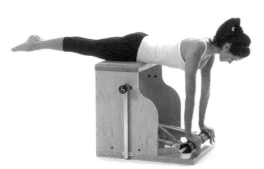

Exhale. Lie prone on the chair with the legs straight and together, parallel to the floor. Place the hands on the pedal, aligning them directly under the shoulders, and straighten the arms. The pedal may be slightly off the base of the chair.

Inhale. Extend the back, lifting the pedal.
Exhale. Lower to the start position.

8

Barrels

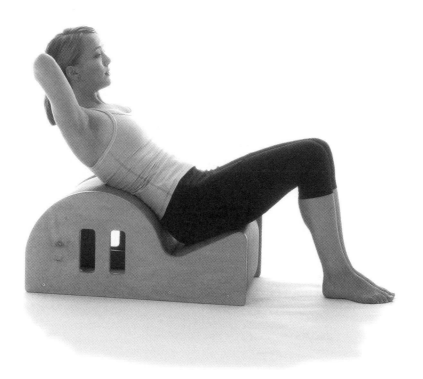

The barrels are as unique in their offerings as they are in appearance. They provide exceptional opportunities for both active and passive back extension at all ability levels. But, of course, they are not limited to back extension. Like the entire lineup of Pilates apparatus, the barrels have endless potential to work the body in every range of motion.

There are two main categories of barrels: The high barrel, also known as the ladder barrel, stands several feet off the ground and is attached to a ladder of the same height. The step barrel, also known as the spine corrector, sits on the floor.

Lighter and more portable versions of the step barrel, such as the half barrel, also known as the arc, are also available. There are many applications for the arc, including placing it on other apparatus like the cadillac and reformer and using it in conjunction with these apparatus. This opens up a world of opportunity for creative and varied repertoire.

The step barrel I prefer using is called the Avalon step barrel. Besides the modifications that have been made to the shape of the barrel to accommodate a wider range of body types, it also offers the option of using springs. In this way resistance can be added to expand the repertoire performed on the barrels, with corresponding benefits. This chapter includes instructions for exercises on the traditional step barrel and, where appropriate, instructions for the Avalon variation.

As I have emphasized throughout this book, spinal extension is crucial to developing back strength and good posture; unfortunately, it is often neglected. The barrels are exceptional tools for strengthening the back extensors and for passively relaxing in a position of spinal extension, thereby stretching the trunk flexors. When doing forward flexion abdominal exercises on the step barrel, the barrel supports the lower back in a neutral position; this is very important in conditions where flexion of the lumbar spine is contraindicated. The barrels also support the trunk during lateral flexion exercises, from fundamental to advanced levels, facilitating improvement of both strength and flexibility. Unique hip and arm work, full-body integration exercises, and stretches can be performed on the barrels, many of which cannot be easily duplicated on other apparatus.

The traditional barrels utilize gravity rather than springs for resistance, a difference that is an important consideration in making exercises less or more difficult. I often add ankle weights or hand weights to the work on the barrels to increase the challenge when developing strength or to facilitate a deeper stretch when doing flexibility exercises. As mentioned previously, a line of the barrels has been developed that integrates springs to facilitate using resistance while doing the barrel exercises.

I highly recommend ending a session by spending a few minutes in relaxation, lying supine over the step barrel, with a cushion supporting the head if need be. It leaves you stretched out, with a delightful *open* feeling.

The order in which the following exercises are presented is not necessarily the sequence in which they would be taught or performed. Typically, we would not do an entire session on the barrels, but would include exercises from the rich and diverse repertoire to fulfill various blocks in a comprehensive session. The exercises are organized by block to make the selection process convenient; for instance the stretches are placed together, the lateral flexion exercises are together, and the back extension exercises are together.

Students often wonder whether they should learn the ladder barrel before the step barrel or vice versa. In my opinion, it does not matter; both have much to offer at every level of work.

Hamstring Stretch

This is a comfortable, relatively easy way to stretch the hamstrings. Although this exercise can be performed on a variety of apparatus (as can the gluteal stretch), the ladder barrel helps keep the body in optimal alignment to achieve an effective stretch of the hamstrings.

Imagery

Visualize the body functioning like a hinge, with the trunk being the top part of the hinge and the pelvis and lower limbs the bottom section. The standing leg and the pelvis are attached to the ladder and remain stable. The other leg is placed on the barrel and is also part of the stable structure. The trunk and pelvis form the upper section of the hinge and move as one piece, closing over the stretching leg and then opening up again.

☐ Keep the back extensors engaged and tilt the pelvis in an anterior direction during the stretch.

☐ Dorsiflex the foot to intensify the stretch.

☐ Extend the trunk further as it is lifted in the final phase.

Muscle Focus
- Hamstrings

Objective
- To stretch the hamstrings

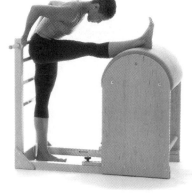

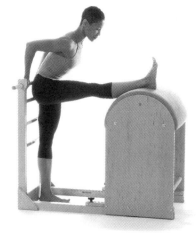

Inhale. Stand on one leg facing the barrel, with the leg straight and positioned against the ladder. Place the other leg on top of the barrel, keeping it as straight as possible (without hyperextending the knee). Hold the ladder with the hands, arms parallel, shoulders externally rotated, and elbows facing backward.

Exhale. Lean forward over the stretching leg, keeping the back as flat as possible. Straighten the arms, pressing them against the ladder while reaching the trunk further over the leg and dorsiflexing the foot to intensify the stretch. Hold this position for three to five breaths.

Inhale. Lift the trunk and return to the start position.

Muscle Focus
- Gluteal muscles

Objective
- To stretch the gluteal muscles

Gluteal Stretch

The gluteal muscles tend to get very tight. In addition, there is often an imbalance in the relative strength of the muscles within this group, with the gluteus medius tending to be weak and the gluteus maximus strong. Any imbalances should be addressed in a comprehensive program. Besides strength, a good stretch is often needed, and the ladder barrel, which places the body in good alignment to maximize the stretch, is a comfortable location to perform it. Note that this position potentially places a great deal of stress on the knee of the stretching leg, particularly when the hip joint is tight and the knee compensates for this tightness. Move into the position with caution, and do not exceed the limits of your own structure. This stretch can be very intense, so remember to breathe!

Imagery

As with all stretches, focus on the stability of the areas above and below the region that is to be stretched, and then visualize the region being stretched becoming soft like rubber, and elongating with each breath.

- ☐ Keep the back extensors engaged, and tilt the pelvis in an anterior direction during the stretch.

- ☐ Stand closer to the barrel to intensify the stretch.

- ☐ Extend the trunk further as it is lifted in the final phase.

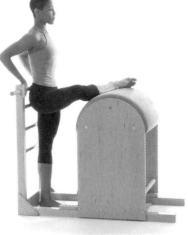

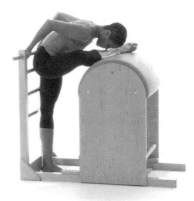

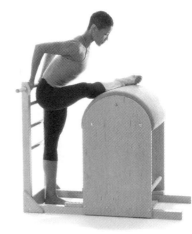

Inhale. Stand on one leg, keeping it straight and positioning the back of the leg against the ladder. Place the lateral aspect of the other leg on the barrel, bend the knee, and externally rotate the hip. Hold the top rung of the ladder with both hands, with the arms parallel, the shoulders externally rotated, and the elbows pointing backward.

Exhale. Lean forward over the stretching leg and keep the back as flat as possible. Straighten the arms, pushing against the ladder while reaching the trunk further over the leg to intensify the stretch. Hold the position for three to five breaths.

Inhale. Lift the trunk and return to the start position.

Adductor Stretch

This stretch is similar to a ballet stretch at the barre. It is most effective when you turn out (externally rotate) the hip of the stretching leg, a position familiar to dancers. The rotation of the hip joint helps keep the pelvis level, so that it doesn't hike up on the stretching side. If this position is not familiar to you, take particular care to achieve correct alignment of the pelvis so that undue stress is not placed on the joints, particularly the hip and knee joints. This exercise also stretches the lateral flexors on the upper side of the trunk and the shoulder adductors on that same side.

Imagery

I like to use the image of a wishbone, with the stretching leg and the trunk creating the two sides of the wishbone. The foot of the stretching leg and the hand of the stretching arm should reach as far as possible in the same direction, with the leg and arm almost parallel when in maximum stretch. Visualize the area between the pelvic crest and the lower ribs on the upper side of the trunk opening and expanding. At the same time, the region under the armpit of the stretching arm also opens, allowing the arm to reach further overhead. Breathing correctly is important in any stretch, but particularly so when stretching the muscles of the trunk. Visualize directing the breath into the upper lung, feeling the trunk expand and the ribs open in moderation and with control.

☐ Keep the pelvis level.

☐ Dorsiflex the foot of the stretching leg to intensify the stretch.

☐ Prevent the ribs from flaring excessively on the upper side of the trunk.

☐ Elongate the trunk as it is lifted in the final phase.

Muscle Focus
- Adductors

Objective
- To stretch the hip adductors, hamstrings, shoulder adductors, and lateral flexors of the trunk

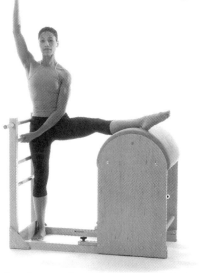

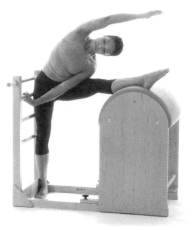

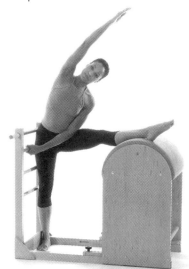

Inhale. Stand on one leg with your side to the barrel. Keep the standing leg straight, in a parallel position against the ladder. Place the stretching leg up on the barrel with the hip externally rotated, keeping the leg as straight as possible (without hyperextending the knee).

Exhale. Reach over the stretching leg with the arm opposite that leg (left arm over right leg, or vice versa), laterally flexing the trunk. Hold onto the ladder with the inside arm (the arm at the bottom of the stretch) as the outside arm stretches overhead. Hold this position for three to five breaths.

Inhale. Lift the trunk and return to the start position.

Muscle Focus

- Oblique abdominals

Objectives

- To strengthen the lateral trunk flexors
- To stretch the lateral trunk flexors
- To develop trunk stabilization

Side Over

This exercise resembles closely the Reformer: Side Over and incorporates many of the same principles. An excellent preparation to both is the Wunda Chair: Side Over. However, performing the exercise on the barrel offers two additional benefits. It requires more balance, which demands deeper activation of the core muscles for stabilization, and the shape of the barrel supports the body in perfect lateral alignment, facilitating a wonderful stretch for the upper side when the body is draped over the barrel.

Imagery

At the start of the exercise a straight energy line runs through the length of the body, highlighting the elongated shape. The next phase in the exercise, lateral flexion, is all about curve and elasticity. Think of the body being draped over the barrel; it conjures up the image of soft, cascading fabric, which is how the body should feel when being lowered over the barrel. Another helpful image is that of a young, green, flexible branch being bent over and then slowly released back to its original straight line. A good visual to help maintain correct alignment of the trunk is to imagine the movement occurring in the coronal plane between two panes of glass.

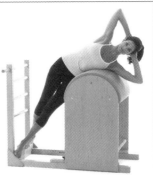

VARIATION

As a preparation for the side over, create a more stable base by placing the lower foot on the bottom rung or cross bar and the other foot directly behind it. Establish the same straight, diagonal line with the trunk. Lower the trunk over the barrel and then lift the trunk. This is essentially the same exercise as the full side over, but the trunk has far more support and is more stable. In addition the lever arm created by the trunk and its distance from the fulcrum is shorter, making the exercise less challenging.

☐ Keep the elbows wide and the fingers interlaced behind the head.

☐ Engage the internal support system (ISS) prior to the movement to stabilize the trunk.

☐ Keep the upper leg stable and avoid pulling up with the foot that is hooked under the ladder.

☐ Elongate the trunk, creating a large arc, as the body is lifted in the final phase.

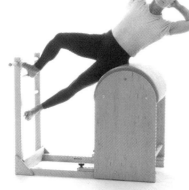

Exhale. Rest one side of the pelvis on the barrel, placing the bottom foot on the first rung of the ladder. Hook the top foot under the top rung, pressing the heel onto the rung below. Externally rotate the upper hip and bend the knee. Establish a straight, diagonal line from the lower foot through the entire body, and place the hands behind the head.

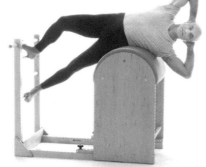

Inhale. Lower the trunk over the barrel with the head following the line of the spine.

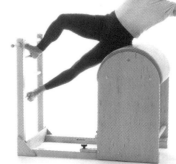

Exhale. Lift the trunk and return to the start position.

Back Extension

In all back extension exercises, it is vital to keep the abdominal muscles engaged throughout the movement. This protects the back, facilitates correct muscle recruitment and body alignment, and distributes the load throughout the back. When setting up the ladder barrel, be aware that the distance between the barrel and the ladder dictates where the work is focused. When the two are close, the fulcrum is lower in the body and the lever arm is longer. In this case the work is focused lower in the back. If the intention is to work the mid- or upper back, set the barrel further from the ladder and place the feet lower down on the ladder. The fulcrum will then be higher on the body, and the lever arm will be shorter. Basically, the closer the barrel is to the ladder, the greater the load on the back extensors, because of the longer lever arm created by the trunk and its distance from the fulcrum. Likewise, the further the barrel is from the ladder, the less the load.

Imagery

I encourage visualizing a reverse spinal articulation, lifting the head and then continuing to articulate into spinal extension down through the spine to the mid-back and finally the lumbar spine and sacrum. Emphasize elongation as opposed to height, reaching out from the tip of the head.

Muscle Focus

• Back extensors

Objectives

• To strengthen the back extensors
• To develop trunk stabilization

VARIATION

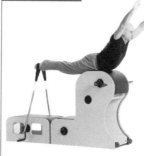

As an alternative, this exercise can be performed on the Avalon Chair and ladder. The most significant difference is that on the ladder barrel the legs are on a stable, fixed base. This allows the legs to do more work than desired, and compensations may appear. On the Avalon the stabilization is dynamic; the legs are supported by springs, which offer only minimal support, encouraging the ISS to ignite. The work is felt deeply and intensely, not only in the back extensors, but also the hip extensors.

☐ Keep the abdominal muscles engaged and the pubic symphysis pressed forward.

☐ Align the head with the spine.

☐ Create a straight line between the legs and the trunk when lifted in extension.

☐ Elongate the trunk further before lowering in the final phase.

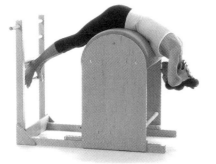

Exhale. Lie prone, with the trunk draped over the barrel. Place the toes on the first rung of the ladder, with the feet in a V position and the heels together. Anchor the heels under the second rung. Place the hands behind the head.

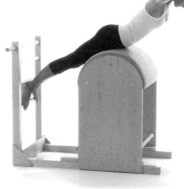

Inhale. Lift the trunk, extending the back.

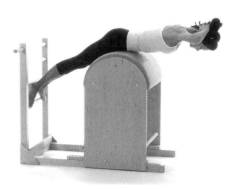

Exhale. Lower the trunk to the start position.

Muscle Focus

- Back extensors

Objectives

- To strengthen the back extensors
- To stretch the hip flexors
- To develop control of the hip extensors

Swan

The swan is one of the most aesthetically beautiful movements in the repertoire and very satisfying to perform. It is an advanced back extension exercise that demands strength, flexibility, and tremendous control. The key to success is integrated and organic movement throughout the body, utilizing the range the movement of the knees, hips, and shoulders in addition to the full range of every vertebral joint in the spine. Many people focus only on the back, specifically the lower back. This results in shearing forces on the lower back and the body *folding over*, rather than arcing from the knees through the trunk to the fingertips.

Engaging the abdominals is critical in order to protect the back and achieve the desired shape. This exercise can help many a gymnast and dancer, who tend to rely almost entirely on flexibility when performing back extension, achieve a healthy balance of strength, flexibility, and control. Note that the barrel should be set relatively close to the ladder so that the thighs are pressing against the barrel. In the final phase of the extension gravity is actually pulling you further into extension, making this exercise not only very advanced, but also potentially dangerous. It is vital to maintain abdominal support throughout.

Imagery

The image of an arc when in full extension is important in creating the correct movement pattern and muscle recruitment sequence. In many of the back extension exercises I like to use the image of an archer's bow being pulled into a taut position, poised to unleash tremendous power.

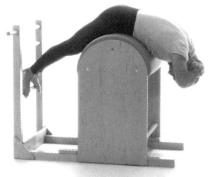

Exhale. Lie prone, with the trunk draped over the barrel and the thighs pressing against it. Place the toes on the first rung of the ladder, with the feet in a V-position and the heels together, anchored under the second rung. Place the hands behind the head.

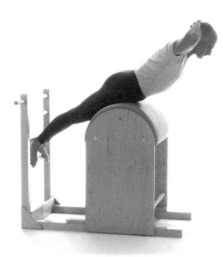

Inhale. Lift the trunk and extend the back, creating a diagonal line with the trunk and the legs.

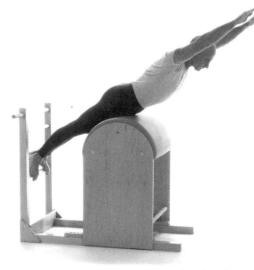

Exhale. Straighten the arms overhead in line with the ears, establishing a long, straight line from the fingers to the toes.

- ☐ Keep the abdominal muscles engaged and push the pubic symphysis forward into the barrel.

- ☐ Bend the knees as the trunk arches back and the hips extend.

- ☐ Distribute the extension of the back through the entire trunk and the hips, adding shoulder flexion to complete the shape.

- ☐ Keep the head aligned with the spine.

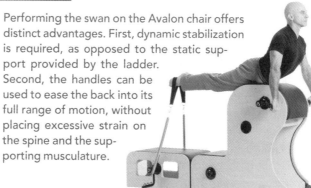

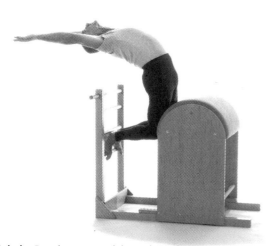

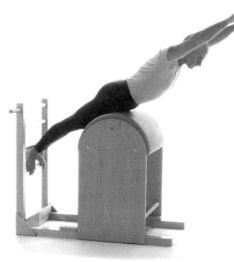

Inhale. Reach up toward the ceiling, drawing a large arc with the body, and prepare for maximum extension of the body.

Continue inhaling as you bend the knees and press the thighs further against the barrel. Extend the hips to the point of maximum extension and take both the trunk and the arms back until they are parallel to the floor, or as close to parallel as possible.

Exhale. Lift the body, reach to the ceiling and then return to the long diagonal line.

Inhale. Place the hands behind the head.

Exhale. Lower the body to the start position.

Muscle Focus
- Abdominal muscles
- Shoulder extensors and flexors

Objectives
- To develop abdominal control
- To stretch the abdominal and shoulder muscles

Reach

This exercise offers a wonderful interplay between deep spinal flexion and spinal extension, with the added bonus of a valuable shoulder stretch. The stretch for the back, particularly the lower back, should be maximized when in the C-curve position, as should the stretch for the shoulders when in the supine position.

Two areas that tend to become tight, particularly in light of today's lifestyle, are the lower back and the shoulders. This exercise homes in on both. In the supine position, the spine should be neutral, the legs straight, and the arms reaching overhead in a straight diagonal line, supported by the barrel. This is an ideal position in which to stretch the shoulders. However, be aware of the tendency to thrust the ribs forward in an endeavor to achieve more range in the shoulders; doing so can result in hyperlordosis and possible stress on the lower back in addition to actually *releasing* the stretch in the shoulders. The ISS must be activated to help maintain a firm, elongated position when supine and to assist when transitioning from supine to sitting and vice versa.

Imagery

Use the image of the two definitive shapes in this exercise: the concave, rounded position of the trunk when sitting followed by the straight line of the body when supine. The visual of a green branch being pulled into an arc with twine tied to each side (like a bow) and then opening out to the straight position conjures up the perfect dynamic for this exercise.

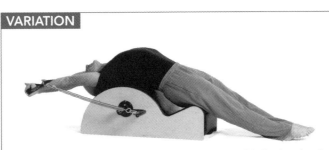

VARIATION

Once good form and control have been established, take the body from the straight line into extension. Rest the back of the head on the barrel, to avoid straining the neck, and continue reaching back with the shoulders. Lift the head and arms, re-establishing a distinct straight line with the body, before returning to the start position. This exercise is demonstrated on the Avalon barrel, which has a gentler curve than the traditional barrel enabling the upper back and head to be supported when in full extension. In addition the Avalon offers the option of using springs to better activate the muscles and develop strength. Also, as the body moves into hyperextension, the springs provide an incredible stretch for the shoulders.

- ☐ Maximize the C curve when in the sitting position.
- ☐ Maintain a straight line with the body when in the supine position.
- ☐ Keep the head aligned with the spine at all times.

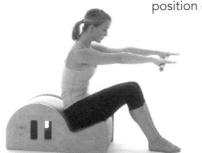

Inhale. Sit in the dip, between the step and the barrel, with the trunk in a C curve (deep spinal flexion). Hold a roll-up pole, approximately 36 inches (90 centimeters) in length, straight in front of you at shoulder height, with the arms shoulder-width apart. Bend the knees, keeping the legs together and the feet firmly on the floor.

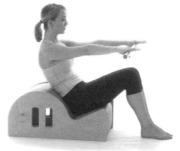

Exhale. Roll down onto the barrel, straightening the legs.

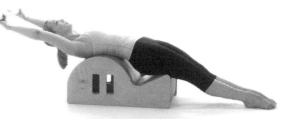

Continue exhaling. Extend the trunk and reach the arms overhead to form a straight line with the legs, trunk, and arms.

Inhale. Stretch the shoulders further.

Exhale. Draw the trunk back into the C curve, bending the legs and bringing the arms forward to the start position.

Overhead Stretch

This exercise resembles the Step Barrel: Reach but offers a more intense stretch for the shoulders and chest. Whereas the reach concludes in a neutral spine position when supine, this stretch takes the trunk into hyperextension. The abdominal muscles must be activated throughout to avoid excessive stress on the lower back in this position. The important role of the abdominal muscles in supporting and protecting the spine, particularly in hyperextension, cannot be overemphasized. The apparatus itself offers valuable support, as it does with many of the exercises on the barrel.

This exercise challenges the mobility of the shoulder, so anyone with shoulder restrictions should approach it with caution. An important element of this exercise is the sequential movement that progresses through the body—starting at the core, the movement proceeds through the spine as you roll down, and then continues to the arms. The arms then circle around and "pick up" the spine again to initiate the roll-up into a sitting C curve. The completion of the exercise is another sequential movement through the spine, transitioning from trunk flexion to sitting upright.

Muscle Focus
- Abdominal muscles
- Shoulder extensors and flexors

Objectives
- To increase shoulder mobility
- To stretch the chest
- To develop abdominal control

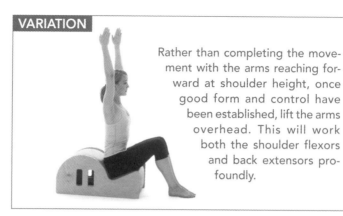

VARIATION

Rather than completing the movement with the arms reaching forward at shoulder height, once good form and control have been established, lift the arms overhead. This will work both the shoulder flexors and back extensors profoundly.

Imagery

The dynamic of this exercise is all-important, and the feeling should be one of a perpetual rolling wave permeating through the body, as it goes through the full spectrum of movement: extension, hyperextension, and flexion.

- ☐ Lower the trunk onto the barrel before circling the arms.
- ☐ Keep the head aligned with the spine, and the neck relaxed.
- ☐ Lift the head and spine sequentially as the arms circle around.

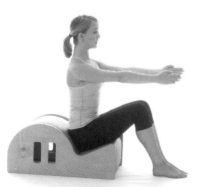

Inhale. Sit in the dip of the barrel, holding the trunk upright, with the arms straight out in front of the body at shoulder height and the palms facing each other. Bend the knees, keeping the legs together and the feet firmly on the floor.

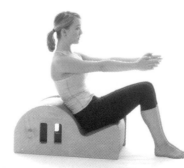

Exhale. Roll down onto the barrel.

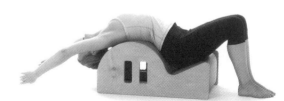

Inhale. Reach the arms overhead and circle them around.

Exhale. Roll up to the sitting C-curve position, with the shoulders over the hips and the spine in flexion. Extend the spine to the start position.

Muscle Focus

- Abdominal muscles

Objectives

- To strengthen and stretch the abdominal muscles
- To stretch the chest

Chest Lift

This exercise on the step barrel is similar to the Mat Work: Chest Lift, with two fundamental differences. First, the range of motion achieved on the barrel is greater, spanning from spinal hyperextension to spinal flexion (as opposed to neutral spine to spinal flexion on the mat). This additional range of motion is very valuable, because the abdominal muscles are seldom strengthened or stretched beyond a neutral position.

Second, the lumbar spine remains in a supported neutral (or close to neutral) position when trunk is lifted. Typically in similar abdominal exercises on other apparatus, the lumbar spine flattens as the trunk lifts into forward flexion. This lumbar support could be important in certain circumstances; for example, if a medical practitioner requests that a patient with a disc problem in the lower back improve abdominal strength but advises against flexion of the lumbar spine. In this version the back remains in a neutral position while supported by the barrel, which protects the spine and minimizes the risk of pressure on the discs. This exercise has the added benefit of a significant stretch for the chest, which most people desperately need, helping overcome or prevent round-shoulder syndrome, kyphotic posture and similar conditions.

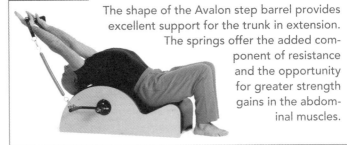

VARIATION

The shape of the Avalon step barrel provides excellent support for the trunk in extension. The springs offer the added component of resistance and the opportunity for greater strength gains in the abdominal muscles.

Imagery

Imagine the lumbar region remaining absolutely stable, as if part of a statue, and the movement occurring from a hinge or pivot point directly below the sternum. In addition, imagine a rubber band connecting the pubic symphysis to the sternum. As the body goes back into extension the rubber band is stretched, but is never released. As the body lifts forward into flexion, the band shortens and assists the abdominals. Visualize the lift beginning from deep within the pelvic bowl.

- ☐ Support the head with the hands. (Rest the head on a cushion when in spinal extension if necessary.)

- ☐ Keep the elbows wide.

- ☐ Maintain contact between the lumbar spine and the barrel throughout.

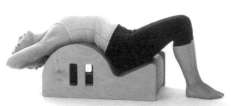

Inhale. Lie supine on the barrel with the pelvis anchored in the valley. Interlace the fingers behind the head and stretch the thoracic spine over the barrel. Bend the knees, keeping the legs together and the feet firmly on the floor.

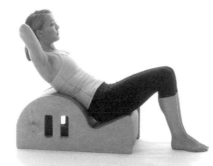

Exhale. Lift the head and chest into spinal flexion.
Inhale. Pause in this position.

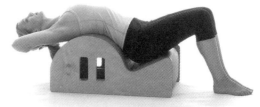

Exhale. Lower the head and chest to the start position.

Opening

The barrel is an excellent place to work the hip adductors, particularly for those with tight hamstrings. The elevated position of the pelvis on the barrel places less stretch on the hamstrings than a supine position on the floor does. As a result, it requires less hip flexor activation to keep the legs lifted (a challenging feat in itself) and allows maximum focus on the hip adductors and on maintaining a stable trunk.

Imagery

Whether using resistance or not, imagine pressing against a huge spring or moving through a heavy gel, creating internal resistance as the legs open and close.

☐ Open the legs as wide as possible, without forgoing control or pelvic alignment.

☐ Pause with the legs perpendicular to the floor after each opening.

☐ Keep the hips externally rotated throughout the movement.

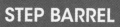

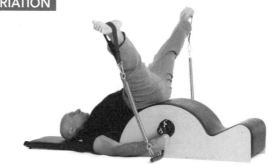

Once excellent control has been achieved, you can add ankle weights to this exercise to facilitate a deeper stretch and develop strength. Alternatively use the Avalon step barrel, which provides resistance via the spring mechanism. Employ extreme caution when using resistance, as it increases the potential danger of pressure on the lower back.

Muscle Focus

- Hip adductors

Objectives

- To increase hip adductor flexibility
- To develop hip adductor control
- To improve pelvic–lumbar stabilization

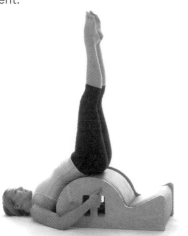

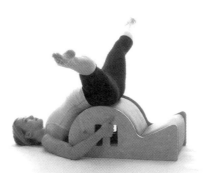

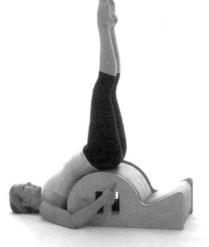

Exhale. Lie with the back and pelvis on the barrel, the legs perpendicular, the hips externally rotated, and the shoulder girdle on the floor. (Place a mat under the shoulder girdle and head to elevate the body in relation to the barrel, if necessary.)

Inhale. Abduct the legs, opening them to a wide V position.

Exhale. Adduct the legs, closing them to the start position. Repeat 10 times.

Muscle Focus

- Hamstrings
- Hip flexors

Objectives

- To increase hamstring and hip flexor flexibility
- To develop hamstring and hip flexor control
- To improve pelvic–lumbar stabilization

Scissors

The scissors provides a wonderful stretch for the hamstrings and hip flexors and develops control of not only these muscle groups, but of all the muscles surrounding the hip joint. The spine is in a hyperextended position and the hip flexors are pulling on the lower back with a very long lever, the legs. Keeping the pelvis stable and maintaining abdominal activation throughout the movement is important. Without abdominal support, you are in danger of placing excessive pressure on the lower back.

Imagery

The name says it all—visualize long scissors opening and closing. The movement is sharp, direct, and precise, just like that of scissors.

- ☐ Pause with the legs perpendicular to the floor after each opening.
- ☐ Create a V shape with the legs, opening them an equal distance to the back and front.

VARIATION

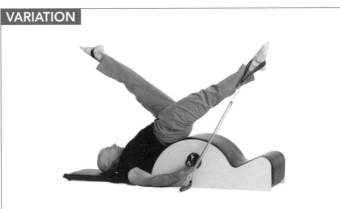

Note also that when using spring the hips are in external rotation (turn out). This allows for a greater range of motion of the hip joint and the springs will not interfere with the movement of the legs.

- ☐ Keep the trunk and pelvis adhered to the barrel throughout.

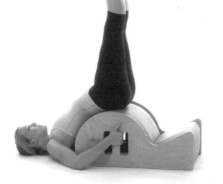

Inhale. Lie supine, with the back and pelvis on the barrel, the legs perpendicular and parallel, and the shoulder girdle on the floor. Place a mat under the shoulder girdle and head to elevate the body in relation to the barrel, if necessary.

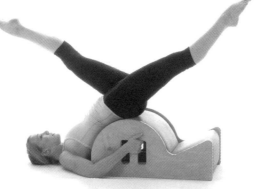

Exhale. Open the legs as wide as possible to the back and front in a scissor-like motion. Pulse twice.

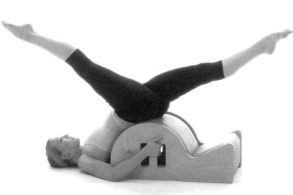

Inhale. Switch the legs, passing through the perpendicular position with each repetition. Repeat 10 times on each leg, finishing in the perpendicular position.

Helicopter

Coordination plays a vital role in this exercise. As the legs move in opposite directions, each leg must move at the same pace, and the range of motion of each should be equal. This exercise combines the Step Barrel: Scissors with Step Barrel: Opening, both being prerequisites.

Imagery

The name of this exercise serves the image well—visualize the blades of a helicopter circling around, preparing for takeoff. (Stay grounded!)

- ☐ Pass through the perpendicular position of the legs after each circle.

- ☐ Touch each point of the circle as the legs move around.

- ☐ Keep the pelvis stable.

Muscle Focus
- Hip flexors
- Hamstrings
- Adductors

Objectives
- To increase hip joint mobility
- To strengthen the muscles of the hip
- To develop pelvic–lumbar stabilization

VARIATION

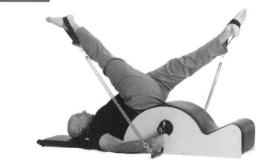

Once excellent control has been achieved, you can add ankle weights to this exercise to facilitate a deeper stretch and develop strength. Alternatively use the Avalon step barrel, which provides resistance via the spring mechanism and has a similar feel to the other Pilates apparatus.

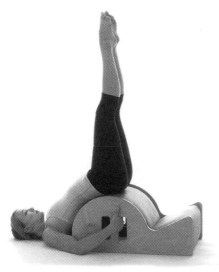

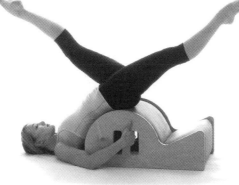

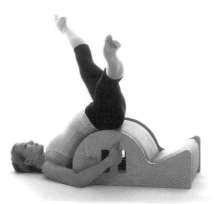

Exhale. Lie with the back and pelvis on the barrel, the legs perpendicular to the floor, the hips externally rotated, and the shoulder girdle on the floor. (Place a mat under the shoulder girdle and head to elevate the body in relation to the barrel, if necessary.)

Inhale. Open the legs as wide as possible to the back and front in a scissoring motion.

Exhale. Circle the legs around, moving them in opposite directions. (The front leg circles to the back; the back leg circles to the front.) Return to the start position. Repeat 5 times in the same direction, and then reverse direction.

Muscle Focus

- Hip flexors
- Hamstrings

Objectives

- To stretch the hamstrings and hip flexors
- To develop hip flexor control

Bicycle

As with the Step Barrel: Helicopter, coordination is possibly the greatest challenge in this exercise. The legs move simultaneously, one bending while the other is straightening. The cycling movement should be as large and elongated as possible. The bicycle includes within it the scissors, and passing through this position is important because it will ensure that the circular motion remains very large and stretches the hip flexors and hamstrings.

As with the Step Barrel: Scissors, which is an excellent preparation for his exercise, the legs are parallel, as opposed to externally rotated, and the path they follow should be close to the center line. This maximizes the stretch of the hip flexors and hamstrings. This version of the bicycle serves as an effective preparation for the Mat Work: Bicycle; here the barrel supports the body, as opposed to the arms having to hold the pelvis in an elevated position. As with the mat version, the movement pattern in this bicycle can be reversed.

Imagery

Imagine cycling a bicycle with very large wheels and pedals. The movement should be circular, not linear, with each leg describing a large circle.

VARIATION

Once excellent control has been achieved, you can add ankle weights to this exercise to facilitate a deeper stretch and develop strength. This particular exercise is not well suited to springs simply because in this position they hamper the smooth, flowing motion. Note that when reversing the movement the foot will not touch the step.

- ☐ Touch the step of the barrel with the foot as the back leg bends to come in.
- ☐ Maintain pelvic–lumbar stabilization throughout the exercise.
- ☐ Keep the legs parallel to each other; avoid splaying the knees as the legs bend.

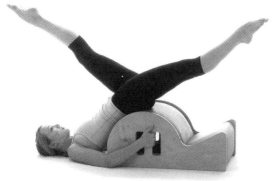

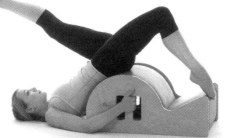

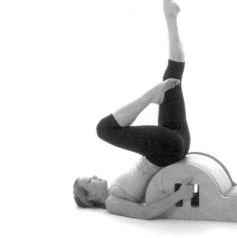

Inhale. Lie with the back and pelvis on the barrel, the legs in a scissors position, the hips in neutral, and the shoulder girdle on the floor. (Place a mat under the shoulder girdle and head to elevate them, if necessary.)

Exhale. Bend the back leg, touching the step with the foot. Simultaneously, begin to extend the front leg, reaching it up to the ceiling.

Still exhaling, draw the bent back leg toward the chest, crossing the other leg, which is now passing through the perpendicular position on its way to the back.

Inhale. Open to the scissors position, straightening what is now the front leg opposite the face. Repeat five times and then reverse direction.

Side Over

The step barrel is exceptionally helpful in accomplishing correct alignment and muscle recruitment for lateral flexion. It supports the body and virtually guides it in the desired direction. This lays a solid foundation for many similar, often more challenging, lateral flexion exercises in the Pilates repertoire, including the Reformer: Side Over and the Ladder Barrel: Side Over. You can address both strength and flexibility of the lateral flexors with this exercise. Although it is possible to start from the "draped over the barrel" position, I recommend building up strength to the point where you can begin with the body in a straight diagonal line, as in the reformer and ladder barrel versions of this exercise.

Keeping the head aligned with the spine and the neck uninvolved in this movement is important. There is a strong tendency to try to lift with the head; clearly this is not the goal. The muscles around the spine support this integrated movement, creating the shape of an elongated arc.

Imagery

Visualize tall grass being blown sideways in a soft breeze; then the breeze subsides and the grass lifts back up. I encourage you to strive for this effortless, soft quality.

VARIATION

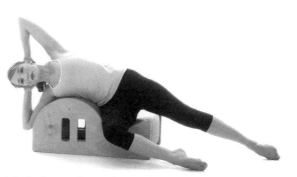

Perform the side over movement pattern, however, rather than placing the hands behind the head, reach the arms overhead. This makes the exercise more challenging, as the center of gravity has been moved further from the fulcrum and a longer lever arm has been created with the arms and trunk. When performing it on the Avalon, a spring can be placed on the straight leg to assist in dynamically stabilizing the body. This facilitates greater lateral flexion of the trunk.

Muscle Focus

- Oblique abdominals

Objectives

- To strengthen the lateral flexors of the trunk
- To stretch the lateral flexors of the trunk

☐ Lift the trunk only as high as the straight diagonal line created by the trunk and the top leg.

☐ Stabilize with the muscles of the core, engaging them prior to the movement.

☐ When lifting, direct the movement up toward the ceiling, rather than crunching sideways.

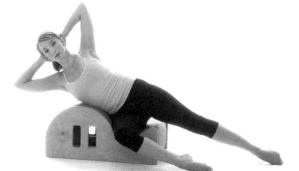

Exhale. Lie on the barrel on one side of the body. Bend the bottom leg to 90 degrees at the hip and knee joints, and rest it in the dip of the barrel. Straighten the top leg, keeping the foot anchored on the floor. Interlace the fingers behind the head.

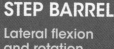

Inhale. Lower the trunk over the barrel.

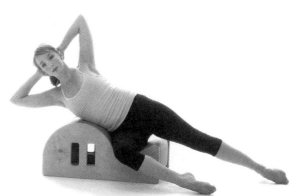

Exhale. Lift the trunk, creating a straight diagonal line with the trunk and the top leg, returning to the start position. After 5 to 10 repetitions, complete the exercise by straightening the arms overhead and relaxing sideways over the barrel, stretching the lateral flexors.

Muscle Focus

- Abdominal muscles
- Hip flexors

Objectives

- To develop abdominal muscle control
- To increase spinal articulation
- To develop hip flexor control
- To stretch the hip flexors, hamstrings and back extensors

Roll-Over

The roll-over on the barrel allows those who find the Mat Work: Roll-Over difficult or impossible (because of tight hamstrings, a tight lower back, weak abdominal muscles, or any other reason) to successfully complete the exercise. The barrel elevates the pelvis, placing it in a position that alleviates the pull on the hamstrings and lower back. It also allows gravity to assist the abdominal muscles in the challenging roll-over phase of the exercise.

Once you have mastered this exercise on the barrel, it is easier to perform it on the mat. Be cautious when bringing the legs, which function as a long lever arm, back to the starting position because the pressure on the lower back can

be excessive, particularly when abdominal support is lacking and the hip flexors are tight. The lower back can easily be pulled into hyperextension because of the body's position on the barrel. The abdominal muscles must be firmly engaged throughout to counteract this danger. However, once excellent pelvic-lumbar stability has been achieved, lowering the legs to a low start position (even to the point of the pelvis and legs being in one straight line) provides an excellent stretch for the hip flexors.

Note that this exercise demands deep spinal flexion and can also place pressure on the cervical spine. Both these aspects of the exercise may be contraindicated in certain

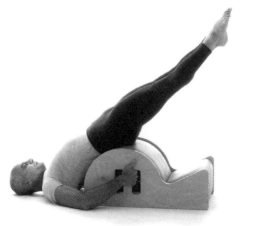

Exhale. Lie supine, with the back and pelvis on the barrel, the shoulder girdle on the floor, and the legs straight on a diagonal line of approximately 60 degrees, or lower if you have adequate pelvic-lumbar stabilization. (Place a mat under the shoulder girdle and head to elevate the body in relation to the barrel, if necessary.)

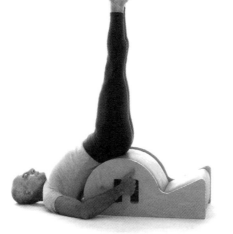

Inhale. Lift the legs to a perpendicular position.

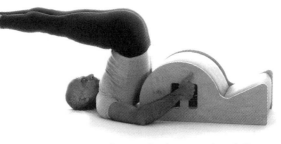

Exhale. Roll over, transferring the legs overhead. Pause with legs parallel to the floor.

circumstances. If in doubt, consult with a medical professional. Ideally, little or no pressure should be placed on the cervical spine; most of the weight should fall on the shoulder girdle. Having the barrel behind the back helps distribute the weight and also assists in controlling the degree of spinal flexion.

Imagery

The visual of the vertebrae being gently lifted off the barrel and then placed back on like a necklace of pearls helps achieve the desired spinal articulation.

☐ Maintain abdominal support throughout the exercise.

☐ Keep the barrel connected to the back.

VARIATION

Once excellent control has been achieved, you can add ankle weights to this exercise to facilitate a deeper stretch and develop strength. Alternatively use the Avalon step barrel, which provides resistance via the spring mechanism and has a similar feel to the other Pilates apparatus. As always, employ extreme caution when using any type of resistance, as it increases the potential danger of pressure on the lower back. Note that the beginning position demands tremendous abdominal and hip flexor control, particularly if the legs and trunk form a straight line.

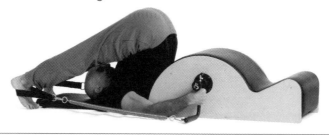

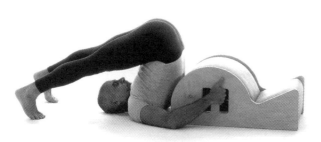

Inhale. Dorsiflex the feet, separate the legs to shoulder-width, and lower the feet to the floor (or as close to it as possible).

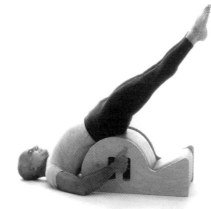

Exhale. Roll down through the spine, placing each vertebra on the barrel until the pelvis is anchored. Continue extending the legs and bring them back together to the start position.

305

Swan

Muscle Focus
- Back extensors
- Hip extensors

Objectives
- To strengthen the back extensors
- To develop hip extensor control

Versions of the swan can be done on almost every piece of Pilates apparatus. The step barrel is an excellent place to teach the positioning, alignment, and muscle recruitment for this popular exercise. The support of the barrel alleviates some of the potential stress on the back and accommodates the perfect bow shape we work hard to achieve. The barrel supports the trunk and the legs, thereby assisting the back extensors and hip extensors. Of course, this does not exempt the abdominal muscles from being active throughout the exercise. They are vital to supporting the movement, achieving the correct form, and protecting the back.

Imagery

The image of an archer's bow being pulled taut works well. This helps you to visualize the position and the dynamic and to integrate the important concept of distributing the work evenly through the back.

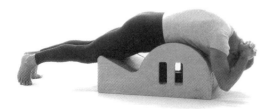

Exhale. Lie prone over the barrel with the knees slightly bent, the hips externally rotated, the feet in a small V-position with the toes anchored on the floor, and the fingers interlaced behind the head.

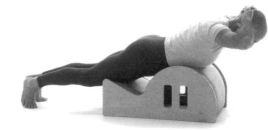

Inhale. Lift the head and trunk, extending the back.

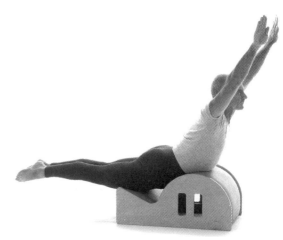

Exhale. Lift the trunk higher as the arms reach forward and up, slightly beyond shoulder-width. Simultaneously lift and straighten the legs while plantarflexing the feet.

- ☐ Glide the scapulae down the back prior to lifting the trunk.

- ☐ Engage the abdominal muscles throughout the exercise.

- ☐ Continue to adduct the legs as they lift into hip extension.

VARIATION

Using the Avalon step barrel for the swan offers the benefit of arm support, which allows you to explore the full range of extension of your spine without placing excess pressure on the lower back. Activate the back extensors and use the arms only for support.

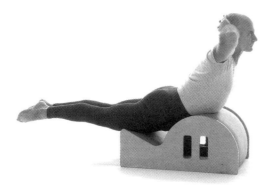

Inhale. Place the hands back behind the head.

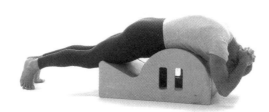

Exhale. Lower to the start position.

Muscle Focus

- Abdominal muscles
- Hip flexors

Objectives

- To develop abdominal and hip flexor control
- To prepare for the many versions of the teaser on all the apparatus

Teaser Prep

The teaser prep assists in building a foundation for the many versions of the teaser performed on almost all the Pilates apparatus, including the step barrel. It also prepares the body well for the pike movements, particularly those performed on the wunda chair. As with all the teasers, although categorized as abdominal work, they in fact involve the entire body, and therefore could also be viewed within the full body integration category. There are three areas of particular focus in all the teasers: abdominals, back extensors, and hip flexors. The barrel provides unique and welcome support for the body: when the body is straight on a diagonal line it is behind the legs and upper back, and when the body is in the pike position it is behind the lower back, allowing the pelvis to sink into the dip behind the step.

Observing the intricate connections between the many exercises in the Pilates method, on all the different apparatus, is fascinating. These connections can be viewed as branches of a large family tree, symbolizing close or more distant relationships. Understanding these multiple relationships helps immensely in preparing the body for the next level, whatever it may be. The teaser prep exercise has proven valuable for the athletes I have worked with over the years, particularly divers and gymnasts.

VARIATION

The movement pattern of the teaser prep on the Avalon step barrel is exactly the same as on the classic step barrel, however springs are used to provide resistance. This challenges the abdominals more and offers the potential for increased strength gains.

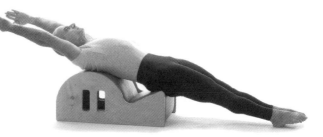

Imagery

Imagine the body opening out and then closing like a switchblade; the action is sharp, precise, and controlled.

- ☐ Keep the head aligned with the spine.
- ☐ Activate the abdominal muscles prior to lifting the legs.
- ☐ Focus the eyes directly forward when in the pike position.

Inhale. Lie supine on the barrel with the coccyx (tailbone) on the edge of the step and the upper back resting on the barrel. Reach the arms overhead, creating a straight diagonal line from the tips of the toes to the tips of the fingers.

Exhale. Lift the arms and trunk forward and simultaneously lift the legs toward the ceiling, creating a deep pike position, with the legs perpendicular to the floor.

Inhale. Lower the trunk and legs to the start position.

9

Ped-a-Pul

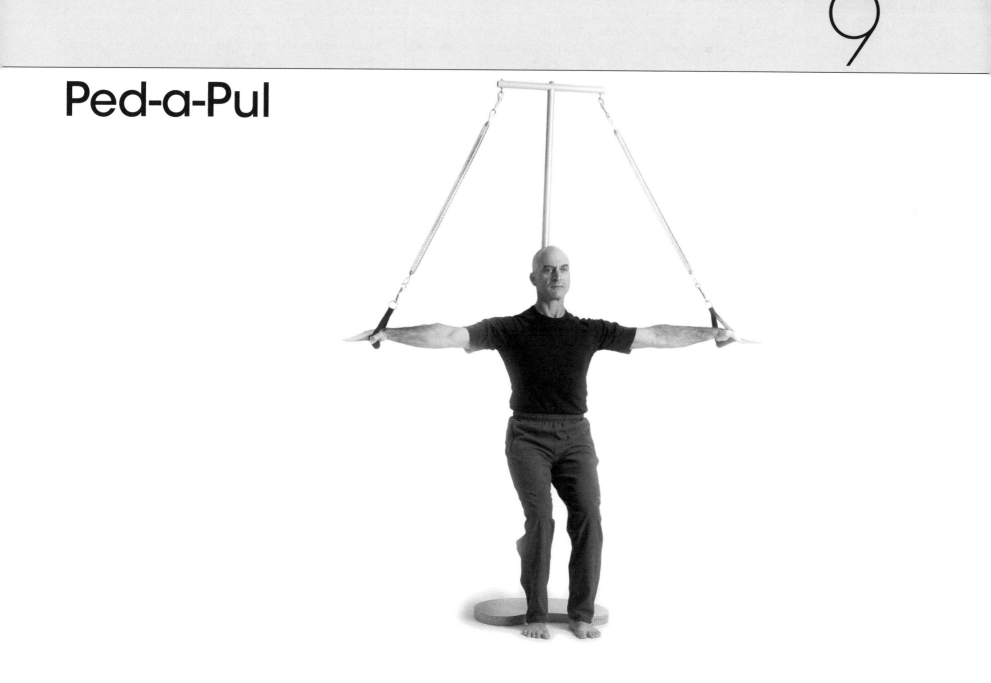

The ped-a-pul is one of Joseph Pilates' original apparatus but, like the arm chair, it is not as commonly used as some of the other pieces, such as the cadillac and the reformer. However, it has unique capabilities that cannot be easily duplicated on the other equipment. The ped-a-pul works the body in a standing position and is excellent for developing upright alignment and balance. In addition, it focuses on the arms and shoulder complex, offering a repertoire that ranges from fundamental to advanced levels.

I have created a series of exercises on the ped-a-pul that work the shoulders below shoulder height. Working at this height is particularly advantageous when teaching scapular stabilization and working with shoulder ailments, such as impingement syndrome. These exercises have proven to be invaluable when rehabilitating the shoulder and for general conditioning of the upper body.

Some ped-a-puls are adjustable, allowing you to vary the resistance to meet individual needs. When working with one that is not adjustable, you can increase the resistance by squatting lower or sitting on a stool. (The lower the body is in relation to the springs, the more resistance there will be.) Sitting on a stool offers more stability, which may be an advantage in certain situations.

Some ped-a-puls are attached to the wall and others are self-standing. Both offer unique benefits for the repertoire presented below. I prefer to attach the ped-a-pul to the wall, unless the base is large and extremely stable—it is safer and presents more possibilities both in terms of repertoire and adding resistance, hence more potential gains in strength.

Extension

This exercise focuses on shoulder extension from shoulder height and below. It develops shoulder extensor control and strength (if there is adequate resistance) in this specific range of motion, utilizing both concentric and eccentric contractions of the shoulder extensors. It is an excellent preparation for shoulder extension together with trunk flexion, a frequently recurring movement pattern in Pilates found in much of the abdominal work, including Mat Work: Hundred and Reformer: Coordination. It also serves as a preparation for shoulder extension together with trunk extension, found in exercises such as Reformer: Pulling Straps I.

The arm work exercises for the ped-a-pul presented here duplicate the supine arm work series on the reformer, however here the body is in an upright position. This upright position is more functional by nature and further challenges the postural muscles.

VARIATION

If it is difficult to maintain the standing position, it is possible to sit on a stool or large ball.

Imagery

Visualize pressing the hands against a big inflated balloon. Alternatively, you can imagine that you are deep underwater and must use only your arms to propel yourself upward.

☐ Maintain scapular stabilization.

☐ Keep the arms straight.

☐ Move the arms in a straight line parallel to each other.

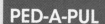

PED-A-PUL

Arm work

FUNDAMENTAL

Muscle Focus
- Latissimus dorsi

Objectives
- To strengthen the shoulder extensors
- To develop scapular stabilization
- To improve trunk alignment

RESISTANCE

Light   Medium   Heavy

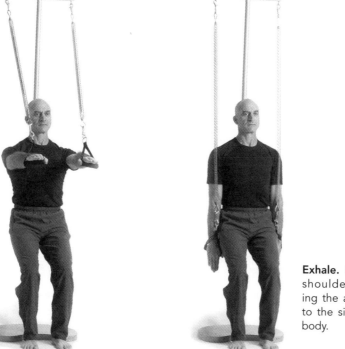

Inhale. Stand with the back against the pole and the feet 12 to 24 inches (30 to 60 centimeters) away from its base. Bend the knees, keeping the legs parallel to each other. Hold the handles and straighten the arms at shoulder height directly in front of the shoulders, palms facing down.

Exhale. Extend the shoulders, lowering the arms down to the sides of the body.

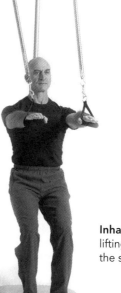

Inhale. Flex the shoulders, lifting the arms and return to the start position.

Muscle Focus

- Latissimus dorsi
- Pectorals

Objectives

- To strengthen the shoulder adductors
- To develop scapular stabilization
- To improve trunk alignment

RESISTANCE

Light | Medium | Heavy

Adduction

This exercise focuses on shoulder adduction from shoulder height and below. Like shoulder extension, shoulder adduction is performed together with the movement of the trunk in many Pilates exercises. It is often accompanied by trunk flexion, as in the case of abdominal work, or back extension, as in the Reformer: Pulling Straps II exercise.

Shoulder adduction is created primarily by the latissimus dorsi and pectoralis major working in concert with each other.

Imagery

Imagine spreading your arms like the wings of an eagle, as they move up and down. This is a powerful image; enjoy the sensation.

☐ Maintain scapular stabilization.

☐ Keep the arms straight and the palms facing the floor.

☐ Maintain a neutral spine position.

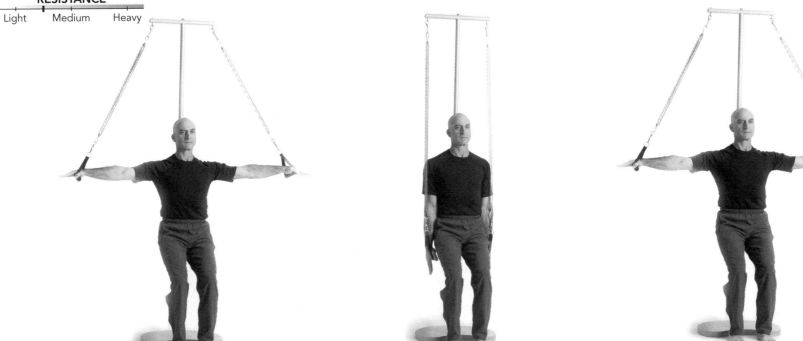

Inhale. Stand with the back against the pole and the feet 12 to 24 inches (30 to 60 centimeters) away from its base, knees bent and legs parallel to each other. Holding the handles, reach the arms out to the sides, establishing a T-position, palms facing down.

Exhale. Adduct the shoulders, bringing the arms down to the sides of the body.

Inhale. Abduct the shoulders, lifting the arms and returning to the start position.

Triceps

This exercise offers extremely focused work for the triceps. Keeping the upper arms stable and close to the sides of the body is key to maximizing the work of the triceps and isolating the movement of the elbow. In addition keeping the wrist perfectly stable and aligned with the arm is very important. When the wrist bends back, as it has a tendency to do, it places excessive pressure on the joint and releases some of the tension from the springs. The lower arm and wrist should be viewed as one solid unit.

Imagery

Imagine the body levitating with each extension of the elbows. The trunk elongates and the scapulae provide a stable base to push off from. The lower arm should feel like a mechanical lever attached at the elbow, and the joint like a well-lubricated hinge.

☐ Maintain scapular stabilization.

☐ Keep the upper arms close to the sides of the body.

☐ Isolate the movement of the lower arm.

Muscle Focus
- Triceps

Objective
- To strengthen the elbow extensors
- To develop scapular stabilization
- To improve trunk alignment

RESISTANCE

Light   Medium   Heavy

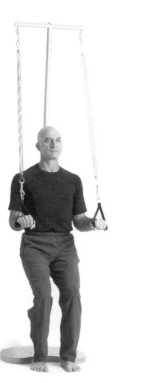

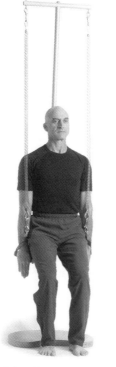

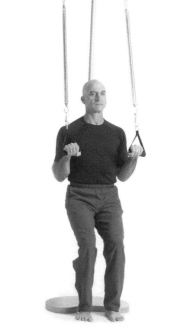

Inhale. Stand with the back against the pole and the feet 12 to 24 inches (30 to 60 centimeters) away from its base. Bend the knees and keep the legs parallel to each other. Hold the handles, either keeping the fingers straight so the line of the arm is continuous, or using a fist grip. Firmly anchor the arms by the sides of the body, with the elbows bent at a 90-degree angle.

Exhale. Extend the elbows, straightening the arms.

Inhale. Flex the elbows, bending the arms beyond the start position to work a greater range of motion.

Muscle Focus

- Latissimus dorsi
- Pectoralis

Objectives

- To strengthen the shoulder adductors and extensors
- To improve shoulder joint mobility
- To improve trunk alignment

RESISTANCE

Light | Medium | Heavy

Circle

The circle exercise combines shoulder adduction and shoulder flexion. When the arms reach the sides of the thighs, and the shoulders rotate with the hands changing from facing the body to facing back, there should be an almost indiscernible pause before the arms lift up again. Controlling the scapulohumeral rhythm (the relationship between the movement of the humerus and the scapula) is a crucial aspect of this exercise and is very important in establishing healthy shoulder mechanics. The scapulae can rotate inward and outward slightly to accommodate the movement of the humerus, however, without scapular elevation.

Performing the circle in both directions, the circle up described here and the circle down described in the variation, is very beneficial in terms of developing coordination and muscular control. In Pilates, we train the muscle in isometric, concentric, and eccentric modes, an approach that is widely supported in the world of exercise science.

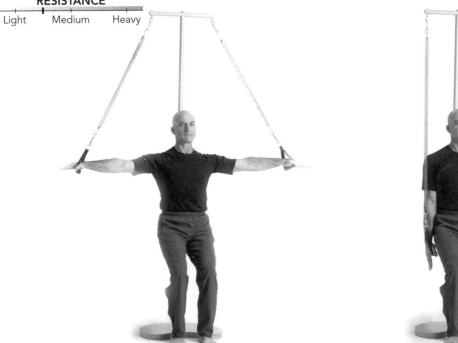

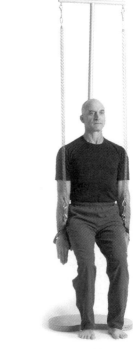

Inhale. Stand with the back against the pole and the feet 12 to 24 inches (30 to 60 centimeters) away from its base. Bend the knees and keep the legs parallel to each other. Holding the handles, reach the arms out to the sides, establishing a T-position, palms facing down.

Exhale. Adduct the shoulders, bringing the arms down to the sides of the body.

At this point rotate the shoulders so that the palms face backward.

Imagery

The feeling should be that of stirring a huge pot of thick porridge. There should be no breaks in the movement, despite the slight pause as the shoulders rotate and the hands change their facing

- ☐ Maintain scapular stabilization.
- ☐ Allow the scapulae to glide and rotate according to the movement of the humerus.
- ☐ Maintain a neutral spine position.

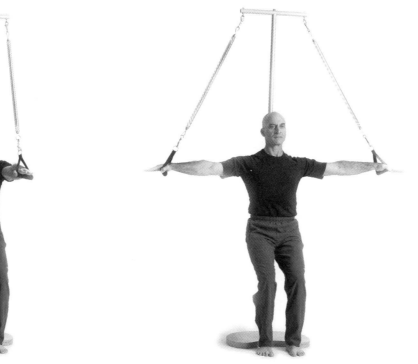

Inhale. Flex the shoulders, raising the arms in front of the body to shoulder height.

Horizontally abduct the shoulders, returning to the T-position.

10

Arm Chair

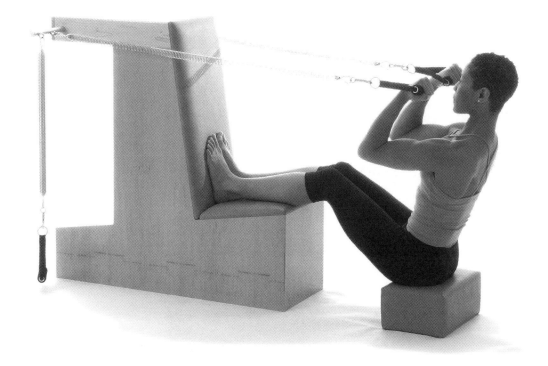

I would find it difficult to run a Pilates studio without the arm chair, yet for some inexplicable reason this piece of equipment is not often used; many Pilates teachers are unaware that it even exists. The arm chair is comfortable, user-friendly, and very convenient for allowing the teacher to offer cueing when teaching arm work. I believe that it has enormous, largely untapped potential.

Several contemporary versions of the arm chair exist, offering a variety of different benefits. Among them is the Avalon Chair, which I designed. A multifaceted apparatus, the Avalon chair addresses the entire body and works it in every conceivable position, range of motion and plane of motion. It is being used in studios, clinics and homes around the globe.

As the name implies, the arm chair in its traditional form is used primarily for the arms and shoulder complex. It is an excellent aid in teaching good shoulder mechanics and the concept of trunk stabilization during arm work. It offers support for the trunk, which is so valuable in the early stages of learning Pilates, specifically the upper body exercises.

As with the wunda chair, it is the simplicity of this apparatus that I find so appealing. The arm chair is relatively small and unassuming, yet it provides abundant opportunities for developing the entire body.

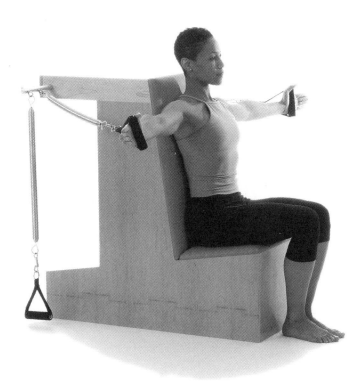

Chest Expansion

The arm chair offers an excellent position for performing this exercise, particularly for those with tight hamstrings who find it difficult to sit upright on the reformer with the legs straight forward (see Reformer: Chest Expansion—Seated). The trunk must be in an optimum position in order to activate the correct muscles and benefit from the exercise. It is surprising how little resistance is required to work the shoulder extensors effectively when the body is aligned correctly.

The most typical compensations or substitution patterns seen in this exercise are shoulder elevation, trunk flexion, and elbow flexion. These compensations occur when the resistance is too high or when body awareness and control are lacking. The arm chair can assist in overcoming these compensations and in laying the foundation for correct movement of the shoulders and arms.

Imagery

The sitting position on the arm chair promotes the feeling of elongation, of reaching down to the floor with the fingertips and up to the ceiling with the crown of the head. I also encourage a slight elevation of the chest, which prompts deeper activation of the mid-back extensors. When I was a young dancer studying Martha Graham technique, I had a

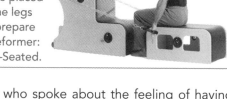

VARIATION

When performing the chest expansion on the Avalon, adjustments can be made to put the body into the optimal position. Note that the box can be moved further back to increase resistance, and the feet can be placed on the seat with the legs straight. This will prepare you well for the Reformer: Chest Expansion—Seated.

wonderful teacher who spoke about the feeling of having a fishhook placed through my sternum with the fishing line pulling me upward to the sky. The image, painful though it sounds, has always stuck with me; I think of it whenever I need to achieve a more upright position.

☐ Keep the range of movement relatively small (approximately 20 degrees forward of the trunk to 5-10 degrees behind the trunk).

☐ Maintain ideal upright alignment of the trunk.

☐ Reach down to the floor with the fingertips, keeping the elbows straight.

Muscle Focus

- Latissimus dorsi
- Triceps

Objectives

- To strengthen the shoulder and elbow extensors
- To develop trunk stabilization

RESISTANCE

Light   Medium   Heavy

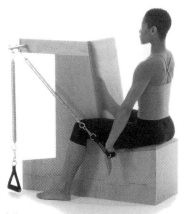

Inhale. Straddle the arm chair, facing the backrest, with the feet firmly on the ground. Hold the handles, with the arms straight against the sides of the body and the palms facing back.

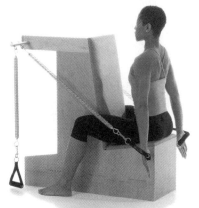

Exhale. Extend the shoulders, pulling the arms straight back.

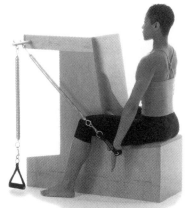

Inhale. Flex the shoulders, bringing the arms forward, and return to the start position, maintaining tension in the springs.

319

Muscle Focus

- Pectoralis major

Objectives

- To strengthen and increase flexibility of the shoulder horizontal adductors
- To develop trunk stabilization

RESISTANCE

Light — Medium — Heavy

Hug-a-Tree

Having the back supported while performing this exercise is invaluable. Not only does the Avalon chair support the trunk in a perfectly upright position as you develop the strength to hold the body in good sitting alignment, it also assists in maintaining good positioning of the scapulae by providing a solid surface to press against. As with the Reformer: Hug-a-Tree, the feeling of reaching out from the fingertips with the arms elongated is important in order to maximize the work in the shoulder region and maintain the resistance from the springs.

Imagery

Although I like hugging, even trees, the image of hugging a tree tends to result in the arms being too rounded. This in turn leads to decreased range of movement, less resistance, and a diminished return as compared with performing the exercise with the arms only slightly bent. You should have a sense of being regal, with the arms opening as if welcoming a dear friend. As you bring the arms toward each other, imagine that you are pressing against a large balloon. Finally, sitting on the chair should feel like sitting on a throne.

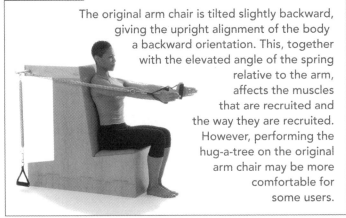

VARIATION

The original arm chair is tilted slightly backward, giving the upright alignment of the body a backward orientation. This, together with the elevated angle of the spring relative to the arm, affects the muscles that are recruited and the way they are recruited. However, performing the hug-a-tree on the original arm chair may be more comfortable for some users.

☐ Keep the back broad and the scapulae stabilized.

☐ Avoid thrusting the ribs forward as the arms open.

☐ Maintain an elongated arm position, without locking the elbows.

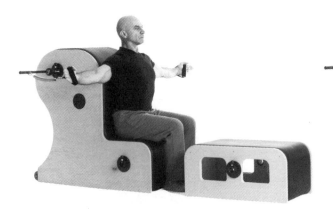

Inhale. Sit with the back against the chair and the legs together or hip-width apart. Hold the arms out in a T position, with the elbows slightly bent (just enough to engage the biceps) and the palms facing forward.

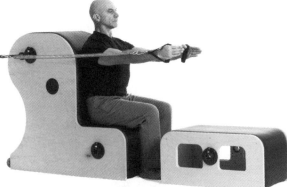

Exhale. Horizontally adduct the shoulders, bringing the arms toward each other until they are parallel.

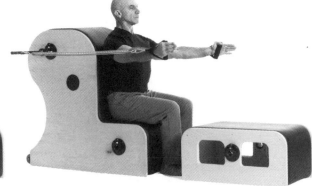

Inhale. Horizontally abduct the shoulders, opening the arms, and return to the start position, maintaining tension in the springs.

Circle

This exercise is an excellent way to promote shoulder control and mobility. Although the movement may appear to place strain on the shoulders, particularly as the arms lift overhead (which would be worrisome if any dysfunction, such as shoulder impingement syndrome, were present), this is not the case. The arms do not lift weight overhead (as they would with dumbbells); they resist the backward pull of the spring therefore using primarily the shoulder horizontal adductors and extensors. In fact, during my rehabilitation after open (as opposed to arthroscopic) rotator-cuff surgery on both of my shoulders, this exercise and the other arm chair exercises in the series presented here assisted me greatly in regaining range of motion without stressing the region.

Shoulder dysfunction is possibly the most common issue that Pilates teachers deal with. We repeatedly give cues regarding correct shoulder mechanics—to release tension, avoid elevating the shoulders, or maintain scapular stabilization.

Imagery

Imagine that the arms are being lifted by a pulley attached to weights. The scapulae are the weights. As the weights are

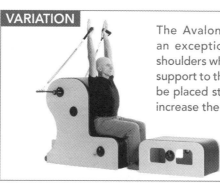

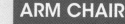
VARIATION
The Avalon's shape facilitates an exceptional stretch for the shoulders while offering excellent support to the trunk. The legs can be placed straight on the box to increase the challenge.

drawn down the back, the arms lift up. The ratio between the weights and the arms is finely balanced; as the arms circle around, the weights move slightly in and out like small pendulums, responding to the movement of the arms. However, they always have a downward orientation, maintaining a feeling of weightlessness in the arms.

- ☐ Keep the back broad and the scapulae stabilized.
- ☐ Maintain abdominal engagement.
- ☐ Avoid thrusting the ribs forward.

Muscle Focus
- Latissimus dorsi
- Pectorals

Objectives
- To increase the range of motion in the shoulder joint
- To develop shoulder control
- To develop trunk stabilization

RESISTANCE

Light   Medium   Heavy

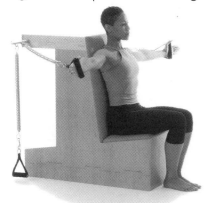

Inhale. Sit with the back against the chair and the legs together or hip-width apart. Hold the arms out in a T-position, with the elbows slightly bent (just enough to engage the biceps) and palms facing forward.

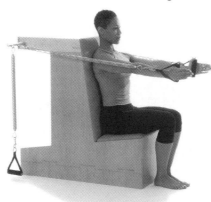

Exhale. Horizontally adduct the shoulders, bringing the arms toward each other until they are parallel.

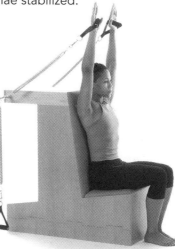

Inhale. Rotate the shoulders so the palms face down. Then lift the arms overhead and circle them around to the T-position (start position). Repeat 5 to 10 times, then reverse the direction, if desired: Starting from the T-position, abduct the shoulders and bring the arms overhead; extend the shoulders and press the arms down to shoulder height; rotate the shoulders so the palms face each other and abduct the shoulders to return to the T-position.

Muscle Focus

- Triceps

Objectives

- To strengthen the elbow extensors
- To develop control of the shoulder horizontal adductors

RESISTANCE

Light — Medium — Heavy

Salute

This exercise is very similar to the Reformer: Salute, and like the other exercises in this series, serves as a good preparation for the more challenging reformer work. Keep tension in the springs throughout the exercise while moving the arms on a slight diagonal line, just above the horizon. Keep the elbows reaching out to the sides.

Imagery

As with the Reformer: Salute, imagine the arms gliding along a ramp slightly above the line of the horizon. The angle is no more than approximately 30 degrees, so that shoulder elevation is minimized, if present at all. Focus on the feeling of an infinite line. As a dancer, I learned the difference between a straight arm that ends at the fingertips and appears short and a line that appears infinite. I always strive for limb and body lines that appear infinite.

VARIATION

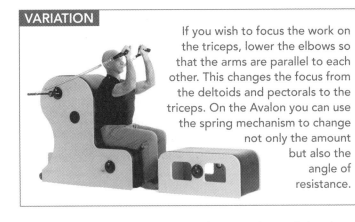

If you wish to focus the work on the triceps, lower the elbows so that the arms are parallel to each other. This changes the focus from the deltoids and pectorals to the triceps. On the Avalon you can use the spring mechanism to change not only the amount but also the angle of resistance.

☐ Keep the back broad and the scapulae stabilized.

☐ Direct the fingers forward throughout the movement.

☐ Avoid rolling the shoulders forward (internally rotating).

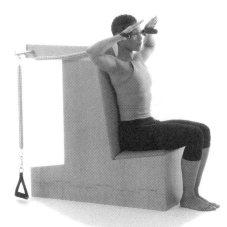

Inhale. Sit with the back against the chair and the legs together or hip-width apart. Place the hands opposite the temples at eyebrow level, palms facing down and fingers facing forward.

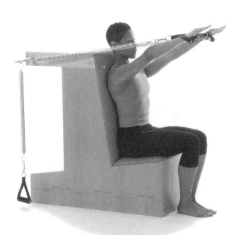

Exhale. Extend the elbows, straightening the arms on a diagonal line emanating from the shoulders.

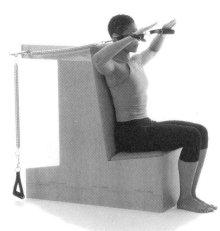

Inhale. Flex the elbows, bending the arms and keeping the fingers pointing in the direction of the movement. Return to the start position, maintaining tension in the springs.

Biceps

I have added this exercise to the classic Pilates repertoire on the arm chair because I wanted a biceps exercise that requires good trunk stabilization, particularly activating the back extensors, but is not hampered by tight hamstrings. The position of the body allows for more resistance than the Reformer: Biceps Curl does, which is an advantage when the goal is to build muscle strength.

Imagery

This exercise should feel like there is an intricate balancing act between the arms and trunk—as the trunk pivots back as one unit, the resistance on the arms can be increased to the point where the trunk feels like it is suspended from the arms and quite weightless.

☐ Keep the back extensors activated.

☐ Keep the arms parallel to each other and prevent the elbows from moving up or down.

☐ Avoid elevating the scapulae.

Muscle Focus
- Biceps

Objective
- To strengthen the elbow flexors
- To develop trunk stabilization

RESISTANCE

Light   Medium   Heavy

VARIATION

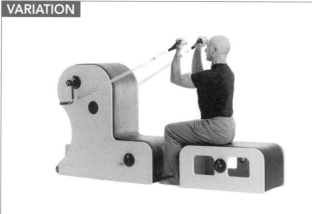

The biceps are often strong in relation to the other muscle groups that are targeted in this series. When performing this exercise on the Avalon chair, you can adjust the amount and angle of the resistance on the muscles.

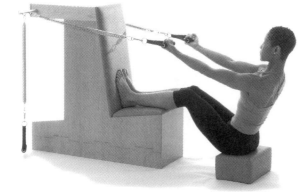

Inhale. Sit on a small box or pad (6-8 inches high), or on the floor if you are tall, facing the chair, with the feet against the backrest. Hold the handles with the arms parallel, directly opposite the shoulders at shoulder height and with palms facing up.

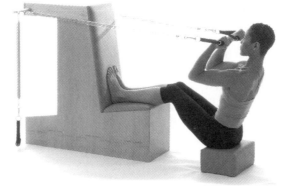

Exhale. Flex the elbows, bending the arms.

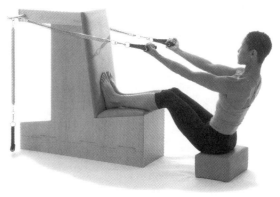

Inhale. Extend the elbows, straighten the arms, and return to the start position.

Muscle Focus

- Deltoid posterior
- Rhomboids

Objective

- To strengthen the shoulder horizontal abductors and scapular adductors

RESISTANCE

| Light | Medium | Heavy |

Rhomboids

This exercise places the body and arms in a different position than in the reformer version (Reformer: Rhomboids—Seated). The arm position emphasizes internal rotation of the shoulder as opposed to the external rotation in the reformer version. Still, these two exercises have a great deal in common. In both versions the position and stability of the trunk are key to successful execution of the exercise. I recommend first isolating the shoulder horizontal abduction and only later adding the scapular adduction and abduction. Doing so isolates the glide of the scapula, rather than combining it with the movement of the arm.

Imagery

The movement of the arms resembles a rowing action, although the trunk, which provides a stable foundation for the movement, remains still. In actual rowing the trunk would move of course. Despite this difference, the image of rowing a boat will assist in achieving the desired action.

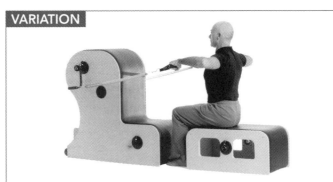

VARIATION

Performing this difficult exercise on the Avalon offers the benefit of a comfortable sitting position, which provides good access for the instructor to monitor and provide appropriate cues.

☐ Keep the back extensors activated.

☐ Move the arms on a horizontal plane.

☐ Keep the elbows high and reaching out and back.

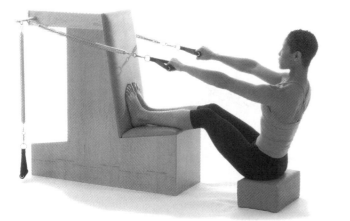

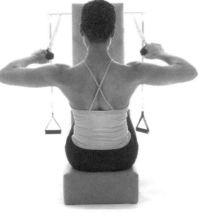

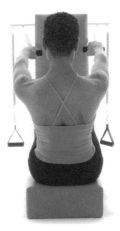

Inhale. Sit on a small box, facing the chair, with the feet against the backrest of the chair, knees bent and legs together. Hold the handles with the arms parallel, directly opposite the shoulders at shoulder height and with palms facing down.

Exhale. Flex the elbows, bending the arms. Reach the elbows out to the sides and back until they cannot move any further without adducting the scapulae. (When you have perfected this movement in terms of form and muscle activation, add the adduction and abduction of the scapulae.)

Inhale. Extend the elbows, straighten the arms, and return to the start position.

11

Magic Circle

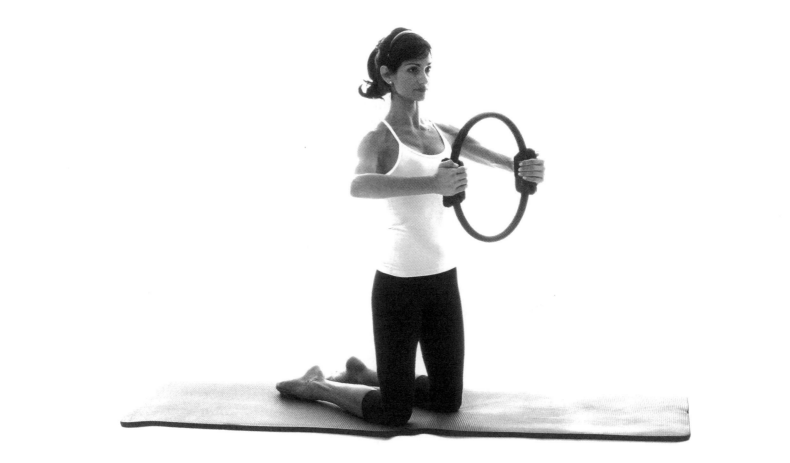

The number of aliases that exist for this simple ring reflects the wide variety of exercises that can be performed with it. It is the perfect travel companion, an ideal complement to the full-apparatus session, and an excellent accessory to use in a mat work class to add challenge and excitement.

The circle can be used simply to keep the body in alignment or the limbs in a desired position; such as holding it between the arms opposite the chest or above the head. Or it can be used to encourage the continuous activation of a certain muscle group, for example, holding it between the legs to help maintain adductor engagement. It can also be used to add resistance to a movement or heighten the level of coordination.

It often amazes me when I see some "new" device that works one or two muscle groups flood the fitness market and sell millions of units; often the magic circle works those same muscle groups and does so much more. For instance, one popular piece of equipment is an inner-thigh apparatus that works the adductors—and that's it!

The magic circle works the adductors just as well, but it also works the abductors, hamstrings, abdominals, back extensors, and arms. The secret is getting out, and magic circles are finally receiving their long overdue credit.

Many types of magic circles are now available in every conceivable packaging. Some offer more resistance than others; some are made of a super-light material and others are heavier. Choose one that suits your lifestyle and needs. In terms of resistance, err toward lighter rather than heavier. If you travel frequently and the circle is to become a travel companion, get the ultra-light version. If it is to be used in a studio and will need to stand up to the demands of continuous use, get one that is made of the most durable materials, even if it is heavier.

The range of motion of the movements performed with the magic circle is very small, if any. It is more like an isometric contraction than an isotonic contraction. The dynamic is a pumping action rather than a slow movement.

Arms Bent

This is a fun, effective exercise to develop the chest muscles, and the pumping action that it requires is well-suited to the magic circle. Be aware of recruiting the pectorals with each pump. Keep the oval shape created by the arms consistent and the wrists firm as you squeeze the arms together.

Imagery

Although this image may seem a little graphic, try to bounce the pectorals with each pump. (This works for both men and women, although women may relate to the image more readily!)

- ☐ Maintain ideal body alignment throughout.
- ☐ Focus on scapular stabilization.
- ☐ Perform small pumping movements.

Muscle Focus
- Pectorals

Objectives
- To strengthen the shoulder horizontal adductors

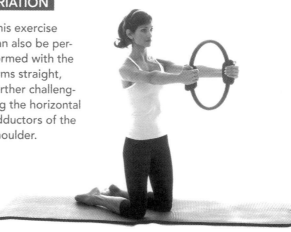

VARIATION

This exercise can also be performed with the arms straight, further challenging the horizontal adductors of the shoulder.

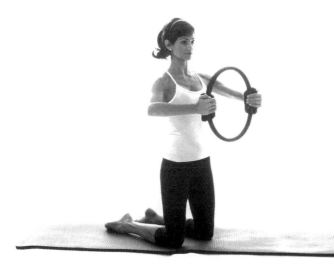

Inhale. While sitting on a large ball, kneeling, or standing upright, hold the circle directly opposite the sternum with the elbows slightly bent.

Exhale. Horizontally adduct the arms, pressing them together.

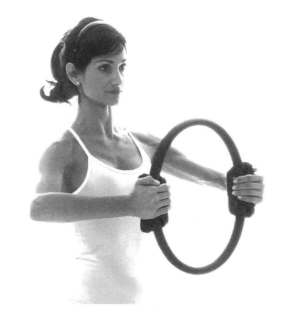

Inhale. Maintain the tension in the circle and continue with small pumps. Return to the start position.

Muscle Focus

- Pectorals

Objective

- To strengthen the pectoral muscles

Arms Overhead

This arm exercise is more difficult than it looks. Maintaining scapular stabilization and avoiding tension in the shoulders and neck are challenging enough. Adding the arm movement makes it even harder. The movement is so challenging that for most people this exercise becomes isometric—the arms remain still as they press together.

Imagery

This exercise never fails to evoke the image of a halo!

☐ Maintain ideal body alignment throughout the exercise.

☐ Focus on scapular stabilization.

☐ Lift the arms only as high as shoulder flexibility allows without elevating the shoulders.

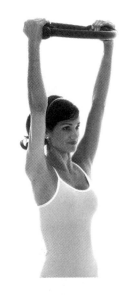

Exhale. Adduct the arms, pressing them together.

Inhale. Maintain the tension in the circle and continue with small pumps. Return to the start position.

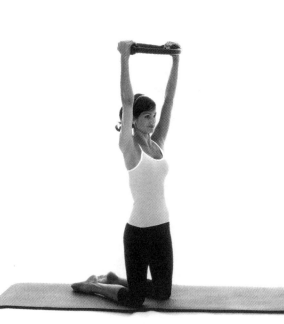

Inhale. Kneeling or standing upright, hold the circle with the arms reaching overhead.

Single-Arm Side Press

This exercise requires that you engage the shoulder adductors, particularly the latissimus dorsi, prior to the pumping action and keep them engaged throughout the sequence. Maintaining scapular stability and a slight bend in the elbow is important; the movement should occur in the glenohumeral joint only.

Imagery

Imagine trying to pat the side of your leg, but the air is thick and gel-like and does not allow you to reach it. But you persist!

☐ Maintain ideal body alignment throughout the exercise.

☐ Maintain scapular stabilization.

☐ Avoid neck and shoulder tension.

Muscle Focus
- Latissimus dorsi
- Pectorals

Objective
- To strengthen the shoulder adductors

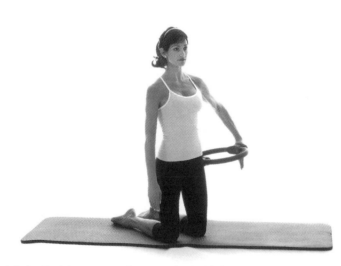

Inhale. Kneeling or standing upright, hold the circle in one hand and rest it against the side of the thigh, directly below the hip joint. The elbow should be slightly bent and the shoulder slightly internally rotated.

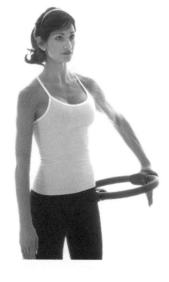

Exhale. Adduct the shoulder, pressing the hand toward the thigh.

Inhale. Maintain the tension in the circle and continue with small pumps. Return to the start position.

Muscle Focus

• Biceps

Objective

• To strengthen the elbow flexors

Single-Arm Biceps

This is a simple yet effective biceps exercise. I added this to the repertoire years ago, when I wanted to provide a more comprehensive workout for the arms and upper body using the circle. Do this exercise slowly, compressing the circle for several seconds before allowing the arm to lift up.

Imagery

This always conjures up an image of Africa, where I grew up. I would see the people, particularly the women, carrying heavy loads on their heads, often balancing them with one hand. Their posture was perfect and strong and they walked gracefully, unencumbered by the enormous load on their heads. This, to me, exemplifies the body in perfect alignment and balance.

☐ Press the circle straight down.

☐ Press down with the palm of the hand, not the fingers.

☐ Find a comfortable place to rest the circle on the shoulder.

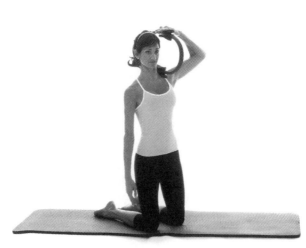

Inhale. Kneeling or standing upright, hold the top of the circle in one hand and rest the lower side on the shoulder, directly above the joint. Bend the elbow and reach it out to the side.

Exhale. Press the hand down toward the shoulder, bending the elbow further.

Inhale. Lift the hand, maintaining tension in the circle, then press down again. Return to the start position.

Above Knees—Seated

This is a straightforward, effective hip adductor exercise. However, you should view it as a full-body exercise, emphasizing the alignment of the trunk, head, pelvis, and feet.

The hip adductor group is made up of several individual muscles originating and inserting at different points. Change the position of the magic circle to work the hip adductors slightly differently; each position engages muscles in its own way.

Imagery

The imagery for the entire series of magic circle hip-adductor exercises, whether performed sitting, prone, or supine, is about the hip joints moving freely without affecting the solid alignment of the rest of the body. The feeling should be like the head of the femur is moving in a soft gel or like a spoon stirring thick porridge.

☐ Find a comfortable location on the inner thighs to place the circle where it will not slip out.

☐ Press equally with both legs.

VARIATION

Try placing the magic circle directly below the knees and also just above the ankles. Placing the circle just above the ankles works the muscles of the feet as well as the hip adductors. The feeling should be one of gliding the legs toward each other with the feet sliding across the floor.

Muscle Focus
- Hip adductors

Objective
- To strengthen the hip adductors

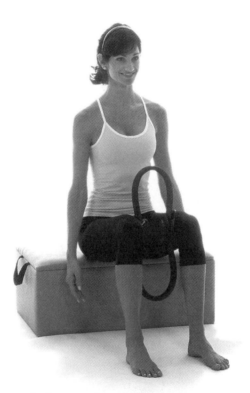

Exhale. Press the legs together, adducting the hips.

Inhale. Maintain the tension in the circle and continue with small pumps. Return to the start position.

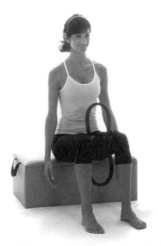

Inhale. Sit upright with the hips and knees at a 90-degree angle. Place the circle between the legs, just above the knees, pressing it with the hip adductors.

Muscle Focus

- Hip adductors

Objectives

- To strengthen the hip adductors
- To develop pelvic–lumbar stabilization

Knees—Supine

Although this exercise is geared toward strengthening the hip adductors, it requires good abdominal strength and exceptional pelvic–lumbar control. In addition, it is an optimal position in which to work the pelvic floor muscles.

If you suspect that you lack the abdominal strength needed for this exercise, perform the variation instead.

Imagery

I like to imagine that the tailbone is a tail that lifts up between the legs, and as it lifts the sit bones are drawn together. Visualize this while hollowing the abdominals and squeezing the legs together. This helps to recruit the pelvic floor and abdominal complex and deepens the work of the hip adductors. However, this should not cause the pelvis to tuck under (posterior tilt).

☐ Maintain good pelvic–lumbar control and spinal alignment.

☐ Keep the hips and knees at a consistent angle.

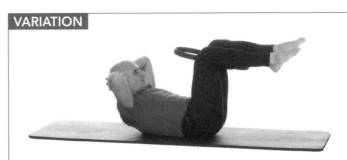

VARIATION

If abdominal strength is limited, keep the lower back flat on the floor instead of maintaining a neutral spine position, even if this results in a slight posterior tilt of the pelvis. If the lower back starts rising off the floor into an arch (hyperlordosis), draw the abdominal muscles in deeper and lift the upper trunk into forward flexion. Place the hands behind the head and interlace the fingers to support the head. If this position places stress on the back, perform the exercise with the feet on the floor.

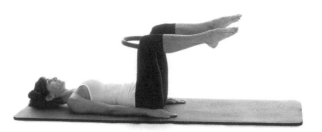

Inhale. Lie supine in a neutral spine position, with the hips and knees at a 90-degree angle (tabletop position). Place the circle between the thighs just above the knees.

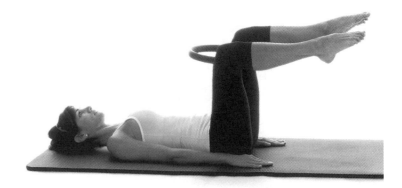

Exhale. Adduct the hips, squeezing the legs together. Maintain the tabletop position, with the hips and knees at a 90-degree angle and the shins parallel to each other and to the floor.

Inhale. Maintain the tension in the circle and continue with small pumps. Return to the start position.

Ankles—Supine

Like the previous exercise, this one strengthens the hip adductors and requires good abdominal strength and exceptional pelvic–lumbar control. Again, it has the benefit of providing an optimal position in which to work the pelvic floor muscles. However, because the legs are straight, the lever arm is longer, magnifying the work of the abdominals and hip flexors and demanding a very high level of control.

Those who lack abdominal strength may benefit from alternative positioning (see "Variation").

Imagery

The tailbone as a tail imagery works well while squeezing the legs together. Recruitment of the pelvic floor muscles and abdominal complex deepens the work of the hip adductors.

☐ Maintain good pelvic–lumbar control and spinal alignment.

☐ Keep the legs at a consistent angle to the floor.

☐ Relax the neck and shoulders

Muscle Focus

- Hip adductors

Objectives

- To strengthen the hip adductors
- To develop pelvic–lumbar stabilization

VARIATION

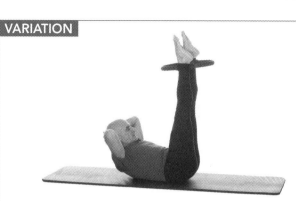

If the low back starts to rise into an arch, draw the abdominal muscles in deeper and lift into trunk flexion, placing the hands behind the head and interlacing the fingers. Lift the legs higher, closer to a 90-degree angle. I encourage experimenting with hip external rotation. Sometimes you can achieve a deeper contraction of the muscles and maintain better spinal support with the legs externally rotated (turned out). If this position proves too challenging, bend the knees slightly.

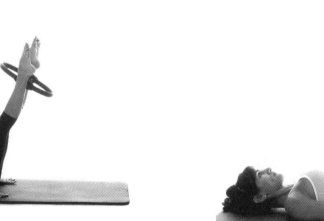

Inhale. Lie supine in a neutral spine position with the legs straight at a 60- to 90-degree angle to the floor (depending on your abdominal strength and pelvic-lumbar stabilization; the lower the legs, the more difficult the exercise becomes). Place the circle between the legs, just above the ankles.

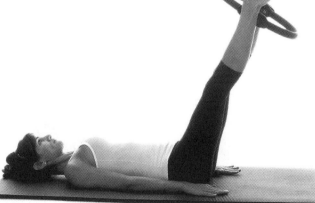

Exhale. Adduct the hips, squeezing the legs together.

Inhale. Maintain the tension in the circle and continue with small pumps. Return to the start position.

Muscle Focus

- Hip adductors
- Hip extensors

Objective

- To strengthen the hip adductors and hip extensors
- To develop pelvic-lumbar stabilization.

Knees Bent—Prone

This exercise is exceptional for building strength in the hip adductors and hip extensors. Keeping the knees bent and lifting the thighs off the mat throughout the exercise maximizes the work of the hip extensors, using both functions of the hamstrings (knee flexion and hip extension). Avoid the tendency to tilt the pelvis anteriorly and hyperextend the lower back, which places stress on this area of the back. This is particularly pertinent when the hip flexors are tight or when the abdominals are not engaged sufficiently to counteract the anterior pull typically exerted by tight hip flexors. The hip flexor that has the most impact in this situation is the rectus femoris. In such cases, draw the abdominals in deeper and emphasize a posterior tilt of the pelvis by pushing the pubic symphysis forward. If necessary, place a small cushion in the abdominal region to assist in achieving a position that is biased toward a posterior pelvic tilt and preventing an anterior tilt of the pelvis.

Imagery

The body should feel like an archer's bow that has been pulled taut. As the feet lift higher toward the ceiling with each squeeze, the bow becomes more taut and the arc is accentuated.

☐ Extend the hips prior to squeezing the legs together, and keep them extended throughout.

☐ Maintain consistent 90-degree flexion in the knees.

☐ Keep the hips parallel as opposed to externally rotated, as the legs squeeze together.

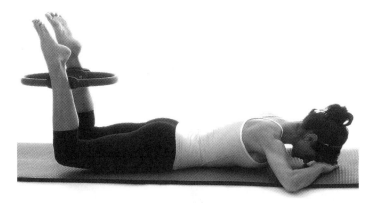

Exhale. Adduct the hips, squeezing the legs together.

Inhale. Maintain the tension in the circle and continue with small pumps. Return to the start position.

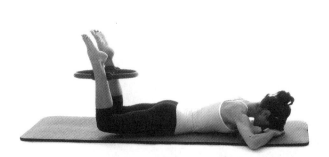

Inhale. Lie prone with the knees bent at a 90-degree angle and the thighs lifted off the mat. Place the circle between the legs just above the ankles. Rest the forehead on the hands.

Knees Straight—Prone

Like the previous exercise, this one is exceptional for building strength of the hip adductors and hip extensors. Keeping the thighs lifted off the mat throughout the movement while contracting the adductors promotes deep hip extensor work. Avoid the tendency to tilt the pelvis in an anterior direction. Although the knees are now straight, which releases the taut hip flexors, the lever arm has been lengthened, challenging the hip extensors and back extensors more, and demanding a very high level of control, potentially placing stress on the lower back.

Imagery

The image of the archer's bow is an excellent one for this exercise. In this case the feeling is one of elongating into the bow shape with each squeeze of the legs, as opposed to lifting high.

- ☐ Extend the hips prior to squeezing the legs together, and keep them extended throughout.

- ☐ Maintain strong abdominal work throughout the exercise.

- ☐ Relax the neck and shoulders.

Muscle Focus
- Hip adductors
- Hip extensors

Objective
- To strengthen the hip adductors and hip extensors
- To develop pelvic-lumbar stabilization.

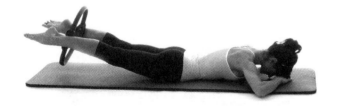

Inhale. Lie prone with the legs straight and the thighs lifted off the mat. Place the circle between the legs, just above the ankles. Rest the forehead on the hands.

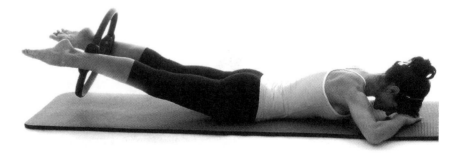

Exhale. Adduct the hips, squeezing the legs together.

Inhale. Maintain the tension in the circle and continue with small pumps. Return to the start position.

Muscle Focus
- Hamstrings

Objective
- To strengthen the hip extensors
- To develop pelvic-lumbar stabilization.

Hamstrings

One of my students came up with this excellent hamstring curl exercise years ago. Since then it has been refined and the element of hip extension has been added to it. A possible disadvantage of this exercise is that the knee moves within a very small range of motion, if at all. However, if the goal is a small range of motion or an isometric contraction, then this will prove to be an advantage. I suggest orienting the pelvis toward a posterior tilt from the outset. That will counter the tendency to tilt it anteriorly, which often results in hyperextension of the lower back. Use a cushion under the abdominal region if necessary to help promote the posterior tilt.

Imagery

Visualize the archer's bow position, and add the hamstring curl that further accentuates the arc shape. Maintain the bow shape with the working leg while the straight leg provides an anchor for the movement. Pressing into the mat with the straight leg will help keep the other leg elevated off the mat.

- ☐ Extend the hip of the bent leg before pressing the heel down, and keep it extended throughout .

- ☐ Avoid externally rotating the working leg and keep the thighs close together.

- ☐ Maintain abdominal activation throughout the exercise.

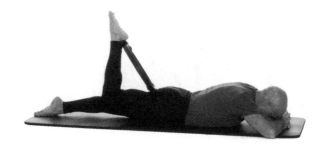

Inhale. Lie prone with one leg straight and the other bent at the knee. Lift the bent leg slightly off the mat. Place the circle below the gluteal muscle and behind the heel of the bent leg. Rest the forehead on the hands.

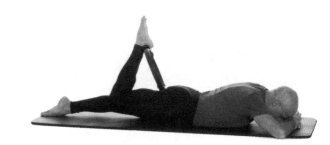

Exhale. Bend the knee further, pressing the heel toward the pelvis.
Inhale. Maintain the tension in the circle and continue with small pumps. Return to the start position.

Swan

This swan exercise focuses on the upper and mid-back as opposed to the lower back. The lower back is often hyperactive, which tends to inhibit the recruitment of the mid and upper-back muscles. Extending the hips and lifting the legs immediately activates the lower back and distracts from the focus of the exercise. For this reason the legs should remain anchored on the floor, uninvolved in the actual movement.

The shoulder flexors feature prominently in keeping the arms aligned with the trunk. Ideally, the arms should line up opposite, or just below the ears. Make sure to keep the head aligned with the spine, avoiding the tendency to lift it to look straight forward rather than looking down and slightly forward.

Imagery

This is a challenging back extension exercise that is wonderful to integrate into a mat work class. I like using the image of the halo, even though the circle is not quite in the halo position.

Muscle Focus
- Back extensors

Objective
- To strengthen the back extensors
- To develop shoulder flexor control

VARIATION

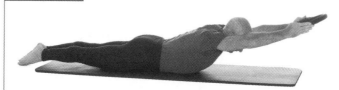

In order to make this exercise a little easier, hold the circle in a horizontal position, parallel to the floor. In this way, the back and shoulders start from a less challenging position and are not required to lift as high.

This image keeps the relationship between the head and the arms consistent.

☐ Adduct the hips throughout the exercise.

☐ Focus on length as opposed to height.

☐ Move the arms, head, and trunk as one unit.

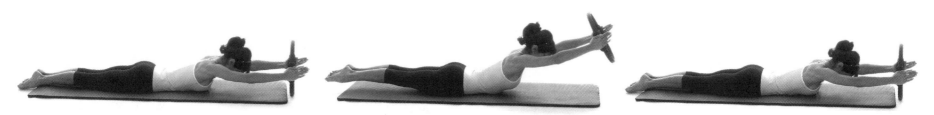

Inhale. Lie prone with the arms straight and reaching overhead. Hold the circle in the palms of the hands.

Exhale. Lift the upper body and legs, pressing the arms together.

Inhale. Maintain the tension in the circle. Return to the start position.

12

Sample Exercise Routines

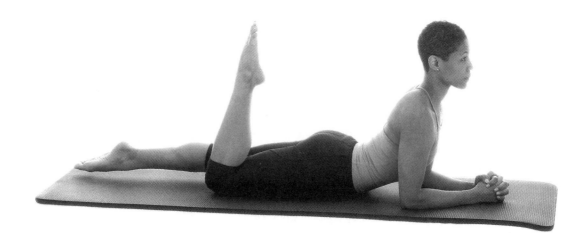

In this chapter, I provide several sample exercise routines for you to use in your Pilates practice. These will help you become acquainted with the exercises and learn how to sequence them effectively within the comprehensive block system described in chapter 3. This in no way implies that the exercises must be practiced in the order I suggest in the following routines. I believe that being able to adapt to different situations is important. But using the block system offers a structure that promotes a positive outcome and opens the door to a myriad of choices. For instance, when deciding which exercises to do for arm work, you can choose upper body exercises from a large pool of exercises that best suit your purpose at the time. In fact you can choose from a selection of *arm series*, compilations of arm exercises which together form a complementary, integrated exercise unit. The same goes for abdominal work, lateral flexion, back extension, and the other blocks—you can choose individual exercises or series of exercises for each block. Practicing set routines (those offered here and others that you devise) so that they become second nature and imprinted in your muscle memory is advantageous. The block system helps guide you in drawing the fine line between reinforcing movement patterns and allowing the work to become mundane and repetitious.

Sequencing Exercises

Once you have learned the exercises, you should then incorporate them into a comprehensive, flowing routine. The mat work particularly lends itself to seamless transitions and unobstructed flow—one continuous movement from beginning to end. It starts with the first breath of the setup and continues to the final breath of the relaxation at the end.

I have been greatly influenced by years of dance and ashtanga yoga, as well as a familiarity with tai chi. These disciplines all share the quality of continuous movement. As explained in chapter 4, my mat work block system incorporates what I call *flow sequences*, and flow is the underlying quality in each exercise, sequence, and routine. Although maintaining the same degree of flow when working on the apparatus is more difficult, you should always experience a feeling of fluidity and continuum, of deep concentration and inner focus. The quality of flow has many benefits. Apart from helping you feel good and look beautiful, it offers physiological benefits: it heightens the cardiovascular effect, elevates the body temperature, and builds muscular endurance. Flow also brings mental benefits, such as concentration and release of tension. Together these characteristics culminate in a state I refer to as *meditation in motion*.

Creating transitions from exercise to exercise to make the sequence flow is a stimulating process. The transitions, on the mat as well as the apparatus, should be choreographed as an integral part of the routine, so that there is no need for stopping, repositioning, and starting again. Separate actions waste energy and break concentration. At the same time, keep in mind that although the transitions are important, they should not dictate the order of the exercises. The order must be determined by physiological principles, addressing the planes of motion, muscle groups, and safe progression. This is the premise of the block system.

The following guidelines will help you compile a session. The same guidelines apply to every session, whether it lasts 10 minutes or 60 minutes, whether it is done on the mat or on the apparatus, and whether it is fundamental or advanced. Keep in mind that to make a program effective and to see continued gains, you must gradually and consistently make the exercises more challenging. Effective cueing, using accessories such as rubber bands, modifying the exercises, adjusting the resistance, and introducing more difficult variations (with a similar muscle focus) can all help achieve this goal.

- Develop the session to progress from less-demanding exercises to more-demanding ones.
- Perform large muscle group exercises earlier in the session.

- Perform lower risk exercises earlier in the session.
- Keep programs progressive in the use of range of motion, resistance, complexity, and speed.
- Address as many muscle groups as possible during a session.
- Practice the various functions of the muscles: stabilization and mobilization.
- Incorporate all types of muscle contraction: isometric, concentric, and eccentric.
- Include all ranges of motion: flexion, rotation, lateral flexion, extension, and combinations of these.
- Balance the exercises according to the primary joints and their movements (such as hip flexion, hip extension, hip abduction, hip adduction, hip rotation).
- Emphasize a particular area based on individual needs while maintaining a good overall balance.
- Include more challenging exercises after an adequate warm-up.
- Add exercises that focus on balance and proprioception when appropriate.
- Work the mind and body together in harmony.

Individualizing a Sequence

Perhaps the most valuable quality of the Pilates method, is its adaptability—it can cater to a broad range of people with differing needs. It is a solution for everyone, from those restricted in mobility to elite athletes. It can accommodate the young, elderly, fit, unfit, dancers, athletes, pregnant women, and the injured and rehabilitating. It is as beneficial for men as for women. I do not believe any other system offers such diversity, and still challenges each person's capabilities to the maximum. Added to this is the calm, trusting, nurturing, and noncompetitive environment that is typical of most Pilates studios. Yet, as I said at the beginning of the book, although Pilates is suited to anyone, not everyone will like this type of work or relate to it.

The extensive body of exercises, along with the choice of apparatus, allows the compilation of a program suited to each individual. The decision to introduce new exercises should be well thought out. Adding challenges is tempting, but new repertoire can be counterproductive if it is not appropriate. You must assess whether an exercise is of a suitable level, whether it will affect any injured areas adversely, whether it will help achieve a desired goal, and whether you (or your student) have adequate training and skills to perform it.

If you are a teacher designing a program, I encourage you to find out as much as possible about the individual you are working with. More important than what to do is what *not* to do, particularly in cases in which taking a certain tack may result in injury or even irreparable damage, such as when working with pregnant women or people suffering from back problems or osteoporosis, to name just a few. Become intricately familiar with the repertoire, be well educated in the science of human movement, know the body you are working with, and then be creative in developing options, never losing sight of the essence of the exercise. When in doubt, err on the side of caution, seek further professional advice (medical and otherwise) as needed—and always be safe, not sorry! When used as it was intended, Pilates can be the answer to anyone's quest for well-being.

Adapting Programs for Select Populations

Select populations is a general term that describes groups that have specific needs. There are two main groups: people for whom you may need to *decrease* the intensity of the work and people for whom you may need to *increase* the intensity of the work. The first group, which includes the elderly, the injured, and people in rehabilitation, typically requires modification of the exercises and the use of assists, such as cushions, rubber bands, and springs. The second group consists of those who may need increased intensity, such as athletes, dancers, and gymnasts, in the form of increased *overload* on the muscles and other measures that make

Fundamentals to Take on the Road

If I told you about the many, and often odd, places I have practiced Pilates, it would surely bring a smile to your face! I do an enormous amount of traveling, and I always take the fundamentals on the road with me. This usually consists of a mat and small accessories such as rubber bands and a magic circle (although the circle has become the cause of growing scrutiny during airport security checks). The beauty of Pilates is that you can compile a program for every occasion and any location as long as you follow the guidelines outlined in this chapter. Remember that consistency is the key, and if you let your Pilates practice lapse while you are traveling, all your hard work is diminished. Besides regular practice will keep you alert, in shape, and on top of your game at all times, even when sunning yourself on a beach in Hawaii!

the exercises more complex. Both groups need specifically tailored programs, often based on vastly different goals. Some populations fit both main categories to varying degrees. Pregnant women, for example, fit into both groups. Their programs need to be continuously modified and intensity must often be decreased to suit their constantly changing bodies, yet, at the same time they are often fit, athletic, and not limited in the same sense as those who are going through rehabilitation.

Even within the main groupings the goals may vary greatly. For instance, athletes often need *specificity-training* in which they work on activity-specific skills and develop the neuromuscular system to improve performance. However, they may also need to improve general balance and enhance their overall conditioning program—in other words, they need *cross-training*. Pilates is exceptional for both forms of training.

It is beyond the scope of this chapter to provide exercise sequences for select populations and modifications and variations to suit every need. However, you can use the routines that appear in this book as a foundation and adapt them to meet your needs or those of your students.

Considering Safety

Whether you are doing mat work or working on the Pilates apparatus, safety is of paramount importance. In addition to following the general safety protocols for any exercise class—warming up, preparing the body for each action, monitoring heart rate and body temperature, and cooling down at the end of the session—you also need to know how to work safely with the full complement of Pilates apparatus. Pilates equipment is generally considered very safe equipment. It is *not*. In fact, it is potentially dangerous *if* not used correctly and with discretion, as the following story shows.

In 1989 I was in Australia, teaching and directing a dance department in a performing arts college where I had introduced a Pilates program. I had a Pilates studio at the college for my work with the students and some amateur and professional dancers and athletes. One morning I was teaching a young dancer, around 12 years old. She was doing mini roll-ups on the cadillac. She was a regular student and had done the exercise many times. She wanted to explain something to me and in so doing let go of the push-through bar, which was attached to two springs. I was standing close by, and the bar flew into my mouth, crushing my four front teeth, sending me tumbling into the wall behind me, and knocking me out. I came around with my hand over my mouth, blood dripping out, and pieces of teeth in my hand.

Today all is fine, other than the fact that I have spent more hours in dentists' chairs since the incident than I wish to recall. Was it anyone's fault? Probably not—just an unfortunate accident that illustrates the potential dangers of the apparatus and the need for students and teachers to be constantly vigilant and respectful. The apparatus was never intended for unsupervised, mass use. Yet given the exposure Pilates is now receiving and some of the modern trends in the way it is taught, this fact is often ignored. Good instruction and proper training are essential.

The features that make the equipment so beneficial to fitness and conditioning also make it potentially harmful—there are springs, straps, and attachments all over the place. The equipment does not support you; you need to support your own body. Each exercise requires recruiting the body's stabilizers, which is one reason this work is so functional. If you do not incorporate good stabilization, you risk not doing the movement correctly, and worse, the possibility of accident and injury.

Starting With Inner Focus

You are now familiar with both the philosophy and the exercises of Pilates and are ready to delve into your practice. I like to begin and conclude each session with a little relaxation or inner focus. If we commence the session with tension, that tension will compound as the body is challenged; then, rather than having a calming and rejuvenating effect and allowing you to achieve the goals of the exercises, the experience will be counterproductive.

A session on the apparatus often commences and concludes with a roll-down, which draws attention to alignment as well as serving as a path to inner-focus, warm-up, and cool-down. After three to five roll-downs, I suggest a short mat work warm-up before moving onto the apparatus. When doing mat work, a session typically begins and ends by going through a brief inner focus period in a standing, sitting, or supine position.

The following is a suggested outline for achieving inner focus when starting a mat work session.

1. Lie down on the mat in a supine position, with the knees bent, legs parallel to each other, and hip-width apart. Spread the feet comfortably on the floor. Place the arms by the sides of the body. Allow the spine to sink into the mat.

2. Relax the feet, the back, and the neck.

3. Engage the adductors slightly to prevent the legs from splaying.

4. Imagine the pelvis floating in space with no forces pulling on it.

5. Visualize an elongated spine, relaxing the muscles of the back.

6. Reach the fingers toward the feet, gliding the scapulae down the back.

7. Elongate the neck, sensing the crown of the head reaching away from the body.

8. Relax the muscles of the face.

9. Be present in the moment, focus on the breath, and feel the lateral expansion of the chest on the mat.

10. Become aware of your body down to the last muscle fiber.

11. Engage the internal support system—you are now ready to move!

Mat Work Sequences

In this section I provide three mat work routines: fundamental, intermediate, and advanced. Each routine builds on the previous one. Practice them while incorporating the principles discussed in this book. Remember, Pilates is about quality, not quantity. Practice the work with integrity and make each movement the best that you possibly can. In the words of Joseph Pilates (in *Return to Life*), "Make a close study of each exercise and do not attempt any other exercise until you first have mastered the current one and know its routine down to the last detail without any reference to the text" (page 32).

Basic Mat Work Program

Exercises: 16 • approximate time: 25 minutes

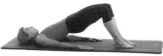

Pelvic Curl, page 49

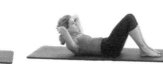

Spine Twist—Supine, page 50

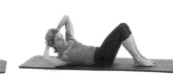

Chest Lift, page 51

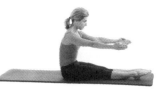

Chest Lift With Rotation, page 52

Roll-Up, page 58

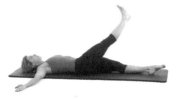

Leg Circle, page 54

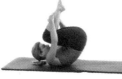

Rolling Like a Ball, page 72

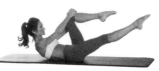

Single-Leg Stretch, page 62

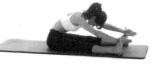

Spine stretch, page 71

Saw, page 102

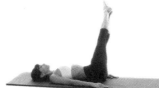

Spine Twist—Sitting, page 101

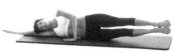

Corkscrew, page 104

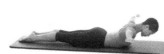

Side Leg Lift, page 96

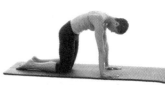

Back Extension, page 111

Cat Stretch, page 112

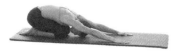

Rest Position, page 118

Exercises: 32 • approximate time: 45 minutes

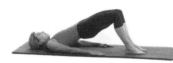

Pelvic Curl, page 49

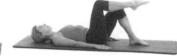

Leg Lift, page 53

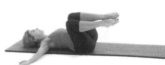

Spine Twist—Supine, page 50

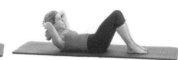

Chest Lift, page 51

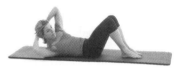
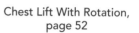

Chest Lift With Rotation, page 52

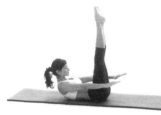

Hundred, page 56

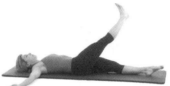

Roll-Up, page 58

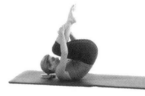

Leg Circle, page 54

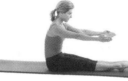

Rolling Like a Ball, page 72

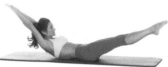

Double-Leg Stretch, page 64

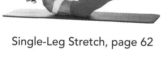

Single-Leg Stretch, page 62

Criss-Cross, page 106

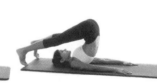

Shoulder Bridge Prep, page 85

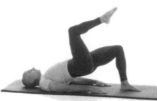

Roll-Over, page 76

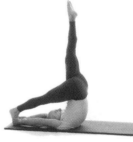

Control Balance, page 75

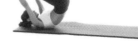

Spine Stretch, page 71

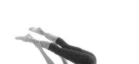

Open-Leg Rocker, page 74

Saw, page 102

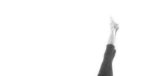

Spine Twist—Sitting, page 101

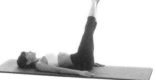

Corkscrew, page 104

> *continued*

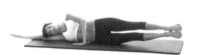

Side Leg Lift, page 96

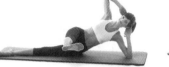

Side Kick, page 97

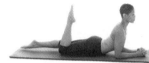

Single-Leg Kick, page 113

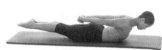

Double-Leg Kick, page 114

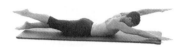

Swimming, page 115

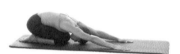

Rest Position, page 118

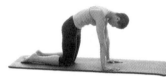

Cat Stretch, page 112

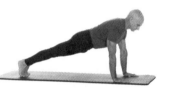

Front Support, page 91

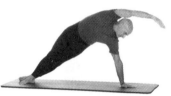

Back Support, page 89

Side Bend, page 98

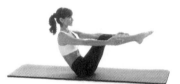

Teaser Prep, page 68

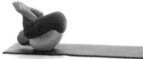

Seal Puppy, page 73

Exercises: 44 • approximate time: 60 minutes

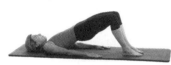

Pelvic curl, page 49

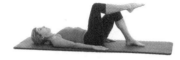

Leg Lift, page 53

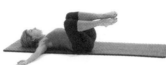

Spine Twist—Supine, page 50

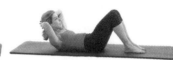

Chest Lift, page 51

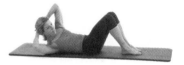

Chest Lift With Rotation, page 52

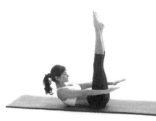

Hundred, page 56

Roll-Up, page 58

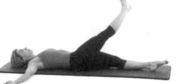

Leg Circle, page 54

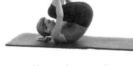

Rolling Like a Ball, page 72

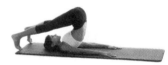

Double-Leg Stretch, page 64

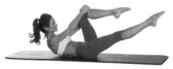

Single-Leg Stretch, page 62

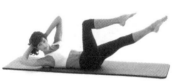

Criss-Cross, page 106

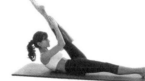

Hamstring Pull, page 66

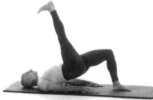

Shoulder Bridge, page 86

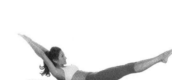

Roll-Over, page 76

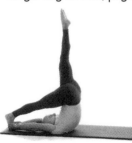

Control Balance, page 75

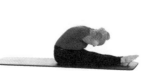

Neck Pull, page 60

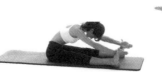

Spine Stretch, page 71

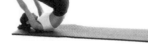

Open-Leg Rocker, page 74

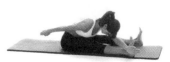

Saw, page 102

> continued
  347

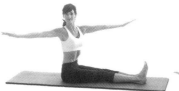

Spine Twist—Sitting, page 101

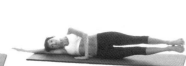

Side Leg Lift, page 96

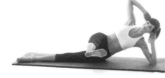

Side Kick, page 97

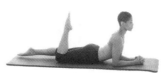

Single-Leg Kick, page 113

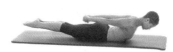

Double-Leg Kick, page 114

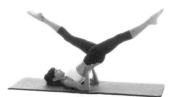

Scissors, page 87

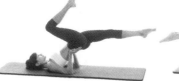

Bicycle, page 88

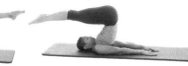

Jackknife, page 78

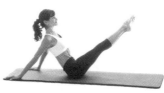

Hip Circle Prep, page 105

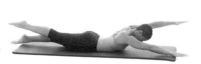

Swimming, page 115

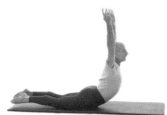

Swan Dive, page 117

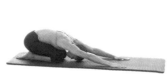

Rest Position, page 118

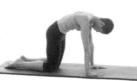

Cat Stretch, page 112

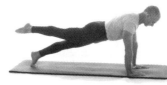

Leg Pull Front, page 94

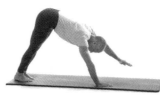

Push-Up, page 92

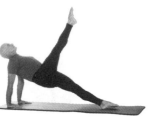

Leg Pull Back, page 90

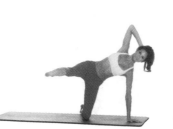

Side Kick—Kneeling, page 100

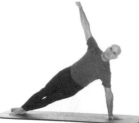

Side Bend, page 98

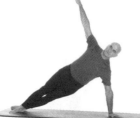

Twist, page 108

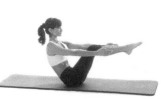

Teaser Prep, page 68

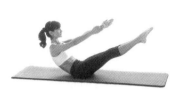 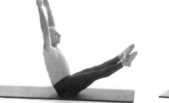 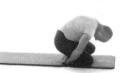 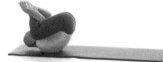

Teaser, page 69   Boomerang, page 80   Crab, page 82   Seal Puppy, page 73

Apparatus Sequences

First and foremost when using any of the apparatus is safety. I cannot stress this point enough. Second, the session should be comprehensive, just as the mat work is. When working on the apparatus people sometimes do only a few exercises, often focusing on one area of the body. Remember, the apparatus are the tools we use, not the system itself. To reap all the benefits that Pilates offers, you must adopt the Pilates approach as well as the repertoire. I have always claimed that I would rather work out using conventional gym equipment with an instructor who uses a Pilates approach than work on Pilates apparatus with a Pilates instructor who does not incorporate the principles of the work. The reason is simple: I know I will achieve better results in the first scenario. The block system ensures that each session you do is a Pilates session and not merely a few exercises done on Pilates apparatus.

I have offered three routines, one from each level, that can be used as frameworks to build on. In addition I have provided several alternative options, illustrating how the repertoire within each block can be interchanged. The possibilities are infinite, and as long as you adhere to the guidelines and principles in this book, you are guaranteed a positive outcome.

Fundamental Apparatus Program

Exercises: 30 • approximate time: 60 minutes

OPTIONAL

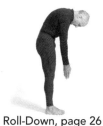

Roll-Down, page 26

WARM-UP

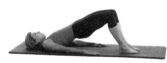

Pelvic Curl (Mat), page 49

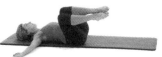

Spine Twist—Supine (Mat), page 50

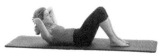

Chest Lift (Mat), page 51

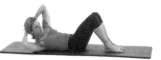

Chest Lift With Rotation (Mat), page 52

FOOT WORK

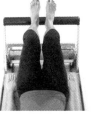

Parallel Heels (Reformer), page 122

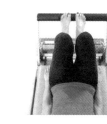

Parallel Toes (Reformer), page 123

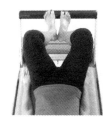

V-Position Toes (Reformer), page 124

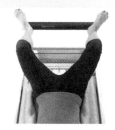

Open V-Position Heels (Reformer), page 125

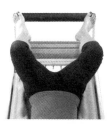

Open V-Position Toes (Reformer), page 126

FOOT WORK

ABDOMINAL WORK

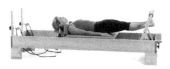

Calf Raise (Reformer), page 127

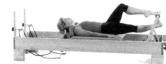

Prance (Reformer), page 128

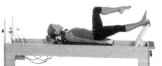

Single-Leg Heel (Reformer), page 130

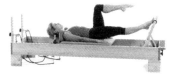

Single-Leg Toes (Reformer), page 131

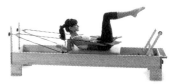

Hundred Prep (Reformer), page 134

HIP WORK

SPINAL ARTICULATION

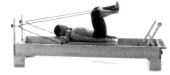

Frog (Reformer), page 149

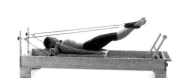

Hip Circle Down (Reformer), page 150

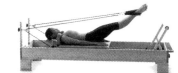

Hip Circle Up (Reformer), page 151

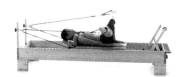

Opening (Reformer), page 152

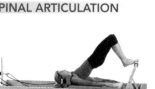

Bottom Lift (Reformer), page 156

> continued 351

STRETCHES

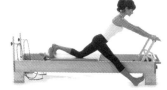

Standing Lunge (Reformer), page 165

FULL-BODY INTEGRATION I

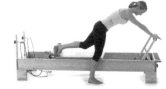

Scooter (Reformer), page 169

ARM WORK

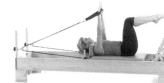

Shoulder Extension—Supine (Reformer), page 182 or (Ped-a-Pul), page 311

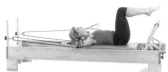

Shoulder Adduction—Supine (Reformer), page 183 or (Ped-a-Pul), page 312

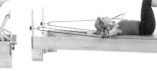

Arm Circle Up—Supine (Reformer), page 184 or (Ped-a-Pul), page 314

ARM WORK

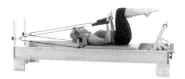

Triceps—Supine (Reformer), page 185, or (Ped-a-Pul), page 313

LEG WORK

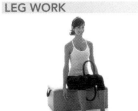

Above Knees—Seated (Magic Circle), page 331

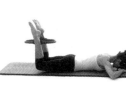

Knees Bent—Prone (Magic Circle), page 334

LATERAL FLEXION & ROTATION

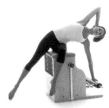

Side Over (Wunda Chair), page 284 or (Step Barrel), page 303

BACK EXTENSION

Basic Swan (Wunda Chair), page 285 or Swan (Step Barrel), page 306

OPTIONAL

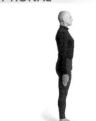

Roll-Down, page 26

Intermediate Apparatus Program

Exercises: 31 • approximate time: 60 minutes

OPTIONAL

Roll-Down, page 26

WARM-UP

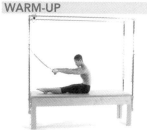

Roll-Up (Cadillac), page 232

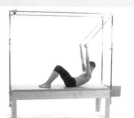

Mini Roll-Up (Cadillac), page 233

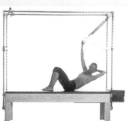

Mini Roll-Up—Oblique (Cadillac), page 236

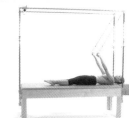

Roll-Up—Top Loaded (Cadillac), page 234

WARM-UP

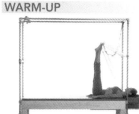

Parallel Heels and Toes (Cadillac), page 225

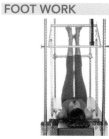

V-Position Toes (Cadillac), page 226

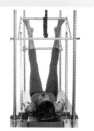

Wide V-Position Heels and Toes (Cadillac), page 227

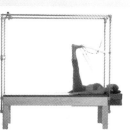

Calf Raise (Cadillac), page 228

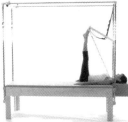

Prance (Cadillac), page 229

FOOT WORK

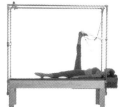

Single-Leg Heel (Cadillac), page 230

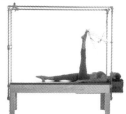

Single-Leg Toes (Cadillac), page 231

HIP WORK

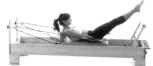

Hundred (Reformer), page 135

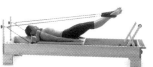

Hip Circle Down (Reformer), page 150

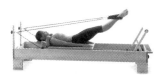

Hip Circle Up (Reformer), page 151

HIP WORK

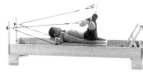

Extended Frog (Reformer), page 153

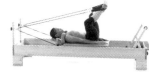

Extended Frog—Reverse (Reformer), page 154

SPINAL ARTICULATION

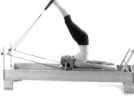

Short Spine (Reformer), page 160

STRETCHES

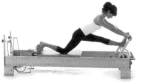

Kneeling Lunge (Reformer), page 166

FULL-BODY INTEGRATION I

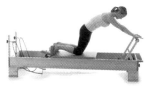

Knee Stretch—Round Back (Reformer), page 170

> continued 353

FULL-BODY INTEGRATION I

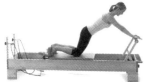

Knee Stretch—Flat Back (Reformer), page 171

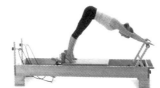

Elephant (Reformer), page 176

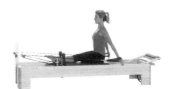

Up Stretch (Reformer), page 177

ARM WORK

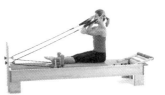

Chest Expansion—Seated (Reformer), page 186

Biceps—Seated (Reformer), page 187

ARM WORK

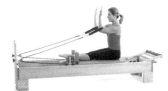

Rhomboids—Seated (Reformer), page 188

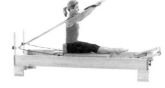

Hug-a-Tree—Seated (Reformer), page 189

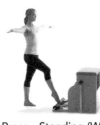

Salute—Seated (Reformer), page 190

LEG WORK

Leg Press—Standing (Wunda Chair), page 282

FULL-BODY INTEGRATION II

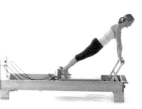

Long Stretch (Reformer), page 178

LATERAL FLEXION & ROTATION

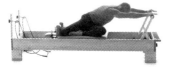

Mermaid (Reformer), page 214

BACK EXTENSION

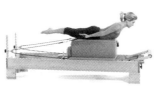

Breaststroke (Reformer), page 219

OPTIONAL

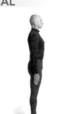

Roll-Down, page 26

Advanced Apparatus Program

Exercises: 41 • approximate time: 60 minutes

OPTIONAL

Roll-Down, page 26

WARM-UP

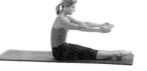

Roll-Up (Mat), page 58

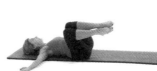

Spine Twist—Supine (Mat), page 50

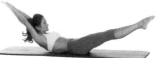

Double-Leg Stretch (Mat), page 64

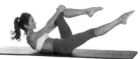

Single-Leg Stretch (Mat), page 62

WARM-UP

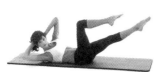

Criss-Cross (Mat), page 106

FOOT WORK

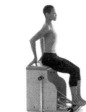

Parallel Heels and Toes (Wunda Chair), page 269

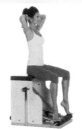

V-Position Toes (Wunda Chair), page 270

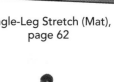

Wide V-Position Heels and Toes (Wunda Chair), page 271

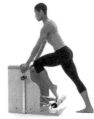

Calf Raise (Wunda Chair), page 272

FOOT WORK

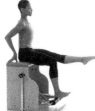

Single-Leg Heel and Toes (Wunda Chair), page 273

ABDOMINAL WORK

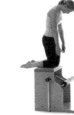

Cat Stretch (Wunda Chair), page 275, or Full Pike (Wunda Chair), page 276

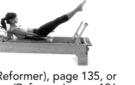
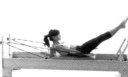

Hundred (Reformer), page 135, or Coordination (Reformer), page 136

HIP WORK

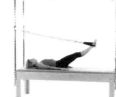

Frog (Cadillac), page 238

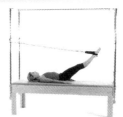

Hip Circle (Cadillac), page 239

HIP WORK

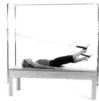

Walking (Cadillac), page 240

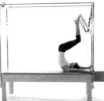

Bicycle and Bicycle—Reverse (Cadillac), page 241

SPINAL ARTICULATION

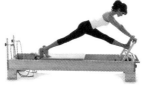

Tower (Cadillac), page 244

STRETCHES

Full Lunge (Reformer), page 167

FULL-BODY INTEGRATION I

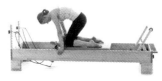

Knee Stretch—Reverse (Reformer), page 174

> *continued* 355

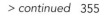

FULL-BODY INTEGRATION I

Down Stretch (Reformer),
page 175

Elephant (Reformer),
page 176

Up Stretch (Reformer),
page 177

ARM WORK

Rowing Back I (Reformer),
page 196

Rowing Back II (Reformer),
page 198

ARM WORK

Rowing Front I (Reformer),
page 200

Rowing Front II (Reformer),
page 202

LEG WORK

Skating (Reformer), page 206

Side Split (Reformer),
page 205

FULL-BODY INTEGRATION II

Balance Control Front
(Reformer), page 179

FULL-BODY INTEGRATION II

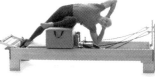

Balance Control Back Prep
(Reformer), page 180

LATERAL FLEXION & ROTATION

Side Over—Short Box
(Reformer), page 212, or
(Ladder Barrel), page 292

BACK EXTENSION

Pulling Straps I (Reformer),
page 220, or Swan (Ladder
Barrel), page 294

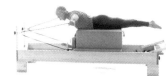

Pulling Straps II (Reformer),
page 221

OPTIONAL

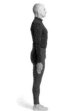

Roll-Down, page 26

As you embark on the practice of Pilates, you can look forward to the delightful and positive changes that lie ahead. For each person, the practice of Pilates means something different and results depend in large part on the goals and the commitment of the individual. Joseph Pilates is quoted as having said, "in 10 sessions, you will feel the difference, in 20, you will see the difference, and in 30, you'll be on your way to having a whole new body." Certain changes—those relating to body awareness and alignment, muscle activation, the release of tension, rejuvenation, and inspiration—can occur immediately. However, for significant physiological changes to take place, the muscles must be challenged consistently for at least six weeks. In *Return to Life Through Contrology*, Joseph Pilates wrote "if you faithfully perform [the] exercises regularly only four times a week for just three months . . . you will find your body development approaching the ideal, accompanied by renewed mental vigor and spiritual enhancement" (pages 18-19). Without consistency and discipline, profound changes are unlikely to occur. Pilates is not a quick, cure-all potion. It is a well-designed system of physical and mental conditioning that, when practiced diligently, brings about the positive changes we strive for and the well-being that we deserve.

As important as consistent practice is, Joseph Pilates intended for his system to be far more than the repetition of exercises. He considered it to be an approach to life that would imbue every daily activity with well-being. I have seen footage in which he went as far as to demonstrate how to shower correctly and wash every part of the body—that was Mr. Pilates, through and through! He was a man of strong opinions, who had unwavering belief in his system and a corresponding determination that it should be practiced universally.

Like the rest of us, Joseph Pilates had his shortcomings. Those who worked with him reported that he could be impatient, egotistical, and something of a show-off. He may have been chauvinistic as well; he intended his method to be practiced mainly by men. It is ironic, therefore, that it is primarily women who have kept the flame alive all these years and that women still represent the majority of Pilates practitioners. As a consequence of the work's popularity with women, the masculinity and athleticism of the work, and even its potential power, has been diminished, or at least partially untapped—although this is changing as more men have begun to teach and practice the work and as more women have become interested in a more athletic approach. Pilates, in its essence, is a wonderful balance of strength and grace that has much to offer men and women.

Above all, Joseph Pilates was a "genius of the body," as renowned choreographer George Balanchine reportedly called him. He embraced the power of the mind–body connection early on, understanding that each human being is a complex entity. He viewed human movement as an intricate sequence of patterns. He was an unshakable idealist who believed that humankind deserved better than the status quo. He spearheaded one of the greatest surges in the history of the fitness industry. He promoted concepts that are only now being truly understood, embraced, and substantiated through research. Joseph Pilates' vast knowledge and creativity, which are even more apparent today than in his own lifetime, are a legacy that we can enjoy and use to enhance our lives.

In bidding farewell, I add my humble wish that we all generously share our knowledge and life experience so that we may all grow as individuals, as a community, and as the human race. By sharing, practicing, and teaching, we keep the essence of Pilates alive. Enjoy this enlightening journey!

Books

Calais-Germain, Blandine. 1993. *Anatomy of movement*. Seattle: Eastland Press.

Calais-Germain, Blandine, and Andrée Lamotte. 1996. *Anatomy of movement exercises*. Seattle: Eastland Press.

Cash, Mel. 1999. *Pocket atlas of the moving body*. London: Ebury Press Random House.

Clippinger, Karen. 2015. *Dance anatomy and kinesiology, 2nd edition*. Champaign, IL: Human Kinetics.

Conraths-Lange, Nicola. 2004. *Survival skills for Pilates teachers*. Ann Arbor, MI: Logokinesis.

Corrigan, Brian, and G.D. Maitland. 1985. *Practical orthopaedic medicine*. Oxford, UK: Butterworth-Heinemann.

Dowd, Irene. 1995. *Taking root to fly: Articles on functional anatomy, 3rd edition*. New York: Dowd.

Dufton, Jennifer. 2003. *The pilates difference*. London: Hamlyn.

Fitt, Sally S. 1988. *Dance kinesiology*. New York: Schirmer.

Franklin, Eric. 2002. *Pelvic power*. Hightstown, NJ: Princeton.

Friedman, Philip, and Gail Eisen. 1980. *The Pilates method of physical and mental conditioning*. Garden City, NY: Doubleday.

Gallagher, Sean P., and Romana Kryzanowska (editor). 2000. *The Joseph H. Pilates archive collection*. Philadelphia: Bainbridge.

Gladwell, Malcolm. 2008. *Outliers*. New York City, NY: Little, Brown and Company.

Gladwell, Malcolm. 2000. *The Tipping Point*. New York City, NY: Little, Brown and Company.

Hessel, Jillian. 2003. *Pilates basics*. Emmaus, PA: Rodale.

Isacowitz, Rael. 2004. *Body arts and science international movement analysis work books: mat, reformer, cadillac, ladder barrel and wunda chair, auxiliary, avalon*. Costa Mesa, CA: Author.

Isacowitz, Rael, and Karen Clippinger. 2011. *Pilates Anatomy*. Champaign, IL: Human Kinetics.

Iyengar, B.K.S. 2001. *The art of yoga*. London: Allen & Unwin.

Juhan, Deane. 1998. *Jobs body: a handbook for body work, 3rd edition*. Barrytown, NY: Station Hill Press.

Kaplanek, Beth, Brett Levine, and William Jaffe. 2011. *Pilates for hip and knee syndromes and arthroplasties*. Champaign, IL: Human Kinetics.

Kendal, Florence P., Elizabeth K. McCreary, and Patricia G. Provance. 1993. *Muscles: Testing and function*. 4th ed. Baltimore: Williams & Wilkins.

Kelly, Suzanne. 2005. *Pilates 4 kidzz*. Bloomington, IN: Authorhouse.

King, Bruce. 1991. *Rule of the bones: Exercise theory and program for correct body usage*. New York: Bruce King Foundation for American Dance.

Kounovsky, Nicholas. 1971. *The joy of feeling fit*. Mattituck, NY: Amereon House.

Lett, Anthony. 2010. *Innovations in pilates*. Eltham, VIC, Australia: Rebus Press.

Lingauer, Gabor. 2002. *Muscle doctor*. Victoria, Canada: Trafford.

Myers, Thomas P. 2001. *Anatomy trains*. London: Harcourt.

Netter, Frank H. 2011. *Atlas of human anatomy, professional edition, 5th edition*. Philidelphia, PA: Saunders/Elsevier.

Pilates, Joseph H. 1945. *Return to life through contrology*. Reprinted 2003. Miami: Pilates Method Alliance.

Pilates, Joseph H. 1934. *Your health: A corrective system of exercising that revolutionizes the entire field of physical education*. Reprinted 1998. Incline Village, NV: Presentation Dynamics.

Robinson, Lynne. 2004. *The body control Pilates pregnancy book*. London: Pan Books.

Tardent, Helen. 2005. *Beautiful pilates*. Camberwell, Australia: Penguin.

Thompson, Cem W. and R. T. Floyd. 2004. *Manual of structural kinesiology*. 15th Edition. St. Louis: Times Mirror/Mosby.

Journals and Magazines

Health Magazine

IDEA Fitness Journal

PilatesStyle

Yoga Journal

Videos and DVDs

Fletcher, Ron. *Ron Fletcher Workshop Tape*. The Ron Fletcher Company.

Isacowitz, Rael. 2003. *Rael Pilates System 7, 17 and 27*. Carlmarsh III Productions.

Gentry, Eve. 1991. *The Eve Gentry Technique*. Institute for the Pilates Method.

Liekens, Bob, Alycea Ungaro, and Peter Fiasca. 2003. *Classical Pilates technique*. Classical Pilates Inc.

Pilates, Joseph H. *Demonstrating the principles of his method with Clara, students and friends, 1932-1945*. From Joseph and Clara Pilates personal collection. Attained by Evelyn de la Tour and bequeathed to Mary Bowen. Mary Bowen made it available to the Pilates community.

Trier, Carola. 1989. *Carola shares . . . A Dadmehr Production*.

Websites

Balanced Body: www.pilates.com

Body Arts and Science International: www.basipilates.com

Body Control UK: www.bodycontrol.co.uk

Dynamic Chiropractic: www.chiroweb.com

Human Kinetics: www.humankinetics.com

Pilates Anytime: www.pilatesanytime.com

Pilates Interactive: www.pilatesinteractive.com

Pilates Style: www.pilatesstyle.com

Pilates Method Alliance: www.pilatesmethodalliance.org

Physician and Sports Medicine: www.physsportsmed.com

National Scoliosis Foundation: www.scoliosis.org

Scoliosis World: www.scoliosis-world.com

Somatics on the Web: www.somatics.com

Index

Note: The italicized *f* following page numbers refers to figures.

Rael Isacowitz is a world-renowned practitioner and teacher of Pilates. With over three decades of Pilates practice and achievement, he is a prominent lecturer and teacher at symposia, universities, colleges, and studios around the globe. He received his bachelor of education degree and teaching credentials from Israel's prestigious Wingate Institute, where he subsequently joined the teaching faculty. He later earned a master of arts degree in dance from the University of Surrey, England.

Rael's early Pilates teachers included Alan Herdman and thereafter several of the first-generation Pilates teachers (known as the Elders), including Kathy Grant, Ron Fletcher, Romana Kryzanowska, Eve Gentry, and Lolita San Miguel.

Rael has mastered all levels of the Pilates repertoire and is noted in the industry for his unique athleticism; synthesis of body, mind, and spirit; and passion for teaching. In 1989 he founded Body Arts and Science International (BASI) Pilates, which has developed into one of the foremost Pilates education organizations in the world. BASI Pilates is currently taught in more than 100 locations spanning 30 countries.

Rael's first edition of *Pilates* (Human Kinetics, 2006) and his *Pilates Anatomy* (coauthored with Karen Clippinger, Human Kinetics, 2011) have received worldwide acclaim and been translated into multiple languages. He has published a series of movement analysis workbooks on all the Pilates apparatus, produced DVDs,

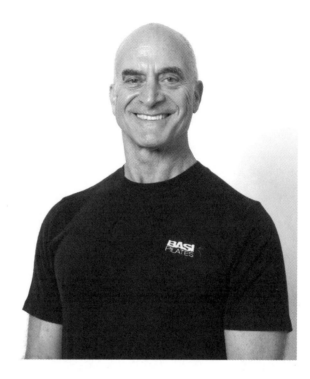

designed the revolutionary Avalon System line of contemporary Pilates equipment, and created the groundbreaking Pilates Interactive software. He is a regular contributor to several industry publications, including *Pilates Style*. Creativity, passion, and energy suffuse his work. Teaching Pilates is, for Rael, the ultimate gift.

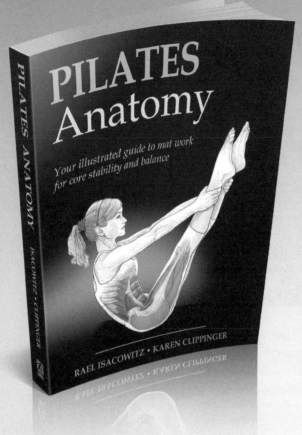